The Interoceptive Mind

The Interoceptive Mind
From Homeostasis to Awareness

Edited by

Manos Tsakiris

Helena De Preester

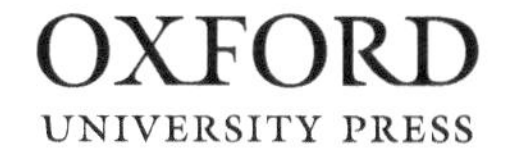

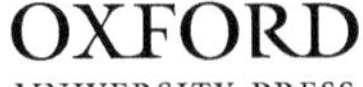

UNIVERSITY PRESS

Great Clarendon Street, Oxford, OX2 6DP
United Kingdom

Oxford University Press is a department of the University of Oxford.
It furthers the University's objective of excellence in research, scholarship,
and education by publishing worldwide. Oxford is a registered trade mark of
Oxford University Press in the UK and in certain other countries

Impression: 1

First Edition published in 2019

Published in the United States of America by Oxford University Press
198 Madison Avenue, New York, NY 10016, United States of America

British Library Cataloguing in Publication Data
Data available

Library of Congress Control Number: 2018945622

ISBN 978–0–19–881193–0

Printed and bound by
CPI Group (UK) Ltd, Croydon, CR0 4YY

Preface

Interoception is the body-to-brain axis of signals originating from the internal body and visceral organs (such as gastrointestinal, respiratory, hormonal, and circulatory systems). It plays a unique role in ensuring homeostasis. Interoception therefore refers to the sensing of the state of the inner body and its homeostatic needs, to the ever-fluctuating state of the body beneath its sensory (exteroceptive) and musculoskeletal sheath. By bringing together the perspectives of experimental psychology and cognitive neuroscience, psychophysiology, psychiatry, clinical psychology, and philosophy, this volume aims to go beyond the known role of interoception for homeostasis in order to ask, and hopefully provide, important insights on the role that interoception plays for our mental life and lived experience, for awareness, affect, and cognition.

The perspectives in the ensuing 17 chapters largely fall within the embodied cognition approach that attempted to ground cognition and the self in the body. Over the last three decades, modern psychology and cognitive neurosciences have focused on the importance of the body as the starting point for a science of the self and the subject. However, this focus concerned the body as perceived from the outside, as, for example, when we recognize ourselves in the mirror, or when the brain integrates sensorimotor information to create our sense of body ownership and agency, or even when we perceive other people's bodies and thereby their mental states via processes of embodied simulation. A first step toward that direction was to consider the role that sensorimotor signals play for the *experience* and the *awareness* of one's self, which goes beyond their well-known role in motor control and sensory perception. For example, research on the sense of agency over one's actions and the sense of ownership of one's body demonstrates how these fundamental experiences rely on specific processes of sensorimotor interaction and multisensory integration, respectively (Haggard, 2005; Tsakiris, 2010). Another, closely related step in that direction was the recognition of the proprioceptive dimension of the body for agency, ownership, and the embodied self (Gallager & Cole, 1995; Bermúdez, Marcel, & Eilan, 1995). In the prolific field of social cognitive neuroscience, similar considerations regarding the role of observable sensorimotor events have been extended to social cognition and our understanding of other minds (Gallese, Keysers, & Rizzolatti, 2004). Such theoretical advances have been instrumental in explaining key aspects of the bodily self and its social cognition.

Notwithstanding the influential research that accumulated in this area, it is clear that our fields have neglected another important dimension of the body, namely the interoceptive body, which is the body as perceived from the inside. This visceral dimension of embodiment has, of course, a long-standing history of predominantly physiological investigations during the last century, but it was only relatively recent that interoception has gained a rapidly expanding interest in the study of human mind. The seminal work of Bud Craig (2009) and Antonio Damasio (1999), despite their differences, placed the visceral milieu, its homeostatic functioning, and our interoceptive awareness thereof at the center stage of self-awareness. In parallel, the development of new methods to measure, not simply interoceptive signaling but our awareness thereof opened up the field of interoceptive research to psychologists and cognitive neuroscientists. In parallel with the exponential increase in the number of publications on the topic, researchers and scholars across physiology, cognitive neuroscience, psychology, philosophy, and medicine are working on interoception without necessarily sharing the same conceptual base or necessarily realizing how their investigations link with the findings and insights of other disciplines and methodologies.

Despite recent advances (Garfinkel et al., 2015; Kleckner et al., 2015), there is consensus that interoception research must develop psychologically relevant and philosophically sound theoretical foundations, a wider and more grounded measurement model and a fuller characterization of the links between different interoceptive dimensions and systems if it is to achieve its appropriate place within the life and mind sciences. This ambitious aim necessitates wide-ranging, dedicated, and systematic theoretical and methodological enquiries into the hierarchical relations in interoceptive processing, the horizontal relations across interoceptive modalities, and the causal relations between interoception and awareness. For example, psychological research into interoceptive awareness has mainly used tasks that quantify our accuracy in detecting single heartbeats. However, as the influential work of Garfinkel, Seth, Barrett, Suzuki, and Critchley (2015) shows, we must be aware of the hierarchical levels of interoception, from interoceptive sensibility, to accuracy and eventual awareness, and how these may impact cognition in health and in illness. Similarly, in relation to horizontal relations, classic approaches to interoception focus on four systems—the cardiovascular, respiratory, gastrointestinal, and urogenital (Adam, 1998; Cameron, 2002), but a fundamental question concerns the interrelation of awareness across different interoceptive systems and the potentially distinctive role that each system plays for cognition. Finally, unlike exteroception, it is particularly difficult to have experimental control over the inputs to the interoceptive system and/or to interfere causally with it, and therefore developing paradigms and theoretical approaches that can probe the causal links between interoception and cognition will accelerate our knowledge.

The contributions collected in this multidisciplinary volume represent an attempt to provide a reference for the conceptualization of this excitingly deep connection between our body and mind. As such it offers an overview of the state-of-art in psychological and neuroscience research, of recent developments in clinical-psychological models for normal and pathological functioning, and of new theories that frame interoception at the intersection between philosophy of mind and the broader context of embodied cognition. To that end, its scope ranges from the psychology and neuroscience of interoception (Part I), to clinical implications of recent research taking into account interoception (Part II), and to theoretical-philosophical frameworks and models of interoception (Part III).

The introductory chapter by Berntson, Gianaros, and Tsakiris goes straight into the heart of the matter by providing the historical context that led to the development of a science of interoception and a state-of-the-art overview of the organizational principles of the interoceptive system. First, it is explained that the autonomic nervous system is not only or even primarily an efferent motor system (historically the predominant view) but constitutes an elaborate afferent system. Second, the authors explain that the interoceptive system does not operate independently of higher brain functions. By addressing the top-down and bottom-up organizational principles that underpin interoception, this introductory chapter sets the stage for the subsequent chapters in the volume.

Part I, Mentalizing interoception: Advances and challenges focuses on recent advances in experimental psychology and cognitive neuroscience that highlight the role that interoceptive signals and awareness thereof play for our mental life, beyond their known role for homeostasis. Allen and Tsakiris consider the implications of the embodied predictive processing account for the conceptualization of interoceptive signals as "first priors" and their role in providing the mind with a biologically plausible model of one's body and self. Babo-Rebelo and Tallon-Baudry review recent electrophysiological studies that extend the role of interoception to show how the cortical processing of cardiac signals may generate a subject-centered reference frame that may underlie different and perhaps distinct facets of the self, such as thought generation and visual consciousness. Wittmann and Meissner discuss the embodiment of subjective time and present evidence to show how the accumulation of physiological signals forms the basis for the subjective impression of time. Aziz and Ruffle delve deeper into the viscera to describe the bi-directional brain–gut axis whose function underpins the generation of "gut-feelings." Such feeling states are important for sensations but also the experience of distinct and often salient experiences such as pain, nausea, and appetite. The last chapter of this first part by Von Morh and Fotopoulou focuses on the homeostatically relevant experiences of pain and pleasure, in particular affective touch, and discuss their peripheral neurophysiological specificity (i.e. bottom-up) and their top-down social modulations within a predictive coding framework.

Part II: From health to disease: Interoception in physical and mental health considers the role of interoceptive processes and their corresponding psychological concepts across a range of clinical conditions, from aberrant emotional processing to anxiety, eating disorders, symptom perception and overall well-being. Recent experimental findings are presented and reviewed in the context of hypotheses about the integration of peripheral afferent signals with central cognitive operations and their role in shaping subjective experience in health and disease.

Quadt, Critchley, and Garfinkel provide an overview of the influence of internal bodily states on emotion. By presenting a predictive coding account of interoceptive predictions errors, they highlight the distinct ways in which deficits in interoceptive abilities may underpin aberrant emotional processes characteristic of several clinical conditions. Khalsa and Feinstein focus on the regulatory battle for control that ensues in the central nervous system when there is a discrepancy between predicted and current bodily states (i.e. when somatic error signals are present). They argue that anxiety disorders are driven by somatic errors that chronically fail to be adaptively regulated. Herbert and Pollatos use a predictive coding framework analogous to the one introduced by Quadt, Critchley, and Garfinkel, and apply it to our understanding of eating behavior. They characterize anorexia and bulimia nervosa as a profound impairment of the "self," with dysfunctional interoception at its core. Yoris and colleagues explore the interoceptive dysfunctions following neurological damage or neurodegeneration and emphasize the significance of interoception to promote a hitherto missing synthesis of simultaneous autonomic, emotional, and social cognition deficits in neurology. Van den Bergh, Zacharioudakis, and Petersen focus on interoception and the perception of bodily sensations in the context of symptom perception, and spell out the consequences of the highly variable relationship between symptoms and physiological dysfunction for the disease model. Farb and Logie focus on the appraisal of interoceptive signals and its consequences for subjective well-being. The modifying role of attention for habitual appraisals of interoceptive signals is presented, along with a novel breathing-focused task for measuring interoceptive awareness.

Part III Toward a philosophy of interoception: subjectivity and experience approaches interoception from a theoretical and philosophical perspective. Because until now the field of interoception has been driven mainly by scientists rather than philosophers, this part represents a highly novel departure for philosophy of mind and subjectivity, often starting from a phenomenological point of view. The relation between subjective experience and physiological processes is an intricate and complicated one. Both the notion of "arousal" in emotion and the experiential dimension of interoception more generally stand in need of descriptive analysis and theoretical framing.

Colombetti and Harrison disentangle the physiology and the experience of "arousal" in emotion and argue for the recognition of the multiple systems and pathways involved in emotional arousal, including not only the autonomic nervous system but also pathways of the endocrine and immune system, somatic sensations, and "background" bodily feelings. Empirical studies in interoception have profound consequences for the way the self or subjectivity is conceived of and conceptualized. The interoceptive dimension of the embodied subject forces us to rethink phenomena such as body ownership and the self, the relation between interoception and exteroception, and the coming about of subjectivity itself. De Vignemont discusses the many ways the notion of interoception is understood, and considers the contribution of interoception for the awareness of one's body as one's own. She approaches body ownership in affective terms and as rooted in self-regulatory interoceptive feelings such as hunger and thirst. Corcoran and Hohwy consider the limitations of homeostasis and favor a reconciliatory position in which homeostasis and allostasis are conceived as equally vital but functionally distinct modes of physiological control to account for the sophisticated regulatory dynamics observed in complex organisms. De Preester focuses on a basis form of subjectivity and its origin in interoceptive processes. She argues that the topographic representation of interoceptive body states in the brain is unfit for explaining the coming about of subjectivity, and offers directions for another model that takes into account the inherent characteristics of subjectivity. Leder closes the volume, offering a phenomenology of inner-body experience and explaining how this experience is influenced by models drawn from the outer world. In line with insights gained in the first and the second part, he points out the importance of inner-body experience for health and well-being.

The different chapters included across the three parts are interrelated in various ways, and the synergy between the chapters crosses the boundaries of the disciplines, opening up opportunities for fruitful dialog between fields that otherwise remain too often separate. For example, attention to subjectivity and subjective experience, to self-awareness and the experience of self, are common threads throughout the volume, together with the intricate role of emotions and their relation to interoception. Similarly, several chapters are motivated by recent predictive coding accounts (Clark, 2013; Friston, 2010) that have been extended from cognition and attention to affect (Critchley & Garfinkel, 2017), bodily self-awareness (Apps & Tsakiris, 2014; Seth, 2013), and mental disorders (Feldman Barrett & Simmons, 2015). A concern for human well-being and human health and suffering is also noticeable in all the chapters, and the capacity to contribute to one's own well-being by paying attention to in-depth bodily signals is a recurrent theme. The chapters thus share a common concern for what it means to experience oneself, for the crucial role of emotions, and for issues of health and well-being, discussed on the joint basis of our bodily existence and interoception, resulting in a more than usual attention for the phenomenology of subjective experience in disciplines outside philosophy. Together, the chapters show that disciplinary specialization is not a hindrance for dialogue but can result into mutual enrichment. We hope that the scholarly research presented in this volume will further motivate the much-anticipated coming of age of interoceptive research in psychology, cognitive neurosciences, and philosophy.

Helena De Preester
Manos Tsakiris

References

Adam, G. (1998). *Visceral Perception, Understanding Internal Cognition.* New York, NY: Springer.

Apps, M. A. J. and **Tsakiris, M.** (2014). The free-energy self: A predictive coding account of self-recognition. *Neuroscience & Biobehavioral Reviews, 41*, 85–97. <https://doi.org/10.1016/j.neubiorev.2013.01.029>

Bermúdez, J. L., Marcel, A. J., and **Eilan, N.** (eds) (1995). *The Body and the Self.* Cambridge, MA: MIT Press.

Cameron, O. (2002). *Visceral Sensory Neuroscience: Interoception.* Oxford: Oxford University Press.

Clark, A. (2013). Whatever next? Predictive brains, situated agents, and the future of cognitive science. *Behavioral and Brain Sciences, 36*, 181–204. <https://doi.org/10.1017/S0140525X12000477>

Craig, A. D. B. (2009). How do you feel—now? The anterior insula and human awareness. *Nature Reviews. Neuroscience, 10*(1), 59–70. <https://doi.org/10.1038/nrn2555>

Critchley, H. D. and **Garfinkel, S. N.** (2017). Interoception and emotion. *Current Opinion in Psychology, 17*, 7–14. doi: 10.1016/j.copsyc.2017.

Damasio, A. (1999). *The Feeling of What Happens: Body, Emotion and the Making of Consciousness.* New York, NY: Harcourt.

Feldman Barrett, L. and **Kyle Simmons, W.** (2015). Interoceptive predictions in the brain. *Nature Publishing Group, 16,* 419–29. <https://doi.org/10.1038/nrn3950>

Friston, K. (2010). The free-energy principle: a unified brain theory? *Nature Reviews. Neuroscience, 11*(2), 127–38. <https://doi.org/10.1038/nrn2787>

Gallagher, S. and **Cole, J.** (1995). Body image and body schema in a deafferented subject. *Journal of Mind and Behavior, 16*(4), 369–89.

Gallese, V., Keysers, C., and **Rizzolatti, G.** (2004). A unifying view of the basis of social cognition. *Trends in Cognitive Sciences, 8,* 396–403.

Garfinkel, S. N., Seth, A. K., Barrett, A. B., Suzuki, K., and **Critchley, H. D.** (2015). Knowing your own heart: Distinguishing interoceptive accuracy from interoceptive awareness. *Biological Psychology, 104,* 65–74. <https://doi.org/10.1016/j.biopsycho.2014.11.004>

Haggard, P. (2005). Conscious intention and motor cognition. *Trends in Cognitive Sciences, 9*(6), 290–5. <https://doi.org/10.1016/j.tics.2005.04.012>

Kleckner, I. R., Wormwood, J. B., Simmons, W. K., Barrett, L. F., and **Quigley, K. S.** (2015). Methodological recommendations for a heartbeat detection-based measure of interoceptive sensitivity. *Psychophysiology, 52,* 1432–40. <https://doi.org/10.1111/psyp.12503>

Seth, A. K. (2013). Interoceptive inference, emotion, and the embodied self. *Trends in Cognitive Sciences, 17*(11), 565–73. <https://doi.org/10.1016/j.tics.2013.09.007>

Tsakiris, M. (2010). My body in the brain: A neurocognitive model of body-ownership. *Neuropsychologia, 48*(3), 703–12. <https://doi.org/10.1016/j.neuropsychologia.2009.09.034>

Acknowledgments

We would like to thank our colleague and friend Ophelia Deroy who introduced us to Martin Baum, Senior Commissioning Editor for Psychology and Neuroscience at Oxford University Press. We are grateful to Martin for supporting and selecting our proposal for this volume among the many high-quality proposals that OUP receives. We are also grateful to April Peake for her assistance during the early stages of preparation and to Charlotte Holloway for her assistance during the final production stages. We would also like to acknowledge the NOMIS Foundation Distinguished Scientist Award to Manos Tsakiris and a research grant from the University College Ghent to Helena De Preester that provided the editors with the time and space of mind needed for the timely development of this volume.

Of course, this volume wouldn't exist without the excellent and timely contributions made by all the authors who fully engaged with our vision for this volume and its multi- and cross-disciplinary emphasis. We also thank the authors for acting as referees for each other's chapters along with Vivien Ainley, Laura Crucianelli, Chris Dijkerman, Karl Friston, Philip Gerains, Rebekka Hufendiek, Peter Reynaert, Roy Salomon, Stefan Sütterlin, and Dan Zahavi who generously devoted their precious time in reviewing several chapters.

Last, but not least, the co-editors would like to thank each other for a seamless mutually enriching and supportive collaboration over the last two years.

Contents

Contributors

Micah Allen
Institute of Cognitive Neuroscience, University College London, United Kingdom
Wellcome Centre for Human Neuroimaging, University College London, United Kingdom

Qasim Aziz
Barts and the London School of Medicine & Dentistry, Queen Mary University of London, United Kingdom

Mariana Babo-Rebelo
Laboratoire de Neurosciences Cognitives, Département d'Etudes Cognitives, Ecole Normale Supérieure (ENS), PSL Research University, INSERM, Paris, France

Gary G. Berntson
Department of Psychology, Ohio State University, United States

Giovanna Colombetti
Department of Sociology, Philosophy and Anthropology, University of Exeter, United Kingdom

Andrew W. Corcoran
Cognition & Philosophy Laboratory, Department of Philosophy, Faculty of Arts, Monash University, Melbourne, Australia

Hugo D. Critchley
Department of Neuroscience, Brighton and Sussex Medical School (BSMS), University of Sussex, Brighton, United Kingdom

Helena De Preester
School of Arts, University College Ghent, Belgium
Department of Philosophy and Moral Sciences, Faculty of Arts and Philosophy, Ghent University, Belgium

Frédérique de Vignemont
Institut Jean Nicod, ENS-CNRS-EHESS, Department of cognitive studies, École Normale Supérieure, PSL, Paris, France

Norman A. S. Farb
Department of Psychology, University of Toronto Mississauga, Mississauga, Canada

Justin S. Feinstein
Laureate Institute for Brain Research, Tulsa, Oklahoma, United States
Oxley College of Health Sciences, University of Tulsa, Tulsa, Oklahoma, United States

Aikaterini Fotopoulou
Research Department of Clinical, Educational and Health Psychology, Faculty of Brain Sciences, University College London, United Kingdom

Adolfo M. García
Laboratory of Experimental Psychology and Neuroscience (LPEN), Institute of Cognitive and Translational Neuroscience (INCYT), INECO Foundation, Favaloro University, Buenos Aires, Argentina
National Scientific and Technical Research Council (CONICET), Buenos Aires, Argentina
Faculty of Education, National University of Cuyo (UNCuyo), Mendoza, Argentina

Indira García-Cordero
Laboratory of Experimental Psychology and Neuroscience (LPEN), Institute of Cognitive and Translational Neuroscience (INCYT), INECO Foundation, Favaloro University, Buenos Aires, Argentina
National Scientific and Technical Research Council (CONICET), Buenos Aires, Argentina

Sarah N. Garfinkel
Psychiatry, Department of Neuroscience, Brighton and Sussex Medical School (BSMS), University of Sussex, Brighton, United Kingdom
Sackler Centre for Consciousness Science, University of Sussex, Brighton, United Kingdom
Sussex Partnership NHS Foundation Trust, United Kingdom

Peter J. Gianaros
Department of Psychology, University of Pittsburgh, United States

Neil Harrison
Department of Neuroscience, Brighton & Sussex Medical School, University of Sussex, United Kingdom
Sussex Partnership NHS Foundation Trust, Swandean, United Kingdom

Beate M. Herbert
Clinical Psychology & Psychotherapy, Department of Psychology, Eberhard Karls University of Tübingen, Germany

Jakob Hohwy
Cognition & Philosophy Laboratory, Department of Philosophy, Faculty of Arts, Monash University, Melbourne, Australia

Agustín Ibáñez
Laboratory of Experimental Psychology and Neuroscience (LPEN), Institute of Cognitive and Translational Neuroscience (INCYT), INECO Foundation, Favaloro University, Buenos Aires, Argentina
National Scientific and Technical Research Council (CONICET), Buenos Aires, Argentina
Universidad Autónoma del Caribe, Barranquilla, Colombia
Center for Social and Cognitive Neuroscience (CSCN), School of Psychology, Universidad Adolfo Ibañez, Santiago, Chile
Centre of Excellence in Cognition and its Disorders, Australian Research Council (ACR), Sydney, Australia

Sahib S. Khalsa
Laureate Institute for Brain Research, Tulsa, Oklahoma, United States
Oxley College of Health Sciences, University of Tulsa, Tulsa, Oklahoma, United States

Drew Leder
Department of Philosophy, Loyola University Maryland, Baltimore, United States

Kyle Logie
Department of Psychology, University of Toronto Mississauga, Mississauga, Canada

Karin Meissner
Institute of Medical Psychology, Ludwig-Maximilian University, Munich, Germany
Division Integrative Health Promotion, University of Applied Sciences, Coburg, Germany

Sibylle Petersen
Health Psychology, KU Leuven–University of Leuven, Leuven, Belgium

Olga Pollatos
Clinical & Health Psychology, Institute of Psychology and Education, Ulm University, Germany

Lisa Quadt
Psychiatry, Department of Neuroscience, Brighton and Sussex Medical School (BSMS), University of Sussex, Brighton, United Kingdom

James K. Ruffle
Centre for Neuroscience and Trauma, Blizard Institute, Wingate Institute of Neurogastroenterology, Barts and the London School of Medicine & Dentistry, Queen Mary University of London, London, United Kingdom

Paula Celeste Salamone
Laboratory of Experimental Psychology and Neuroscience (LPEN), Institute of Cognitive and Translational Neuroscience (INCYT), INECO Foundation, Favaloro University, Buenos Aires, Argentina
National Scientific and Technical Research Council (CONICET), Buenos Aires, Argentina

Lucas Sedeño
Laboratory of Experimental Psychology and Neuroscience (LPEN), Institute of Cognitive and Translational Neuroscience (INCYT), INECO Foundation, Favaloro University, Buenos Aires, Argentina
National Scientific and Technical Research Council (CONICET), Buenos Aires, Argentina

Catherine Tallon-Baudry
Laboratoire de Neurosciences Cognitives, Département d'Etudes Cognitives, Ecole Normale Supérieure (ENS), PSL Research University, INSERM, Paris, France

Manos Tsakiris
Lab of Action & Body, Department of Psychology, Royal Holloway University of London, United Kingdom
The Warburg Institute, School of Advanced Study, University of London, United Kingdom

Omer Van den Bergh
Health Psychology, KU Leuven–University of Leuven, Leuven, Belgium

Mariana von Mohr
Research Department of Clinical, Educational and Health Psychology, Faculty of Brain Sciences, University College London, United Kingdom

Marc Wittmann
Institute for Frontier Areas of Psychology and Mental Health, Freiburg, Germany
Institute of Medical Psychology, Ludwig-Maximilian University, Munich, Germany

Adrián Yoris
Laboratory of Experimental Psychology and Neuroscience (LPEN), Institute of Cognitive and Translational Neuroscience (INCYT), INECO Foundation, Favaloro University, Buenos Aires, Argentina
National Scientific and Technical Research Council (CONICET), Buenos Aires, Argentina

Nadia Zacharioudakis
Health Psychology, KU Leuven–University of Leuven, Leuven, Belgium

PART I

Introduction

Chapter 1

Interoception and the autonomic nervous system: Bottom-up meets top-down

Gary G. Berntson, Peter J. Gianaros, and Manos Tsakiris

1.1 Introduction

Interoception is a multidimensional construct, broadly encompassing the processing of afferent (sensory) information arising from internal organs, tissues, and cells of the body. This afference contributes to the regulation of homeostatic reflexes, and, as we will see in this chapter and throughout this volume, more broadly to the generation and regulation of cognitive and emotional behaviors.

Interoception can be encompassed by the broader construct of bodily afference. The latter includes both visceral afference and somatic afference. We use the term visceral afference to refer to the processing of internal sensory information derived from interoceptors that are located in the organs and tissues of the main cavities of the body (i.e. the viscera), as well as from olfactory and gustatory receptors, all being generally associated with the limbic system and the autonomic nervous system. We use the term somatic afference to refer to the processing of sensory information (e.g. proprioceptive input and tactile sensitivity) derived from components of the somatic system (e.g. muscles, joints, skin). This distinction between somatic and visceral afference does not imply a complete independence. Indeed, in many cases, there is an integration of multiple modes of bodily or somatosensory information derived, for example, from metabolic changes in active muscle tissue. Hence, the term somatovisceral afference is more appropriately applied to integrated, multimodal, or otherwise nonspecific internal sensory input from within the body (e.g. see Yates & Stocker, 1998). In these regards, the construct of interoception itself is more specifically aligned with that of visceral afference, referring to the processing of sensory information from interoceptors that are located within the visceral organs and from interoceptors located elsewhere in the body that provide for local energy needs. Thus, in contrast to exteroceptors, interoceptors are tuned to sense internal events (Cameron, 2002).

The so-called general visceral afferents (GVAs) that relay internal sensory information from interoceptors are carried by several cranial nerves, the most notable being the vagus nerve. These afferents carry information (e.g. pressor receptor activity from blood vessels) originating from the gut and the viscera more generally (i.e. organs and tissues located in the thoracic, abdominal, and pelvic cavities, as well as blood vessels and muscles). By comparison, special visceral afferents (SVAs) convey gustatory senses (i.e. taste) and olfaction (i.e. smell and pheromonal senses). Although the SVAs detect environmental stimuli, they do so by virtue of those stimuli impinging on the internal bodily environment. Hence, they differ from exteroceptors; for example, conveying information related to touch or audition. Furthermore, the visceral senses have common central projections to cell groups in the brainstem, including the nucleus tractus solitarius (NTS), midbrain, and thalamus, that are distinct from those of somatic exteroceptors, and they link anatomically and functionally with a distinct set of central neural systems and processes (Craig, 2014; Saper, 2002). Moreover, they share biochemical markers in common with GVAs and with autonomic neurons (see Squire et al., 2012). There are other classes of sensory systems, such as proprioceptors, that sense joint position, and vestibuloceptors, that sense body orientation in gravitational space. These might be considered interoceptors as they are internal to the body. Yet, they are closely linked with somatic motor systems anatomically and functionally, and they have biochemical markers more in concert with somatic motor systems. Hence, they are sometimes considered within the unique class of proprioceptors, or otherwise just included within the general class of exteroceptors.

What is important to consider is that both exteroceptive and interoceptive information can powerfully influence cognitive and emotional processes, and, importantly, vice versa. Moreover, as will be developed later in this chapter, visceral afferents carrying interoceptive information have a constitutional link with central neural systems underlying cognitive and emotional processes, and they thus impact these behavioral processes (e.g. Tsakiris & Critchley, 2016a; see also the entire Theme issue, Tsakiris & Critchley, 2016b). This is clearly apparent in the positive and negative (e.g. disgust) hedonic effects of tastes and smells. As detailed in the remaining chapters of this volume, it is thus doubtful that interoception can be meaningfully parsed or dissociated from cognitive, emotional, and behavioral processes. Indeed, a recent meta-analysis of fMRI (functional MRI) studies revealed considerable overlap in systems co-activated by interoceptive signaling, emotional regulation and low-level social cognition, and convergent results were found for the effects of lesions (Adolfi et al., 2017).

1.2 **Historical perspectives**

Claude Bernard is generally credited with developing the concept of the "fixity" or relative stability of the internal fluid matrix (*milieu intérieur*) as a necessary condition for what he termed the free and independent life (Bernard, 1878). Walter Cannon, chair of the Department of Physiology at Harvard around the turn of the twentieth century, further elaborated on this concept and coined the term homeostasis (Cannon, 1932/1939). He believed that the autonomic nervous system (ANS) plays an important part in maintaining this homeostatic stability. Although Cannon recognized the importance of visceral afferents in homeostatic reflexes, the predominant view of the ANS was as an efferent, lower-level, reflexive motor system. Cannon further asserted that the ANS is termed "'autonomic' because it acts automatically, without direction from the cerebral cortex" (Cannon, 1939, p. 250). This misconception was perhaps understandable, as it would be another half century before the existence of direct, monosynaptic projections from cortical and other telencephalic areas to lower brainstem autonomic source nuclei and reflex substrates would be documented (e.g. Barbas et al., 2003; Cechetto & Saper, 1990; Dum, Levinthal, & Strick, 2016; Neafsey, 1990).

In retrospect, this misconception is also somewhat surprising in view of the work of Cannon's friend, contemporary, and Nobel Laureate, Ivan Pavlov (see Figure 1.1). Here, it is often underappreciated that much of Pavlov's work on learning centered on the modification of an autonomic and homeostatic reflex that involves the processing of interoceptive information in preparation for digestion—the cephalic vagal reflex, or the cephalic phase insulin release to a stimulus which had previously been paired with food. Indeed, this work contributed to a foundation for understanding how interoceptive phenomena can be powerfully related to learning and other processes instantiated in higher brain systems that can jointly influence visceral control, including systems within the cerebral cortex. This includes experience-based acquired responses that can both modulate

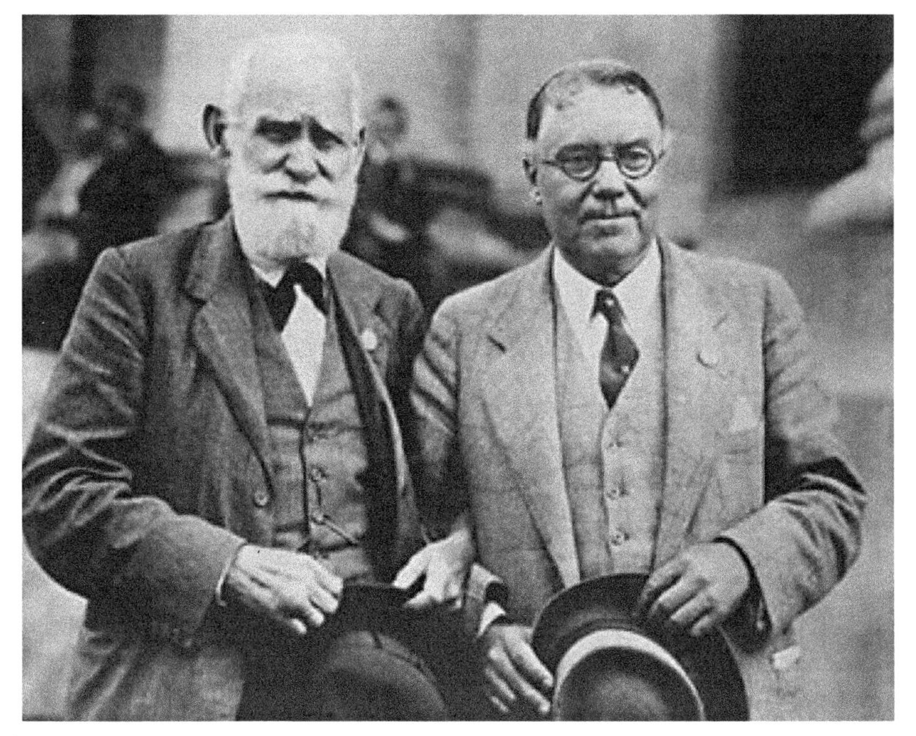

Figure 1.1 Walter B. Cannon with Ivan Pavlov at the 1929 International Physiological Congress. Photograph reproduced with the acquiescence of the curator (Harvard Medical Library in the Francis A. Countway Library of Medicine).

ongoing visceral processes as well as anticipate and prospectively guide adaptive autonomic, cognitive, and emotional responses (Cameron, 2002; Dworkin, 1993).

Well before the existence of long descending pathways linking brain and viscera had been established, functional studies revealed autonomic representations in multiple higher-level diencephalic and telencephalic areas of the forebrain. The 1949 Nobel Laureate, Walter Hess, for example, had reported striking autonomic responses elicited by stimulation of telencephalic (e.g. the amygdala and septal area) and diencephalic structures, including the hypothalamus, which Hess considered the head-ganglion of the autonomic nervous system (Hess, 1954; see also Ranson, Kabat, & Magoun, 1935). The Canadian neurosurgeon, Wilder Penfield, also reported autonomic responses to cortical stimulation in conscious human patients (Penfield & Jasper, 1954). At this point, we recognize a broad central autonomic network comprising a number of forebrain areas, including the insular cortex, cingulate cortex, medial prefrontal cortex, amygdala, and hippocampus, as well as caudal cell groups in the midbrain periaqueductal gray, pons, cerebellum, and medulla (Benarroch, 1993; Cechetto & Saper, 1990; Critchley, 2005; Dampney, 2015; Loewy, 1991; Neafsey, 1990; Saper, 2002; Shoemaker & Goswami, 2015). This network highly overlaps and interacts with systems implicated in complex cognitive, skeletomotor, and affective processes (Annoni et al., 2003; Critchley, 2005; Myers, 2017; Saper, 2002).

Another legacy from the Cannon era that did not survive the test of time is the view that the ANS is primarily an efferent motor system, with minimal visceral afferents necessary to support homeostatic reflex functions. In his influential book, *The Wisdom of the Body*, Cannon stated: "The nerve fibers of the autonomic nervous system, which are mostly efferent, pass out of the central nervous system" (Cannon, 1939, p. 252). Similarly, John Newton Langley, who coined the term autonomic nervous system[1] (Langley, 1898) viewed the ANS largely as a motor system, although he recognized that one might "consider as afferent autonomic fibers those which give rise to reflexes in autonomic tissues . . . [but are] . . . incapable of directly giving rise to sensation" (Langley, 1903, p. 2). As early as the mid-1930s, however, there were quantitative studies demonstrating that the majority of fibers in the vagus are sensory (Foley & DuBois, 1937; Heinbecker & O'Leary, 1933). This is consistent with contemporary estimates that 70–90% of vagal fibers, about 2–20% of fibers in the splanchnic (sympathetic) nerves, and about 2% in spinal nerves are visceral afferents[2] (Berthoud & Neuhuber, 2000; Cameron, 2002; Jänig & Morrison, 1986).

Historically, there were also notable conceptual challenges to the notion that the ANS is primarily a motor system. In contrast to the view that emotions precede and trigger bodily reactions, William James (1884) proposed that exciting events induce bodily

[1] "We propose the term 'autonomic nervous system,' for the sympathetic system and the allied nervous system of the cranial and sacral nerves, and for the local nervous system of the gut" (p. 270).

[2] Although some of these afferents run with parasympathetic and sympathetic efferents, it is not appropriate to consider them "parasympathetic" and "sympathetic" afferents (Freire-Maia & Azevedo,1990; Jänig & Häbler, 1995). They are general visceral afferents that are not strictly coupled to an autonomic branch.

changes (including autonomic responses) and that our subsequent feeling of these changes constitutes the emotion. Shortly thereafter, Carl Lange (1885) independently proposed a vascular theory of emotion, which held that vasomotor responses are the primary effects of affectations, and subjective sensations of emotion arise secondarily. Both of these perspectives converged into a view of visceral afference as fundamental for the generation and experience of emotion.

This view came under severe assault from two notable figures: Walter Cannon (1927, 1931), often considered the "father of the autonomic nervous system" and Sir Charles Sherrington (1900)—a notable turn-of-the-century physiologist and a recipient of the Nobel Prize in Physiology or Medicine (1932) for "discoveries regarding the functions of neurons." At least the strong form of the James–Lange concept (emotions as the mere perception of visceral feedback) was largely discredited at that time. There were a number of arguments against the James–Lange perspective. Cannon, for example, argued that the viscera have few afferents and are relatively insensate. However, it is now recognized that visceral afferents in fact outnumber efferents. Additionally, it was argued that (a) visceral responses are too slow to underlie emotion; (b) similar visceral changes may occur across different emotions and even non-emotional states; (c) inducing autonomic responses does not necessarily invoke emotions; and (d) that autonomic denervations of various types do not prevent emotional reactions. None of those are particularly telling arguments unless one wants to assert an identity relationship between visceral afference and emotion. James (1884), in fact, viewed emotions as being multiply determined, and to include cognitive contributions. He stipulated in his 1884 article that the only emotions that he will "consider here are those that have a distinct bodily expression" (p. 189)—the so-called coarser emotions. It is well established that there are multi-level hierarchical and heterarchical representations in neurobehavioral systems and central autonomic networks (see Berntson, Cacioppo, & Bosch, 2016; Norman, Berntson, & Cacioppo, 2014), and there are multiple determinants of affective processes. What will become apparent through the chapters of this volume is that there are powerful interactions between cognitive and emotional processes, somatic and autonomic outflows, and interoceptive feedback. Consequently, the effects of interoceptive feedback would not be expected to be invariant but to show notable brain-state and context dependencies (e.g. see Cacioppo, Berntson, & Klein, 1992).

1.3 **A case report**

Visceral afference can powerfully modulate cognitive and emotional processes, as illustrated by the following case report on MM (personal communication). MM is a graphic artist and videographer who was working on a documentary about a historical kidnapping and murder. She had extensively researched and documented the story and had located and interviewed most of the characters involved (except for the perpetrator, who had killed himself). The story was ready for filming (January 2007), but, alas, filming never happened:

> I handed the story back to the producer when it became clear that I could not work the script (kept repeating the same scenes), as I was able to keep it all in my head for only about 3 pages—few

> minutes, and no amount of colour coordinated storylines and Post-It notes were going to save me when I was not able to make a simple decision on spot (calculating what days we had available for shooting whom . . . etc.).

What led to this transformation (February 2007)? It was *endoscopic thoracic sympathectomy* (ETS), the surgical destruction or disabling of the upper spinal sympathetic (autonomic) nerve trunk, for hyperhidrosis (excessive sweating). Thereafter, MM's life (she was 39 years old at the time) was dramatically changed[3]:

> It is my experience that following this surgery there is a shift in personality and how emotions are experienced. It is, however, not only emotional blunting but also an impaired impulse control and disinhibition (as if a grown-up brain has been replaced by a primitive, and at times manic brain, that affects higher functioning). I am not sure how to describe it really . . . There is an indifference and striking lack of fear . . . I witnessed within myself once I got into my car and started driving around, or in general danger situations any urbanite encounters. My emotions are blunted, and there is an unsettling deadness and indifference towards my prior life and aspirations, goals. This indifference and emotional blunting was present as soon as I woke up from the surgery and has not left me since.
>
> . . .
>
> In general, the procedure led to a personality change, in some aspects subtle, in others a profound shift that I find exceedingly difficult to accept—a kind of physiological expression of how I was feeling, zombie-like.
>
> . . .
>
> I was described by one (video) critic as a human seismograph, recording the finest shifts in mood/tone . . . (now) I have problems in social settings, where I generally might appear antisocial. I force myself to ask questions and engage in "banter", but more often I forget. I would say that it has changed how I relate to people: I do not relate.

Tragically, this outcome was not unique to MM. There is a considerable literature documenting a range of post-sympathectomy complications including cognitive deficits, altered mood, emotional blunting, fatigue, and neuropathic complications (e.g. Furlan, Mailis, & Papagapious, 2000; Goldstein, 2012; Mailis & Furlan, 2003). Indeed, a support group, the Sympathetic Association (FfSo), was formed in Karlstad, Sweden, by people who found themselves disabled by serious side effects of sympathectomies (<http://home.swipnet.se/sympatiska/index3.htm>). We will return to the case of MM in section 1.4.2.

1.4 Central visceral pathways and the visceral cortex

An important integrative site in the forebrain for visceral afference is the insular cortex, which could be considered a primary visceral cortical site. The insula, in turn, is highly interconnected with cortical and subcortical areas involved in cognition, emotion, and

[3] There was no pre-surgical history of psychopathology. The patient elected the procedure to reduce excessive sweating, and to some extent, this was achieved. However, as is common with ETS (Furlan et al., 2000), she did experience periodic "compensatory" sweating.

motivation, including the prefrontal cortex, the cingulate cortex, and the amygdala (Allen et al., 1991; Augustine, 1996; Nieuwenhuys, 2012; Oppenheimer & Cechetto, 2016). The insula receives input from all visceral afference and, as will be seen throughout this volume, contributes to the integration of this afference with neurobehavioral processes (Tsakiris & Critchley, 2016a), and anomalies in insular function are associated with a wide range of cognitive, emotional, and behavioral disturbances (Gasquoine, 2014).

1.4.1 Special visceral afferents: The chemical senses—Olfaction and gustation

Olfaction is a special visceral sense closely linked with both positive and negative hedonics. This is especially true in lower animals where it plays a central role in guiding behavior. The olfactory system is closely linked with a medial central brain network that was historically referred to as the rhinencephalon (nose brain). Paul Broca (1878) referred to the medial central components of the brain as the great limbic lobe (*le grand lobe limbique*) because they arch around the central encephalon ("*limbique*" in French translates as "hoop" or "curve"). Papez (1937) proposed that limbic areas and associated structures are an important central network in emotion (often referred to as Papez circuit). This concept was further developed by Paul MacLean (1954) who coined the term "limbic system" and viewed this system as an evolutionary heritage (the paleomammalian brain) that regulates emotion, motivation, and survival-related behaviors, as well as links these phenomena with vulnerability to chronic health conditions (e.g. hypertension, asthma). Olfactory afferents play an important role in emotion, motivation, and survival-related behavioral processes. Although the olfactory system more directly projects to a number of cortical areas, olfactory information is also relayed via the thalamus and other cortical areas to the insular cortex (which itself is often considered to be a part of the limbic system). Odors can modulate mood, cognition, and behavior, and many of these effects appear to be mediated by the insula (for reviews see Miranda, 2012; Saive, Royet, & Plailly, 2014; Soudry et al., 2011).

The primary gustatory cortex lies in the anterior insula. Gustatory afferents (cranial nerves VII, IX, and X) terminate in a medullary nucleus, the NTS, and then are relayed via the midbrain parabrachial nucleus to the ventroposteromedial thalamus, which issues direct projections to the anterior insula (Saper, 2002). A similar functional pattern emerges in the literature to that of olfaction (Rolls, 2015). There are potent insular contributions to the processing of taste hedonics and attentional and memorial processes associated with taste, and insular cortex abnormalities are associated with disturbances in these processes (Frank, Kullmann, & Veit, 2013; Maffei, Haley, & Fontanini, 2012).

1.4.2 General visceral afferents

As is the case with gustatory afferents, all GVAs in cranial nerves project to the NTS in the brainstem, to the parabrachial nucleus in the midbrain, and then via the ventroposteromedial (VPM) nucleus of the thalamus to the insular cortex. In his classic studies, Wilder Penfield reported that electrical stimulation of the insula induced a variety of visceral sensory experiences (Penfield & Jasper, 1954; Penfield & Faulk, 1955). In addition to cranial nerves, GVAs carrying nociceptive, temperature, and chemosensory information from the body enter the spinal cord via dorsal spinal roots and terminate in the dorsal horn (especially in lamina I). Until around the turn of the twenty-first century, the general belief was that small-diameter nociceptive (i.e. sensory information about tissue damage)/temperature afferents were part of the somatosensory system and were ultimately relayed to the somatosensory cortex in the parietal lobe. Indeed, this view persists. In their 2016 textbook on neuroscience, Bear, Connors, and Paradiso assert that the "spinothalamic pathway is the major route by which pain and temperature information ascend to the cerebral cortex" (2016, p. 444). In fact, it is now well established that the small diameter fibers carrying nociceptive, temperature, and chemical senses project from the VPM not to the somatosensory cortex but to the insula (Craig, 2014; Saper, 2002). This accounts for the fact that in Wilder Penfield's studies, patients never reported pain on stimulation of the somatosensory cortex (Penfield & Jasper, 1954; Penfield & Faulk; 1955). Moreover, surgeons do not extirpate the somatosensory cortex for pain syndromes. In contrast, however, Mazzola and colleagues (2012) report induced pain with stimulation of the insular cortex, and painful "somatosensory" seizures appear to arise not from the somatosensory cortex but from the opercular-insular cortex (Montavont et al., 2015).

This general visceral afference, and the top-down and bottom-up integration of insular cortical systems, underlie the cognitive-emotional processes that reflect the broad integrative contributions of the insula (Tsakiris & Critchley, 2016a). Insula lesions, for example, result in diminished emotional arousal to affective pictures, and a reduced ability to even recognize the affective picture content (Berntson et al., 2011). Although the literature on insular involvement in emotion and emotional processing is quite consistent (Uddin, Nomi, & Hébert-Seropian, 2017), there appears to be some diversity in the effects of insular lesions.[4] In addition to its role in emotion and motivation, the insula appears to play a pivotal role in the sense of self, agency, and indeed, consciousness (Craig, 2014; Strigo & Craig, 2016; Tsakiris & Critchley, 2016a, b; see also Chapters 2, 3, and 16 in the present volume). Thus, insula activation is correlated with the sense of body ownership and agency (Farrer, Franck, & Georgieff, 2003; Tsakiris et al., 2007). In accord, lesions of the insula can lead to a disturbed sense of body ownership, including somatoparaphrenia or the denial of body ownership (Cogliano et al., 2012; Gandola et al., 2012; Karnath & Baier, 2010; Moro et al., 2016).

These findings and further results addressed in the present volume indicate that visceral afferent input to the insula appears to be critical in cognitive and emotional processes.

[4] Garcia and colleagues (2016) report minimal cognitive or socio-emotional deficits in a single case report after extensive vascular lesion damage, including the insular cortex. The authors, however, emphasize how unusual this case was as there were also minimal disturbances in sensorimotor and other functions. The literature on disgust, especially, is quite variable, but Uddin and colleagues (2017) report consistent socio-emotional deficits with insular lesions, but they also emphasize the considerable functional heterogeneity in this brain region.

However, one may see similar deficits with disrupted visceral afference in the absence of frank insular impairments. Patients with pure autonomic failure, and the associated blunting of autonomic activity and visceral afference, have been reported to show deficits in cognitive processing, empathy and emotional reactivity (Chauhan, Mathias, & Critchley, 2008; Critchley, Mathias, & Dolan, 2001; Tsakiris et al., 2006). In this regard, returning to our case study, although MM did not have a direct insular insult, the surgical sympathectomy would have as a necessary consequence a diminution of both sympathetic and parasympathetic visceral afference, and this may have contributed to the cognitive and emotional sequelae she experienced. Critchley and colleagues (2001, p. 207) asserted that "body state changes, particularly those mediated by the autonomic nervous system, are crucial to the ongoing emotional experience of emotion," and Goldstein (2012) reported that partial cardiac denervation was associated with fatigue, altered mood, blunted emotion, and decreased ability to concentrate. The findings that meditation can increase insular activity, connectivity, gray and white matter volume raise a question as to a potential therapeutic strategy in visceral denervation syndromes (Gotink et al., 2016; Hernandez et al., 2016; Laneri et al., 2016).

1.5 Current applications and implications

The central autonomic network (CAN) and neurobehavioral substrates more generally become re-represented and elaborated with the evolutionary development of higher-level neural systems (Jackson, 1884). This has significant implications for the functional understanding of the autonomic nervous system, visceral afference, and the multi-level representations in the CAN. To elaborate, lower-level autonomic reflexes, such as those studied by Cannon, are relatively hardwired and highly regulated by local visceral afference contributing to the feedback regulation of homeostasis. The baroreceptor reflexes, for example, are visceral homeostatic control loops that constrain short-term variations in blood pressure via rapid autonomic adjustments. The afferent limb of the baroreflexes encompasses interoceptors positioned in the heart and great arteries. Increases in blood pressure cause a distortion of their free nerve endings, leading to an increase in afferent firing and associated afferent input to the NTS. Via relays in the rostral and caudal ventrolateral medulla, this NTS afferent input results in a subsequent reflexive reduction in sympathetic and an increase in parasympathetic control of the heart and cardiovascular system, culminating in an associated compensatory reduction in blood pressure. The sensitivity of the homeostatic baroreceptor heart rate reflex can be quantified by the slope of the function relating heart rate to blood pressure. This slope reflects in part the servocontrol of blood pressure by heart rate decreases with increasing blood pressure (decreasing cardiac output) and heart rate increases with decreasing blood pressure (increasing cardiac output). It was Cannon's student, Philip Bard, however, who noted that the slope of the baroreflex function could be decreased (flattened) by a typical laboratory stressor (reflecting a decrease in sensitivity of the baroreflex). That is to say, stressors "inhibit" the homeostatic control over blood pressure by the baroreflex, which presumably enables heart rate and blood pressure to rise simultaneously and rapidly to provide hemodynamic and metabolic support for adaptive action or stressor coping. Although stressor-evoked effects on the baroreflex have been widely seen across species, such effects raise a number of basic questions insofar as they reflect “anti-homeostatic” actions that appear to be implemented by higher levels of the CAN. That is, while homeostasis is an important contribution of the ANS, ANS effects are not always homeostatic across behavioral states (see Berntson, Cacioppo, & Bosch, 2016). Indeed, it may be maladaptive to maintain a “fixity” of the internal milieu by lower reflex substrates of the CAN. In this way and in the face of adaptive challenges, higher levels of the CAN may modulate or “reset” lower substrates for reflex control to implement contextually appropriate, anticipatory, or otherwise “adaptive” increases in both blood pressure and heart rate (Dampney, 2017).

Sterling and Eyer (1988) and later Schulkin (2003) introduced the concept of allostasis to reflect the fact that homeostasis is not necessarily static, but can assume different regulatory levels (setpoints), to adapt to survival challenges. An example of this is fever, which unlike the “anti-homeostatic” baroreflex effects of stress, represents a true adoption of a higher regulatory setpoint, which is monitored and actively defended both physiologically and behaviorally. Bruce McEwen (2012) subsequently introduced the concept of allostatic load to reflect the fact that while short-term allostatic adjustments may be adaptive, sustained, long-term allostatic adjustments may have cumulative and deleterious health consequences. However, deviations from homeostasis may not always entail simply an altered setpoint level. Berntson, Cacioppo, and Bosch (2016) advanced the concept of heterodynamic regulation in which higher level CAN and neurobehavioral substrates, integrating somatovisceral afference, cognitive and emotional processing, can dynamically regulate autonomic outflows and therefore somatovisceral afference in a flexible, dynamic fashion to achieve more optimal adaptive outcomes that are appropriate to given behavioral contexts.

These considerations suggest that classical concepts of the autonomic nervous system, which focus on autonomic reflexes and homeostasis, are inadequate for a full understanding of the contributions of the ANS and its afference to neurobehavioral processes. An illustration of the latter point is evident in contemporary perspectives on the role of interoceptive processes in physiological stress reactivity and recovery. More precisely, physiological stress reactivity and recovery have received widespread and long-standing attention because of their presumptive relationships with aspects of physical and mental health across the lifespan (Cohen , Gianaros, & Manuck, 2016). For example, people with phenotypes to exhibit exaggerated and prolonged rises in heart rate and blood pressure that are mediated by the autonomic nervous system are at elevated risk for hypertension, stroke, myocardial infarction, and early death (Ginty, Kraynak, Fisher,et al., 2017).

The central substrates for such patterns of stressor-evoked physiological reactivity and recovery have been studied for over a century in human and non-human animal studies. Notwithstanding, a historically neglected dimension of these substrates is how they are influenced by stressor-evoked interoceptive information encoded in peripheral physiology (Gianaros & Wager, 2015). To elaborate, stressors are thought to engage higher neural substrates of the CAN, including the insula and anterior cingulate cortex (ACC), which may appraise stressors and in turn issue descending visceral motor commands for rapid autonomic adjustments to cardiovascular physiology. These centrally determined and stressor-evoked adjustments may entail simultaneous rises in blood pressure and heart rate, with accompanying modifications to the baroreflex, to provide metabolic support for behavioral action and stressor coping (Gianaros et al., 2012). This central linkage of behavior with metabolically supportive changes in cardiovascular physiology is exemplified in the cardiac-somatic coupling hypothesis of Obrist (1981) and the "central command hypothesis" within the field of exercise physiology (Fisher et al., 2015). More recent perspectives on this linkage now emphasize that central substrates for peripheral stress reactivity most likely issue visceral motor commands in a predictive fashion, providing metabolic support for behavior that is anticipated in the future (Ginty et al., 2017; Gianaros & Jennings, 2018). Moreover, these substrates may also predict patterns of expected visceral (interoceptive) feedback in a way that serves to calibrate peripheral physiology with behavior and the metabolic demands of a given context (Barrett & Simmons, 2015).

Understood in this way, "mismatches" between actual and predicted metabolic demands can be viewed as visceral prediction errors. These errors may manifest in the magnitude or patterning of stressor-evoked changes in peripheral physiology. For example, a rise in blood pressure in excess of 40 mmHg in preparing for a public speech can be seen as a visceral prediction error—insofar as it is a hemodynamic change that is disproportionate to the actual metabolic needs of the context. Likewise, sustained or prolonged changes in cardiovascular physiology that far outlast the ending of a given stressor can be viewed as metabolically disproportionate or otherwise contextually unnecessary and inappropriate. Visceral prediction errors of these types may be quantified by integrating laboratory stress reactivity testing with methods of exercise physiology, wherein changes in cardiovascular physiology that are in excess of oxygen consumption and metabolic requirements of a context can be computed (see Ginty et al., 2017; Gianaros & Jennings, 2018).

The presumptive bases for visceral prediction errors may partly involve the resetting or modulation of homeostatic functions by substrates of the central autonomic network, allowing for context-dependent changes in visceral control via the autonomic nervous system. Visceral prediction errors underlying observable patterns of stress physiology may also involve insensitivity to interoceptive and visceral feedback as well (Ginty et al., 2017; Gianaros & Jennings, 2018; see also Chapter 17 in the present volume). For example, as a result of such insensitivity, the visceral feedback provided by baroreceptors about "exaggerated" and stressor-evoked rises in blood pressure may not serve to minimize future visceral prediction errors that manifest as exaggerated stress reactivity. Moreover, interoceptive information from stressor-evoked changes in cardiovascular physiology (e.g. relayed by the baroreceptors) is capable of powerfully shaping the appraisal of threatening and painful information (Garfinkel & Critchley, 2016; see also Chapter 7 in this volume). Put simply, stressor-evoked changes in peripheral physiology do not happen in a vacuum, having "bottom-up" effects on higher neural substrates. Open questions in this domain extend to other parameters of physiology beyond the cardiovascular system that change with stress (e.g. immune and neuroendocrine functions), as well as how visceral feedback from multiple physiological parameters are integrated by higher neural substrates to shape behavioral states as they unfold across contexts.

1.6 From interoception to interoceptive awareness

The multiple reciprocal links between interoception and psychological function, as highlighted in the preceding sections, do not necessarily imply a conscious awareness or intervention. However, several research strands across psychological sciences and cognitive neuroscience have recently focused on our ability to become aware of interoceptive states and the importance that such states of interoceptive awareness have for the awareness of the self and of others. Earlier psychological research has shown how higher levels of interoceptive accuracy that is typically quantified in behavioral tasks that require participants to pay attention to interoceptive states such as heartbeats (Schandry, 1981), respiration (Daubenmier et al., 2013), or feelings of fullness and gastric sensitivity (Herbert et al., 2012) influence emotional processing. For example, higher levels of interoceptive accuracy are associated with more intense emotional experiences and better emotion regulation (see Critchley & Harrison, 2013)

Capitalizing on such findings, more recent studies have expanded their focus to ask questions about the role that interoceptive awareness may play for body representations (for reviews see Craig, 2009; Tsakiris, 2010). Historically, the perception of one's own body from the outside (e.g. self-recognition) and the perception of the body from within (e.g. of signals coming from the visceral organs) have largely been studied independently. For example, the question of how the brain produces the experience of body ownership has focused mainly on multisensory integration. In the Rubber Hand Illusion (RHI), one of the most influential experimental models of embodiment, watching a rubber hand being stroked synchronously with one's own unseen hand causes the rubber hand to be experienced as part of one's body (Botvinick & Cohen, 1998; Tsakiris, 2010). These results speak in favor of an exteroceptive model of the self within which self-awareness is highly malleable, subject to the perception of the body from the outside. However, exteroceptive input represents only one set of channels of information available for body awareness. We are also interoceptively aware of our body.

To address how interoceptive signals are integrated with exteroceptive signals to create an integrated sense of the bodily self, Tsakiris, Tajadura-Jiménez, and Costantini (2011) measured and quantified Interoceptive Accuracy (IAcc) with the heartbeat-counting task and compared this with the change in body ownership caused by multisensory stimulation, using the RHI as a paradigmatic case of the exteroceptive self. Participants with lower IAcc experienced a stronger illusory sense of body ownership, suggesting that in the absence of accurate interoceptive representations one's model of self is predominantly exteroceptive. While others had shown how a change in the body ownership during RHI affects homeostatic regulation (Moseley et al., 2008), we now had evidence showing that both the experience of body ownership, and subsequent changes in homeostatic regulation, depend partly on levels of IAcc. Consistent with these behavioral findings, neuroimaging and neuropsychological observations on the critical role of the insular cortex for body awareness support the view that the ways in which we perceive our body from the inside interact with our perception of the body from the outside. Right anterior insula activity correlates with performance in interoceptive accuracy tasks (Critchley et al., 2004). A rare single-case study shows that heartbeat awareness decreased after insular resection (Ronchi et al., 2015), and Couto and colleagues (2015) report impaired interoceptive awareness with insular cortical or white matter lesions. Right mid-posterior insula activity correlates with the body ownership experienced during the Rubber Hand Illusion, a paradigm that uses exteroceptive input (e.g. vision and touch) to study, in a controlled way, the bodily self (Tsakiris et al., 2007). This same area seems to be the critical lesion site for somatoparaphrenia—a striking loss of body ownership (Karnath & Baier, 2010). These findings suggest that the interoceptive and the exteroceptive representations of the body are integrated from the posterior to anterior subregions across the insular cortex (Farb, Segal, & Anderson, 2013; Simmons et al., 2013). Moreover, this integration appears to underpin the experience of my body as mine—an experience that is the hallmark of the bodily self (Gallagher, 2000).

Such approaches paved the way for a large number of psychophysiological and neuroimaging studies (Aspell et al., 2013; Blefari et al., 2017; Crucianelli et al., 2017; Park et al., 2017; Ronchi et al., 2017; Schauder et al., 2015; Sel, Azevedo, & Tsakiris, 2016; Shah, Catmur, & Bird, 2017; Suzuki et al., 2013; Tajadura-Jiménez & Tsakiris, 2014) that corroborate the basic hypothesis about the crucial psychological role that interoception plays for self-awareness and awareness of other people (see also Chapter 2 in the present volume). Across different domains, from emotion processing (Dunn et al., 2010; Pollatos et al. 2007) to body image (see Badoud & Tsakiris, 2017 for a review), and social cognition (Shah et al. 2017), the representation that one has of her internal body seems to be crucial for the representation of the "material me", as Sherrington would put it, in relation to others (Fotopoulou & Tsakiris, 2017).

1.7 Future perspectives

The complexity of the central autonomic network, its vast interconnectivity with other brain systems, and the broad functional impact of visceral afference all pose challenges to progress in the interoceptive canon. Although there may certainly be a place for studies of single interoceptive dimensions or measures, a full understanding is most likely to require the consideration of multiple parameters and physiological patterns, from a multi-system, multi-level interacting (top-down and bottom-up) perspective. Thus, important directions for the future include a focus on multiple interoceptive dimensions, interdisciplinary perspectives (cognitive/behavioral, neural, physiological, etc.) and interactions among interoceptive processes and a broader range of affective-cognitive processes. An illustration of this point comes from the literature on autonomic specificity of emotions and the role of visceral afference.

Consider Cannon's arguments against the James–Lange view, that: (a) visceral responses are too slow to underlie emotion; (b) similar visceral changes may occur across different emotions and even non-emotional states; (c) inducing autonomic responses does not necessarily invoke emotions; and (d) that autonomic denervations of various types do not prevent emotional reactions. There clearly is not a simple isomorphism between autonomic responses and emotions, but that really should not be expected; there are multiple determinants of emotion and multiple levels of organization in affective substrates and the central autonomic network. Emotions can be triggered cognitively, as well as from external stimuli and context. These may well have different patterns of activation within central networks. The arguments that visceral responses are too slow and that autonomic denervations do not eliminate emotions would only be arguments against the view that visceral afference is the only determinant of emotion. We now know this not to be the case. Moreover, visceral afference is also likely to be "fast" enough to exert influences along the lines of what James and Lange envisioned. Neurally mediated baroreflex influences on heart rate and blood pressure control, for example, happen within milliseconds. These influences extend to the processing of and reactivity to affective and nociceptive stimuli on a heartbeat-to-heartbeat basis (Garfinkel and Critchley, 2016).

Canon's two remaining arguments, that autonomic arousal may not lead to emotional states and that similar autonomic responses may be associated with different emotions, are also not compelling. As noted earlier, the effects of visceral afference are likely to be varied and brain-state dependent (e.g. see also Chapter 10 in the present volume). A given pattern of visceral afference in one context (be that environmental, psychological, or neurophysiological) may well have quite distinct effects. How we perceive a stimulus or context is very much determined by expectations, goals, and attentional focus, in the same way that classic visual illusions (e.g. the old woman/young woman illusion; Boring, 1930) depend on attentional focus, expectations, priming, or other variables.

A given pattern of visceral afference, for example, may be functionally perceived, and have different outcomes depending on the context or neurobiological or neurobehavioral (brain) state. This has been termed the somatovisceral model of emotion (SAME) wherein the same pattern of visceral afference may be associated with different emotions (see Cacioppo et al., 1992; Norman et al., 2014). As with research on interoception, there is consensus that research on interoceptive awareness must develop a wider and more grounded measurement model, a richer theoretical framework that is at the same time biologically plausible and psychologically meaningful, and a fuller characterization of the links between different interoceptive systems and across interoceptive and exteroceptive systems. This contextual and brain-state dependency needs to be considered in interpreting and understanding visceral afference and our awareness of it, across different fields, from basic research to clinical applications and from theoretical and computational perspectives. The chapters included in this volume intend to address at least some of these aims.

References

Adolfi, F., **Couto, B.**, **Richter, F.**, **Decety, J.**, **Lopez, J.**, **Sigman, M.**, et al. (2017). Convergence of interoception, emotion, and social cognition: A twofold fMRI meta-analysis and lesion approach. *Cortex*, **88**, 124–42. doi:10.1016/j.cortex.2016.12.019.

Allen, G. V., **Saper, C. B.**, **Hurley, K. M.**, and **Cechetto, D. F.** (1991). Organization of visceral and limbic connections in the insular cortex of the rat. *Journal of Comparative Neurology*, **311**, 1–16.

Annoni, J. M., **Ptak, R.**, **Caldara-Schnetzer, A. S.**, **Khateb, A.**, and **Pollermann B. Z.** (2003). Decoupling of autonomic and cognitive emotional reactions after cerebellar stroke. *Annals of Neurology*, **53**, 654–8.

Aspell, J. E., **Heydrich, L.**, **Marillier, G.**, **Lavanchy, T.**, **Herbelin, B.**, and **Blanke, O.** (2013). Turning body and self inside out: Visualized heartbeats alter bodily self-consciousness and tactile perception. *Psychological Science*, *24*, 2445–53. <https://doi.org/10.1177/0956797613498395>

Augustine, J. R. (1996). Circuitry and functional aspects of the insular lobe in primates including humans. *Brain Research Reviews*, **22**, 229–44.

Badoud, D. and **Tsakiris, M.** (2017). From the body's viscera to the body's image: Is there a link between interoception and body image concerns? *Neuroscience & Biobehavioral Reviews*, **77**, 237–46. doi:10.1016/j.neubiorev.2017.03.017.

Barbas, H., **Saha, S.**, **Rempel-Clower, N.**, and **Ghashghaei, T.** (2003). Serial pathways from primate prefrontal cortex to autonomic areas may influence emotional expression. *BMC Neuroscience*, **4**, 25.

Barrett, L. F. and **Simmons, W.K.** (2015). Interoceptive predictions in the brain. *Nature Reviews Neuroscience*, **16**, 419–29.

Bear, M.F., **Connors, B.W.**, and **Paradiso, M. A.** (2016). *Neuroscience: Exploring the Brain*. Philadelphia, PA: Wolters Kluwer.

Benarroch, E. E. (1993). The central autonomic network: Functional organization, dysfunction, and perspective. *Mayo Clinic Proceedings*, *68*(10), 988–1001.

Bernard, C. (1878). *Les Phénomènes de la Vie*. Paris: Ballière.

Berntson, G. G., **Bechara, A.**, **Damasio, H.**, **Tranel, D.**, **Norman, G.J.**, and **Cacioppo, J.T.** (2011). The insula and evaluative processes. *Psychological Science*, **22**, 80–6.

Berntson, G. G., **Cacioppo, J. T.**, and **Bosch, J. A.** (2016). From homeostasis to allodynamic regulation. In J. T. Cacioppo, L. G. Tassinary, and G. G. Berntson (eds). *Handbook of Psychophysiology*, 4th edn. Cambridge: Cambridge University Press, pp. 401–26.

Berthoud, H. R. and **Neuhuber, W. L.** (2000). Functional and chemical anatomy of the afferent vagal system. *Autonomic Neuroscience*, **85**, 1–17.

Blefari, M. L., **Martuzzi, R.**, **Salomon, R.**, **Bello-Ruiz, J.**, **Herbelin, B.**, **Serino, A.**, et al. (2017). Bilateral Rolandic operculum processing underlying heartbeat awareness reflects changes in bodily self-consciousness. *European Journal of Neuroscience*, *45*(10), 1300–12. <https://doi.org/10.1111/ejn.13567>

Boring, E. G. (1930). A new ambiguous figure. *The American Journal of Psychology*, **42**, 444.

Botvinick, M. and **Cohen, J.** (1998). Rubber hands "feel" touch that eyes see. *Nature*, *391*, 756. doi:10.1038/35784.

Boucher, O., **Rouleau, I.**, **Lassonde, M.**, **Lepore, F.**, **Bouthillier, A.**, and **Nguyen, D. K.** (2015). Social information processing following resection of the insular cortex. *Neuropsychologia*, **71**, 1–10. doi:10.1016/j.neuropsychologia.2015.03.008.

Broca, P. (1878). Anatomie comparée des circonvolutions cérébrales: Le grand lobe limbique et la scissure limbique dans la série des mammifères. *Revue d'Anthropologie*, **1**, 385–498.

Cacioppo, J. T., **Berntson, G. G.**, and **Klein, D.J.** (1992). What is an emotion? The role of somatovisceral afference, with special emphasis on somatovisceral "illusions". *Review of Personality and Social Psychology*, **14**, 63–98.

Cameron, O. G. (2002). *Visceral Sensory Neuroscience: Interoception*. Oxford: Oxford University Press.

Cannon, W. B. (1927). The James–Lange theory of emotions: A critical examination and an alternative theory. *American Journal of Psychology*, **39**, 106–24.

Cannon, W. B. (1931). Again, the James–Lange and the thalamic theory of emotion. *Psychological Review*, **38**, 281–95.

Cannon, W. B. (1932/1939). *The Wisdom of the Body*. London: Kegan Paul, Trench, Trubner & Co.

Cechetto, D. F. and **Saper, C. B.** (1990). Role of the cerebral cortex in autonomic function. In: A. D. Loewy and K. M. Spyer (eds), *Central Regulation of Autonomic Functions*. New York, NY: Oxford University Press, pp. 208–33.

Chauhan, B., **Mathias, C. J.**, and **Critchley, H. D.** (2008). Autonomic contributions to empathy: Evidence from patients with primary autonomic failure. *Autonomic Neuroscience*, **140**, 96–100.

Cogliano, R., **Crisci, C.**, **Conson, M.**, **Grossi, D.**, and **Trojano, L.** (2012). Chronic somatoparaphrenia: A follow-up study on two clinical cases. *Cortex*, **48**, 758–67

Cohen, S., **Gianaros, P.J.**, and **Manuck, S.B.** (2016). A stage model of stress and disease. *Perspectives on Psychological Science*, **11**, 456–63.

Couto, B., **Adolfi, F.**, **Sedeño, L.**, **Salles, A.**, **Canales-Johnson, A.**, **Alvarez-Abut**, et al. (2015). Disentangling interoception: Insights from focal strokes affecting the perception of external and internal milieus. *Frontiers in Psychology*, **6**, 503. doi:10.3389/fpsyg.2015.00503.

Craig, A. D. (2009). How do you feel-now? The anterior insula and human awareness. *Nature Reviews Neuroscience*, *10*, 59–70

Craig, A. D. (2014). *How Do You Feel? An Interoceptive Moment with Your Neurobiological Self*. Princeton, NJ: Princeton University Press.

Critchley, H. D., **Mathias, C. J.**, and **Dolan R. J.** (2001). Neuroanatomical basis for first- and second-order representations of bodily states. *Nature Neuroscience*, **4**, 207–12.

Critchley, H. D. (2005). Neural mechanisms of autonomic, affective, and cognitive integration. *Journal of Comparative Neurology*, **493**, 154–66.

Critchley, H. D., **Wiens, S.**, **Rotshtein, P.**, **Ohman, A.**, **Dolan, R. J.**, **Öhman, A.**, et al. (2004). Neural systems supporting interoceptive awareness. *Nature Neuroscience*, *7*(2), 189–95. <https://doi.org/10.1038/nn1176>

Critchley, H. D. and **Harrison, N. A.** (2013). Visceral influences on brain and behavior. *Neuron*, *77*, 624–38. <https://doi.org/10.1016/j.neuron.2013.02.008>

Crucianelli, L., **Krahé, C.**, **Jenkinson, P. M.**, and **Fotopoulou, A.** (2017). Interoceptive ingredients of body ownership: Affective touch and cardiac awareness in the rubber hand illusion. *Cortex*. <https://doi.org/10.1016/j.cortex.2017.04.018>

Daubenmier, J., **Sze, J.**, **Kerr, C. E.**, **Kemeny, M. E.**, and **Mehling, W.** (2013). Follow your breath: Respiratory interoceptive accuracy in experienced meditators. *Psychophysiology*, *50*(8), 777–89. <https://doi.org/10.1111/psyp.12057>

Dampney, R. A. (2015). Central mechanisms regulating coordinated cardiovascular and respiratory function during stress and arousal. *American Journal of Physiology. Regulatory, Integrative and Comparative Physiology*, **309**, R429–43.

Dampney, R. A. (2017). Resetting of the baroreflex control of sympathetic vasomotor activity during natural behaviors: Description and conceptual model of central mechanisms. *Frontiers in Neuroscience*, **11**, 461. <https://doi.org/10.3389/fnins.2017.00461>

Dum, R. P., Levinthal, D. J., and **Strick, P. L.** (2016). Motor, cognitive, and affective areas of the cerebral cortex influence the adrenal medulla. *Proceedings of the National Academy of Sciences*, **113**(35), 9922–7.

Dunn, B. D., Galton, H. C., Morgan, R., Evans, D., Oliver, C., Meyer, M., et al. (2010). Listening to your heart. How interoception shapes emotion experience and intuitive decision making. *Psychological Science*, *21*(12), 1835–44. <https://doi.org/10.1177/0956797610389191>

Dworkin, B. R. (1993). *Learning and Physiological Regulation*. Chicago, IL: University of Chicago Press.

Farb, N. A. S., Segal, Z. V., and **Anderson, A. K.** (2013). Attentional modulation of primary interoceptive and exteroceptive cortices. *Cerebral Cortex*, *23*(1), 114–26. <https://doi.org/10.1093/cercor/bhr385>

Farrer, C., Franck, N., Georgieff, N., Frith, C. D., Decety, J., and **Jeannerod** M. (2003). Modulating the experience of agency: A positron emission tomography study. *Neuroimage*, **18**, 324–33.

Fisher, J. P., Young, C. N., and **Fadel, P. J.** (2015). Autonomic adjustments to exercise in humans. *Comprehensive Physiology*, **5**, 475–512.

Foley, J. O. and **DuBois, F. S.** (1937). Quantitative studies of the vagus nerve in the cat. I. The ratio of sensory to motor fibers. *Journal of Comparative Neurology*, **67**, 49–64.

Fotopoulou, A. and **Tsakiris, M.** (2017). Mentalizing homeostasis: The social origins of interoceptive inference. *Neuropsychoanalysis*, **19**, 3–28

Frank, S., Kullmann, S., and **Veit, R.** (2013). Food related processes in the insular cortex. *Frontiers in Human Neuroscience*, **7**, 499.

Freire-Maia, L. and **Azevedo, A. D.** (1990). The autonomic nervous system is not a purely efferent system. *Medical Hypotheses*, **32**, 91–9.

Furlan, A. D., Mailis, A., and **Papagapiou, M.** (2000). Are we paying a high price for surgical sympathectomy? A systematic literature review of late complications. *Journal of Pain*, **1**, 245–57.

Gandola, M., Invernizzi, P., Sedda, A., Ferrè, E.R., Sterzi, R., Sberna, M., et al. (2012). An anatomical account of somatoparaphrenia. *Cortex*, **48**, 1165–78.

Gallagher, S. (2000). Philosophical conceptions of the self: Implications for cognitive science. *Trends in Cognitive Sciences*, *4*, 14–21.

García, A. M., **Sedeño, I., Murcia, E. H., Couto, B.,** and **Ibáñez, A.** (2016). A lesion-proof brain? Multidimensional sensorimotor, cognitive, and socio-affective preservation despite extensive damage in a stroke patient. *Frontiers in Aging Neuroscience*, **8**, 335.

Garfinkel, S. N. and **Critchley, H. D.** (2016). Threat and the body: How the heart supports fear processing. *Trends in Cognitive Science*, **20**, 34–46.

Gasquoine, P. G. (2014). Contributions of the insula to cognition and emotion. *Neuropsychology Review*, **24**, 77–87.

Gianaros, P. J., Onyewuenyi, I. C., Sheu, L. K., Christie, I. C., and **Critchley, H. D.** (2012). Brain systems for baroreflex suppression during stress in humans. *Human Brain Mapping*, **33**, 1700–16.

Gianaros, P. J. and **Wager, T. D.** (2015). Brain–body pathways linking psychological stress and physical health. *Current Directions in Psychological Science*, **24**, 313–21.

Gianaros, P. J. and **Jennings, J. R.** (2018). Host in the machine: A neurobiological perspective on psychological stress and cardiovascular disease. *American Psychologist*. doi:10.1037/amp0000232.

Ginty, A. T., Kraynak T. E., Fisher J. P., and **Gianaros P. G.** (2017). Cardiovascular and autonomic reactivity to psychological stress: Neurophysiological substrates and links to cardiovascular disease. *Autonomic Neuroscience*. doi:10.1016/j.autneu.2017.03.003.

Goldstein, D. S. (2012). Neurocardiology. *Cardiovascular Therapeutics*, **30**, e89–e106.

Gotink, R. A., Meijboom, R., Vernooij, M. W., Smits, M., and **Hunink, M. G.** (2016). 8-week mindfulness based stress reduction induces brain changes similar to traditional long-term meditation practice—A systematic review. *Brain and Cognition*, **108**, 32–41.

Heims, H. C., Critchley, H. D., Martin, N. H., Jäger, H. R., Mathias, C. J., and **Cipolotti, L.** (2006). Cognitive functioning in orthostatic hypotension due to pure autonomic failure. *Clinical Autonomic Research*, **16**, 113–20.

Heinbecker, P. and **O'Leary, J.** (1933). The mammalian vagus nerve—afunctional and histological study. *American Journal of Physiology*, **106**, 623–46.

Herbert, B. M., Muth, E. R., Pollatos, O., and **Herbert, C.** (2012). Interoception across modalities: On the relationship between cardiac awareness and the sensitivity for gastric functions. *PLoS One*, *7*(5), e36646.

Hernández, S. E., Suero, J., Barros, A., González-Mora, J. L., and **Rubia, K.** (2016). Increased grey matter associated with long-term sahaja yoga meditation: A voxel-based morphometry study. *PLoS One*, **11**(3).

Hess, W. R. (1954). *Diencephalon: Autonomic and Extrapyramidal Functions.* New York, NY: Grune & Stratton.

Jackson, J. H. (1884). On the evolution and dissolution of the nervous system. Croonian Lectures 3, 4 and 5 to the Royal Society of London. *Lancet*, **1**, 555–739.

James, W. (1984). What is emotion. *Mind*, **9**, 188–205.

Jänig, W. and **Morrison, J. F. B.** (1986). Functional properties of spinal visceral afferents supplying abdominal and pelvic organs with special emphasis on visceral nociception. In: F. Cervero and J. F. B. Morrison (eds). Visceral sensation. *Progress in Brain Research*, **67**, 87–114.

Jänig W. and **Häbler, H.-J.** (1995). Visceral-autonomic integration. In: G. F. Gebhart (ed.). *Visceral pain. Progress in Pain Research and Management*, Vol. **4**. Seattle, WA: IASP Press, pp. 311–48.

Karnath, H.-O. and **Baier, B.** (2010). Right insula for our sense of limb ownership and self-awareness of actions. *Brain Structure and Function*, *214*(5–6), 411–17. <https://doi.org/10.1007/s00429-010-0250-4>

Lange, C. G. (1885). *Om sindsbevaegelser: et psycho-fysiologisk studie.* Copenhagen: Jacob Lunds.

Laneri, D., Schuster, V., Dietsche, B., Jansen, A., Ott, U., and **Sommer, J.** (2016). Effects of long-term mindfulness meditation on brain's white matter microstructure and its aging. *Frontiers in Aging Neuroscience*, 7, 254.

Langley, J. N. (1898). On the union of cranial autonomic (visceral) fibers with the nerve cells of the superior cervical ganglion. *The Journal of Physiol*ogy, **23**, 240–70.

Langley, J. N. (1903). The autonomic nervous system. *Brain*, **26**, 1–26.

Loewy, A. D. (1991). Forebrain nuclei involved in autonomic control. *Progress in Brain Research*, **87**, 253–68.

MacLean, P. D. (1954). *Psychosomatic Medicine.* Alphen aan den Rijn: Wolters Kluwer Health, Inc.

Maffei, A., Haley, M., and **Fontanini, A.** (2012). Neural processing of gustatory information in insular circuits. *Current Opinion in Neurobiology*, **22**, 709–16.

Maffei, A. M., Haley, M., Fontanini, A., and **Miranda, M. I.** (2012). Taste and odor recognition memory: The emotional flavor of life. *Review of Neuroscience*, **23**, 481–99.

Mailis, A. and **Furlan, A.** (2003). Sympathectomy for neuropathic pain. *The Cochrane Database of Systematic Reviews*, **2**, CD002918.

Mazzola, L., Isnard, J., Peyron, R., and **Mauguière, F.** (2012). Stimulation of the human cortex and the experience of pain: Wilder Penfield's observations revisited. *Brain*, **135**, 631–40.

McEwen, B. S. (2012). Brain on stress: How the social environment gets under the skin. *Proceedings of the National Academy of Sciences of the USA*, **16**, 109 Suppl 2, 17180–5.

Montavont, A., Mauguière, F., Mazzola, L., Garcia-Larrea, L., Catenoix, H., Ryvlin, P., et al. (2015). On the origin of painful somatosensory seizures. *Neurology*, **84**, 594–601.

Moro, V., Pernigo, S., Tsakiris, M., Avesani, R., Edelstyn, N. M., Jenkinson, P.M., et al. (2016). Motor versus body awareness: Voxel-based lesion analysis in anosognosia for hemiplegia and somatoparaphrenia following right hemisphere stroke. *Cortex*, **83**, 62–77.

Moseley, G. L., Olthof, N., Venema, A., Don, S., Wijers, M., Gallace, A., et al. (2008). Psychologically induced cooling of a specific body part caused by the illusory ownership of an artificial counterpart. *Proceedings of the National Academy of Sciences of the USA*, *105*(35), 13169–73. <https://doi.org/10.1073/pnas.0803768105>

Myers, B. (2017). Corticolimbic regulation of cardiovascular responses to stress. *Physiology & Behavior*, **172**, 49–59.

Neafsey, E. J. (1990). Prefrontal cortical control of the autonomic nervous system: Anatomical and physiological observations. *Progress in Brain Research*, **85**, 147–65.

Nieuwenhuys, R. (2012). The insular cortex: A review. *Progress in Brain Research*, **195**, 123–63.

Norman, G. J., Berntson, G. G., and **Cacioppo, J. T.** (2014). Emotion, somatovisceral afference and autonomic regulation. *Emotion Review*, **6**, 113–23.

Obrist, P. A. (1981). *Cardiovascular Psychophysiology: A Perspective*. New York, NY: Plenum Press.

Oppenheimer, S. M. and **Cechetto, D. F.** (2016). Insular cortex and the regulation of cardiac function. *Comprehensive Physiology*, **6**, 1081–133.

Papez, J. (1937). A proposed mechanism of emotion. Reprinted in *Journal of Neuropsychiatry and Clinical Neuroscience* (1995) 7, 103–12.

Park, H.-D., Bernasconi, F., Salomon, R., Tallon-Baudry, C., Spinelli, L., Seeck, M., et al. (2017). Neural sources and underlying mechanisms of neural responses to heartbeats, and their role in bodily self-consciousness: An intracranial EEG Study. *Cerebral Cortex*, *116*, 1–14. <https://doi.org/10.1093/cercor/bhx136>

Penfield, W. and **Jasper, H.** (1954). *Epilepsy and the Functional Anatomy of the Human Brain*. New York, NY: Little, Brown & Co.

Penfield, W., and **Faulk, M. E.** (1955). The insula; further observations on its function. *Brain*, **78**, 445–70.

Pollatos, O., Gramann, K., and **Schandry, R.** (2007). Neural systems connecting interoceptive awareness and feelings. *Human Brain Mapping*, *28*(1), 9–18. <https://doi.org/10.1002/hbm.20258>

Ranson, S. W., Kabat, H., and **Magoun, H. W.** (1935). Autonomic responses to electrical stimulation of hypothalamus, preoptic region and septum. *Archives of Neurology & Psychiatry*, **33**, 467–77.

Rolls, E. T. (2015). Taste, olfactory, and food reward value processing in the brain. *Progress in Neurobiology*, **127–8**, 64–90.

Ronchi, R., Bello-Ruiz, J., Lukowska, M., Herbelin, B., Cabrilo, I., Schaller, K., et al. (2015). Right insular damage decreases heartbeat awareness and alters cardio-visual effects on bodily self-consciousness. *Neuropsychologia*, *70*, 11–20. <https://doi.org/10.1016/j.neuropsychologia.2015.02.010>

Ronchi, R., Bernasconi, F., Pfeiffer, C., Bello-Ruiz, J., Kaliuzhna, M., and **Blanke, O.** (2017). Interoceptive signals impact visual processing: Cardiac modulation of visual body perception. *NeuroImage*, *158*, 176–85. <https://doi.org/10.1016/j.neuroimage.2017.06.064>

Saive, A-L, Royet, J-P, and **Plailly, J.** (2014). A review on the neural bases of episodic odor memory: From laboratory-based to autobiographical approaches. *Frontiers in Behavioral Neuroscience*, **8**, 240.

Saper, C. B. (2002). The central autonomic nervous system: Conscious visceral perception and autonomic pattern generation. *Annual Review of Neuroscience*, **25**, 433–69.

Schandry, R. (1981). Heart beat perception and emotional experience. *Psychophysiology*, *18*(4), 483–8.

Schauder, K. B., **Mash, L. E.**, **Bryant, L. K.**, and **Cascio, C. J.** (2015). Interoceptive ability and body awareness in autism spectrum disorder. *Journal of Experimental Child Psychology, 131*, 193–200. <https://doi.org/10.1016/j.jecp.2014.11.002>

Schulkin, J. (2003). *Rethinking Homeostasis: Allostatic Regulation in Physiology and Pathophysiology.* Cambridge, MA: MIT Press.

Sel, A., **Azevedo, R. T.**, and **Tsakiris, M.** (2016). Heartfelt self: Cardio-visual integration affects self-face recognition and interoceptive cortical processing. *Cerebral Cortex.* <https://doi.org/10.1093/cercor/bhw296>

Shah, P., **Catmur, C.**, and **Bird, G.** (2017). From heart to mind: Linking interoception, emotion, and theory of mind. *Cortex.* April 28. Pii, S0010-9452(17)30060-6. doi:10.1016/j.cortex.2017.02.010.

Sherrington, C. S. (1900). Experiments on the value of vascular and visceral factors for the genesis of emotion. *Proceedings of the Royal Society (London) B*, **66**, 390–403.

Shoemaker, J. K. and **Goswami, R.** (2015). Forebrain neurocircuitry associated with human reflex cardiovascular control. *Frontiers in Physiology*, **6**, 240. doi:10.3389/fphys.2015.00240. <https://www.frontiersin.org/articles/10.3389/fphys.2015.00240/full>

Simmons, W. K., **Avery, J. A.**, **Barcalow, J. C.**, **Bodurka, J.**, **Drevets, W. C.**, and **Bellgowan, P.** (2013). Keeping the body in mind: Insula functional organization and functional connectivity integrate interoceptive, exteroceptive, and emotional awareness. *Human Brain Mapping, 34*, 2944–58. <https://doi.org/10.1002/hbm.22113>

Soudry, Y., **Lemogne, C.**, **Malinvaud, D.**, **Consoli, S.-M.**, and **Bonfils, P.** (2011). Olfactory system and emotion: Common substrates. *European Annals of Otorhinolaryngology, Head and Neck Diseases, 128(1)*, 18–23.

Squire, L., **Berg, D.**, **Bloom, F. E.**, **du Lac Anirvan, S.**, **Nicholas, G.**, and **Spitzer, C.** (2012). *Fundamental Neuroscience.* Oxford: Elsevier.

Sterling, P. and **Eyer, J.** (1988). Allostasis: A new paradigm to explain arousal pathology. In: S. Fisher and J. Reason (eds), *Handbook of Life Stress, Cognition and Health.* New York, NY: John Wiley & Sons, pp. 629–49.

Strigo, I. A. and **Craig, A. D.** (2016). Interoception, homeostatic emotions and sympathovagal balance. *Philosophical Transactions of the Royal Society of London. Series B, Biological Sciences*, **371**, 1708.

Suzuki, K., **Garfinkel, S. N.**, **Critchley, H. D.**, and **Seth, A. K.** (2013). Multisensory integration across exteroceptive and interoceptive domains modulates self-experience in the rubber-hand illusion. *Neuropsychologia, 51*, 2909–17. <https://doi.org/10.1016/j.neuropsychologia.2013.08.014>

Tajadura-Jiménez, A. and **Tsakiris, M.** (2014). Balancing the "inner" and the "outer" self: Interoceptive sensitivity modulates self-other boundaries. *Journal of Experimental Psychology: General, 143*(2). <https://doi.org/10.1037/a0033171>

Tsakiris, M., **Hesse, M. D.**, **Boy, C.**, **Haggard, P.**, and **Fink, G. R.** (2007). Neural signatures of body ownership: A sensory network for bodily self-consciousness. *Cerebral Cortex, 17*, 2235–44.

Tsakiris, M. (2010). My body in the brain: A neurocognitive model of body-ownership. *Neuropsychologia, 48*(3), 703–12. <https://doi.org/10.1016/j.neuropsychologia.2009.09.034>

Tsakiris, M., **Tajadura-Jiménez, A.**, and **Costantini, M.** (2011). Just a heartbeat away from one's body: Interoceptive sensitivity predicts malleability of body-representations. *Proceedings. Biological Sciences/The Royal Society, 278*, 2470–6. <https://doi.org/10.1098/rspb.2010.2547>

Tsakiris, M. and **Critchley, H.** (2016a). Interoception beyond homeostasis: Affect, cognition and mental health. *Philosophical Transactions of the Royal Society of London. Series B, Biological Sciences*, **371**, 1–6.

Tsakiris, M. and Critchley, H. (eds) (2016b). Theme issue: "Interoception beyond homeostasis: Affect, cognition and mental health". *Philosophical Transactions of the Royal Society of London. Series B*, **371**, issue 1708.

Uddin, L. Q., Nomi, J. S., Hébert-Seropian, B., Ghaziri, J., and **Boucher O.** (2017). Structure and function of the human insula. *Journal of Clinical Neurophysiology*, **34**, 300–6. doi:10.1097/WNP.0000000000000377.

Yates, B. J. and **Stocker, S. D.** (1998). Integration of somatic and visceral inputs by the brainstem: Functional considerations. *Experimental Brain Research*, **119**, 269–75.

PART II

Mentalizing interoception

Advances and challenges

Chapter 2

The body as first prior: Interoceptive predictive processing and the primacy of self-models

Micah Allen and Manos Tsakiris

2.1 Introduction

Behind every human experience lies a tapestry of embodied sensations; the beating of the heart, air filling the lungs, or the skin of the chest pulling taught with each breath are all instances of such sensations. Fascinatingly, although the sensations of the living, moving body are ever-available, they can also go easily unnoticed; in reading the previous sentence, you probably became more aware of them. Our heartbeat is usually silent unless we have exerted physical effort; in which case, its thrumming beat comes to dominate, however briefly, our self-awareness. In this sense, one can characterize our embodiment as a kind of ever-present, yet just behind-the-scenes kind of experience. What can cognitive neuroscience reveal about this special relationship between the body and our conscious mind?

Phenomenologists typically describe the transparency of the body as a preconditioning factor for awareness of the self, world, and others, emphasizing that all experience takes place from within this embodied subjective frame (Gallagher & Zahavi, 2013; Heidegger, 1996; Merleau-Ponty, 1996). Until recently however, the foundational role of embodied sensations in shaping our perceptual, cognitive, and socio-affective activity has been largely neglected by cognitive and computational neuroscience. This neglect may be in part due to a paucity of mechanistic theories equipped to generate testable hypotheses concerning the neural integration of visceral and exteroceptive bodily sensations. Now, resurgent interest in Bayes-inspired neuroscience is driving an explosion of empirical data and theoretical models which places the visceral milieu, its homeostatic functioning, and our interoceptive awareness thereof back on center stage. In this chapter, we provide an overview of the latest developments in this area, considering the developing notions of bodily precision and computational "self-models." At the core of our approach is the hypothesis that homeostatic priors are "first priors" in the sense that, given the impetus for the organism to maintain homeostasis, they are afforded a privileged status within the cortical hierarchy. Having explained their privileged status for ensuring the stability of organism, we then turn to the psychological importance that interoceptive priors and precision have for self-awareness, in particular for our understanding of domain-specific (i.e. body-awareness) as well as more global self-models (i.e. metacognition).

2.2 Predictive processing and the hierarchical optimization of precision

New developments in computational and cognitive neuroscience drive an increased emphasis on top-down, prediction-based theories of mind and brain function. These collectively describe the brain as a "prediction engine" which embodies or implements a statistically generative model describing the hidden causes of sensory inputs (Clark, 2013; Friston, 2010; Hohwy, 2013). Although so-called predictive processing (PP) approaches have a long history in neuroscience, beginning with early models of motor control (for review, see Miall & Wolpert, 1996), this renewed interest is driven in part by their recent generalization to domains such as social (Friston & Frith, 2015; Gallagher & Allen, 2016; Koster-Hale & Saxe, 2013), affective (Barrett & Simmons, 2015; Joffily & Coricelli, 2013; Seth, 2013), and embodied cognition (Ainley et al., 2016; Allen & Friston, 2016; Apps & Tsakiris, 2014). In particular, this new wave emphasizes the role of the visceral body in maintaining homeostasis as a fundamental aspect of the predictive mind.

The essential elements of the PP framework have been elaborated in numerous articles (Clark, 2013; Friston, 2005, 2010; Hohwy, 2014; see also Chapter 15 in the present volume); here we rehearse the basic elements to inform a discussion of their application to interoception and embodiment. The most general, formally articulated theory of predictive processing is found in the Free Energy Principle (FEP) as developed by Karl Friston (Friston, 2009, 2010, 2013). The FEP dictates that an organism can only survive by minimizing the entropy of internal states. That is, an entity which is subject to unbounded entropy—such as a snowflake—will not survive for very long. In contrast to the snowflake, which can only increase in entropy over time, a living organism like you and me, or an amoeba, can take self-sustaining (or autopoietic) actions which, for a time, resist entropy. This entails that an organism is fundamentally comprised of a Markov Blanket, constituted by an interlocking causal web of self-sustaining actions, new sensations, and an internal model interlinking the two. The Markov Blanket thus demarcates internal from external states and enables an organism to resist entropy both by acting on the world so as to render it closer to one's predictions (active inference) or through updating one's internal states (perceptual inference). In this way, the FEP furnishes a basic normative principle by which to guide our understanding of the embodied mind; biological organisms persist by virtue of their ability to maintain a stable autopoietic self, and to predict the impact of future actions on that homeostatic imperative. However, understanding how this *normative* principle plays out in specific neurobiological *process* theories requires specifying a particular architecture; for example, at what level of the cortical hierarchy do signals conveying successful homeostasis exert their influence on cognition, and in what manner, precisely?

Here it is useful to appeal to the varieties of Bayesian Predictive Coding (BPC) found in the predictive processing literature. As a general process theory, BPC-based approaches describe the brain as a hierarchical network implementing a distributed Bayesian inference scheme. Within this network, "top-down" signals encode a prior probability distribution (prediction); incoming sensory data are understood as a statistical likelihood, and the precision-weighted posterior difference between these two inputs—the prediction error—is passed upward to the next level of the hierarchy.[1] Neurobiologically, this scheme is thought to be accomplished by a canonical microcircuit motif, in which deep (infra-granular) pyramidal cells receive prediction errors from lower levels and superficial (agranular) cells encode predictions. This motif is assumed to be replicated across the brain[2] such that the prediction error originating from the deep layer of, for example, primary visual cortex (V1) will be integrated with a prediction originating from the superficial layer of secondary visual cortex (V2), and so on. As higher-order circuits must integrate increasingly multimodal and abstract inputs (e.g. multisensory parietal areas), the predictions and prediction errors at each level become subsequently more removed from the fast temporal dynamics of sensory stimulation, and more intrinsically self-related.[3]

Thus, each canonical microcircuit integrates top-down expectations and bottom-up sensory prediction errors according to a cascading application of approximate Bayesian inference. This entails that top-down predictions and bottom-up prediction errors are neurobiologically encoded in such a way as to reflect their precision (i.e. confidence or inverse variance), with the interaction between the two governed by whichever input is more precise (Feldman & Friston, 2010; Kanai et al., 2015; Moran et al., 2013). As an intuitive example of how precision-weighting works, consider a scientist, Daisy, who sets out to test the hypothesis that the average height of Dutch people is 182 cm (6 ft). If Daisy is unsure about her prediction—perhaps previous studies have had divergent results, or there is a lack of prior data—then she will assign a lower prior precision.[4] Conversely, if Daisy visits Holland and only manages to sample very few individuals, or perhaps uses an unreliable measurement device, then the precision of the sensory data (or likelihood) will be very low. Bayes' law captures the intuitive notion then that one should update one's theory or belief according to whichever aspect of inference—prior knowledge or empirical observations—is more reliable.

The hierarchical optimization of precision naturally motivates an account of both endogenous and exogenous attentional spotlight effects (Fardo et al., 2017; Feldman & Friston, 2010). For example, the classical Posner cueing task has been modeled as inducing an expectation of enhanced expected precision on the right versus left visual hemifield (Feldman & Friston, 2010). Here, descending neuromodulation encoding

[1] The distinction of likelihood vs prediction error is here relative to the hierarchical level one describes; the prediction error at level 1 becomes the inferential likelihood at level 2, and so on (see Figure 2.1).

[2] Or plausibly, within a particular hierarchy if one does not subscribe to radically predictive processing (i.e. the notion that all systems everywhere in the brain are predictive).

[3] In the sense of describing increasingly intrinsic (as opposed to extrinsic) processes: level B describes Level A, level C describes levels A and B, and so on.

[4] Statistically, the prior probability distribution will have a wider variance or standard deviation.

expected precision enhances the precision of sensory prediction errors on the expected field, causing them to dominate in perception, while simultaneously reducing the precision of stimuli presented to the unattended visual field, weakening their ability to attract attention. Similarly, exogenous attentional effects, or "salience," are also well-captured by the model, as bottom-up changes in stimulus intensity will drive stronger post-synaptic depolarization, increasing bottom-up gain to result in highly precise prediction errors which can override top-down predictions. Thus, according to most BPC-related schemes, both expected (top-down) and sensory precision play a crucial role in dictating the priority of information processing in the brain.

These computational tools give us a fresh window into understanding both visceral perception itself and the integration of visceral signals within a more general self-model. For example, respiratory or cardiac control, awareness, and disruptions thereof can be related to various levels of a predictive coding hierarchy in visceromotor brain areas (Faull, Hayen, & Pattinson, 2017; Stephan et al., 2016). Visceral awareness in general has been proposed to depend upon the precision (or confidence, more on this later) of the interoceptive hierarchy (Ainley et al., 2016). As any hierarchical network will necessarily encode more abstract, supramodal representations at higher levels, others have emphasized a more general role of interoceptive predictions in emotion, self-awareness, and motor control (Seth, 2013; Seth, Suzuki, & Critchley, 2012). The homeostatic axioms of the FEP have further led to increased emphasis on the global priority of visceral predictive codes in conditioning cortical representations and self-awareness (Allen & Friston, 2016; Barrett & Simmons, 2015). To improve our understanding of these views, we now introduce the concept of "embodied precision" (see also Ainley et al., 2016; Fotopoulou, 2013) and the related notion of homeostasis in predictive processing.

2.3 Embodied precision and homeostatic "first priors"

The FEP sets homeostatic and allostatic function as the defining core of organismic life (Friston, 2013). This emphasis on an imperative to maintain internal states in the face of uncertainty renders FEP-based process theories embodied in the first order. For the free-energy minimizing agent, "value" or "optimality" should be understood as an imperative to maintain homeostasis (Friston et al., 2015). This is accomplished not by subserving some external economic principle but instead through modelling the self, the world, and their interaction in such a way as to maximize the chance of survival. In this sense, it might be said that the autopoetic principle at the basis of FEP acts as a kind of "first prior"; Bayesian inference is always bootstrapped from within the subjective needs of the agent and its embodied econiche within the world (Bruineberg, Kiverstein, & Rietveld, 2016; Bruineberg & Rietveld, 2014).

In terms of a more specific process theory, there are multiple ways in which visceral, tactile, and proprioceptive bodily signals might be afforded some privileged status within the cortical hierarchy. The FEP dictates that organisms are themselves "models of the world" (in the cybernetic sense); those models are then passed on through phylogenetic evolution as genetic "priors" which constrain every aspect of biological function from the DNA-driven development of synaptic weights and cortical networks to the very morphology of the agent itself. In this sense, the priors one is born with[5] are also imbued with an inherited prior precision.[6] Interoceptive signaling, perception, and control are perhaps the phylogenetically oldest of all sensory motor systems; all vertebrates possess the basic homeostatic biomechanics of pumping blood, respiratory oxygenation, and so on. Further, in terms of importance for organism survival, the stability and reliability of our visceral function is vital. Quite literally, if our internal organs become unreliable, the immediate result is death. It makes sense then that evolutionarily speaking, the afferents of the interoceptive hierarchy are likely to be afforded the highest expected precision of any sensorimotor channel.

There are several rather profound implications of this observation. Recall that the optimization of precision across the hierarchy can be unpacked as a mechanism for both top-down, endogenous attention and bottom-up saliency (Feldman & Friston, 2010). Here, salience is nothing more than the relative precision of incoming prediction errors. If the visceral body is afforded, a priori, the highest expected precision then interoceptive prediction errors should dominate the perceptual hierarchy (see Figure 2.1). This means that perceptual and value-based salience are, for the homeostatic organism, always relative to the impact some stimulus or decision has on the organisms' visceral prediction.

Note that this account goes much further than previous theories such as the somatic marker hypothesis (Damasio, 1999). The somatic marker hypothesis states in essence that subjective value is determined by adding or weighting some bodily representation to a value computation. Instead, according to our account, salience is literally defined by whatever has the most (or least) impact on visceral and autonomic homeostasis. Visceral sensations here are the dominant basis to which perceptual- and value-based computations are added; through active inference, cognition is enslaved to embodiment, rather than the other way around. In the perceptual domain, the implication is that unexpected deviations in heart rate, gut response, or other systems may literally change the way we perceive the world and our metacognitive uncertainty about such percepts. Indeed, it has recently been shown that unexpected disgust signals can reverse the impact of sensory precision on the exteroceptive perception of uncertainty itself (Allen et al., 2016), demonstrating the priority of visceral surprise as dictated by homeostatic prior precision.

The presumed a priori hyper-precision of visceral channels may explain a variety of classical cognitive phenomenon, beginning with substantive work done by mid-century Soviet psychologists who, inspired by the pioneering work of Pavlov and Sokolov, exhaustively investigated "interoceptive conditioning" and its relationship to the orienting reflex (Razran, 1961; Sokolov, 1963). In an impressive body of work combining various means of stimulating cardiac, respiratory, and enteric nervous systems with classical conditioning

[5] For example, consider the tendency to perceive certain conjunctions of circles as "faces" with an inherently social meaning, or to inhabit certain environments.

[6] Also known as "hyper-priors,"—priors dictating an expected level of sensory precision.

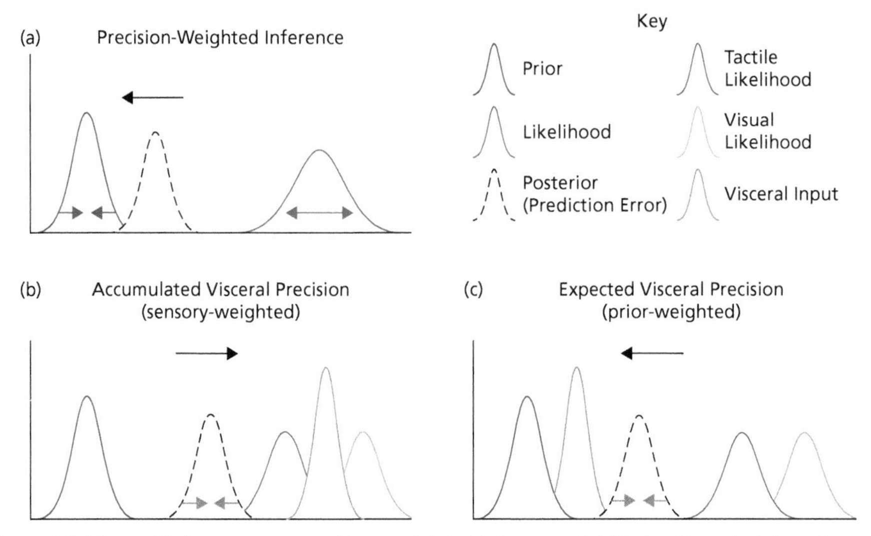

Figure 2.1 Visceral influences on precision-weighted inference. **(a)** Under the principles of Bayesian Inference, prediction errors are weighted by their statistical confidence (i.e. inverse variance or precision). Both "top-down" predictions and "bottom-up" prediction errors can be more or less precise. In this example, a precise prior belief (in red, relative to likelihood or sensory precision, in blue) has shifted a perceptual prediction error (dotted black line) towards the prediction. Note that the precision of the prediction error itself is the product of both prior and sensory precision; some models posit that an additional system must read out the precision of prediction errors to guide subjective sensitivity and/or confidence. **(b)** This example is expanded to consider how visceral information may enter a low-level multisensory "self-model" combining prior beliefs (red) with visual (green) and tactile (blue) sensory inputs. In this example, visceral signals are inherently more precise than other signals (see text), causing sensory signals to overwhelm prior expectations. **(c)** Here, highly precise visceral signals strengthen the influence of prior beliefs rather than feed-forward prediction errors. Note that in both examples, the hypothetical hyper-precision of visceral signals causes the prediction error to be highly stable, regardless whether prior or likelihood are weighted.

paradigms and biophysiological recording, these scientists sought to understand how visceral processes contribute to both implicit and explicit cognitive processes. This approach enabled them to study how exteroceptive unconditioned stimuli could be transferred to conditioned interoceptive responses, and vice versa. This revealed not only that subjects could quickly learn to associate internal sensations with exteroceptive phenomena but also that interoceptive learning itself was much faster to acquire and harder to extinguish than purely external learning.

This is exactly what one would expect if the brain affords higher a priori precision to internal changes than to external stimuli. This enhanced precision would lead to prediction errors on the interoceptive channel dominating how we learn about various cues, particularly when those highly precise prediction errors are integrated with other sensory channels. In a sense, this can be recast as an account of how interoceptive signals themselves provide a source of reliability in our self-perception and conscious awareness.

Interoceptive signals rise and fall according to a highly predictable pattern of slowly oscillating circadian and hormonal biorhythms. This low volatility, high precision stream of prediction errors may therefore provide a natural kind of "pacemaker" by which the brain can bind together a more coherent, potentially conscious stream of experience from the more noisy, unpredictable exteroceptive senses (see also Chapter 3 in the present volume).

In the brain, this mechanism of enhanced interoceptive precision neatly explains both phenomena within the laboratory, such as the interoceptive conditioning findings outlined earlier, but also more relatable real-world experiences. Nearly everyone has had the unfortunate experience of eating some food which has gone off, and then suffered through a day of food poisoning. Typically, this will result in a strong, lasting preference never to eat that food again—a form of highly precise learning which is often quite general as well. For example, if a bad bit of venison burger makes you sick, you are likely never to look at any burger (even a veggie one) in quite the same way again.

From the brain's point of view, this sudden surge in highly precise interoceptive prediction errors represents a potentially fatal event and affords for an equally precise alteration of internal models. To overwhelm the precise interoceptive prediction errors, the brain must essentially engage in "one-shot learning," sending an equally precise cascade of predictions to alter the global neural networks governing appetite, aversion, and eating behavior. Through interoceptive active inference, the brain thus ensures that the next time you see a burger, or anything even closely related to it, you immediately feel some revulsion or perhaps even "see" the meat as green.

Interoceptive signals thus play a very important role in regulating the cortical hierarchy and how we learn from aversive, potentially life-threatening events. However, not all is bad within the domain of the viscera. Indeed, highly pleasurable sensations can be obtained from the interoceptive encoding of social touch and sexual intercourse. It is interesting to note here the parallel between how the precision of visceral pain or distress may subserve the evolutionary priority to stay alive, and a potentially equal a priori precision for affective or sexual sensations may subserve the principle of doing whatever makes one more likely to reproduce, and therefore ensure the survival of one's "species model" (see Chapter 6 in the present volume). Also, of course, beyond aversive or affective interoceptive prediction errors associated with specific experiences, interoceptive signals, as first priors, may provide, as we explain in the following sections, the necessary basis for the experience of "the same body always there" as James aptly put it, the experience, in other words, of body ownership which seems to be central feature of the bodily self.

2.4 Self-models and interoceptive predictions

An important emerging extension of the predictive coding literature is its application to the notion of a predictive self-model (Allen & Friston, 2016; Apps & Tsakiris, 2014) that can explain fundamental aspects of selfhood such as body ownership and agency. At least two predominant self-model process theories can be motivated from EPP approaches; a more domain-constrained model which specifies how exteroceptive and interoceptive sensations are bound together to identify a sensation as originating from "me" (i.e. having to do with body ownership and agency), and a more global or emergent concept emphasizing the role of the hierarchical brain in iteratively predicting its own neural activity. We discuss these in turn.

2.4.1 The multisensory self and body ownership

One of the first attempts towards a predictive coding self-model focused strictly on the domain of body awareness, namely the sense of body ownership (Apps & Tsakiris, 2014). This model is posited entirely within the multisensory integration of bodily and exteroceptive sensations and thus describes a lower-order self-model situated between the integrative and sensori-motor layers. The Rubber Hand Illusion (RHI), one of the most influential and well-studied experimental paradigms of body ownership of embodiment, illustrates how predictions and predictions errors are used to compute the probability that a body part belongs to me. In the RHI, watching a rubber hand being stroked synchronously with one's own unseen hand causes the rubber hand to be experienced as part of one's body (Tsakiris, 2010 for a review). The illusion and its striking effects (for review see Tsakiris, 2010) illustrate how multisensory stimulation can lead to changes in how one's body is processed, leading to an update of what is experienced as "my body."

How can a predictive coding account of the self explain changes in body ownership that are driven by multisensory stimulation? During the induction of the illusion there is considerable bottom-up sensory surprise evoked in one's sensory system. The somatosensory experience of touch on one's hand that is temporally congruent with the vision of touch on the rubber hand is surprising, as prior to stimulation participants cannot see the touch on their own hand and would not predict that touch on the rubber hand would evoke a sensation of touch. Instead they would predict that the vision of touch and felt touch should come from the same single body part. This surprise will be explained away by top-down effects from multisensory areas where the relative precision weighting of vision over touch may explain away the prediction error, updating the prediction of what and where my "real" hand now is. In turn, perceptual learning processes will update representations of one's body, such that the probabilistic representation of one's body is different after synchronous multisensory stimulation. Therefore, one's body, at least as perceived exteroceptively, seems to be processed in a probabilistic manner as "the most likely to be me" (Apps & Tsakiris, 2014). Such probabilistic representations are created through the integration of top-down predictions about the body with bottom-up prediction errors from unimodal sensory systems that are explained away by priors. These results speak in favor of an exteroceptive model of the self, within which body ownership, a key aspect of self-awareness, is highly malleable, subject to the perception of the body from the *outside*. However, exteroceptive input represents only one set of channels of information available for self-awareness. We are also *interoceptively* aware of our body (Craig, 2002).

What is then the role of the interoceptive and bodily hierarchies in such predictive self-models? As one's body is not simply perceived exteroceptively but is also felt interoceptively, a unifying model of the self must account for the integration of these modalities. For example, during the RHI, the exteroceptive evidence suggests that what I am looking at (i.e. the rubber hand) is *my* hand. However, if this is my hand, then there are interoceptive prediction errors between how my *true* hand feels (i.e. interoceptive prediction) and the fact that I cannot feel the rubber hand interoceptively. Therefore, exteroceptive and interoceptive streams must be integrated to explain away these prediction errors before the body can be represented as "self."

Beyond the domain of predictive processing, numerous theorists have emphasized a foundational role of visceral-sensory integration in providing a basis for the "embodied subjective frame" in the notion of interoceptive first priors (see section 2.3). In an attempt to address the apparent dichotomy that existed in the field between a purely exteroceptively driven model of the self (Apps & Tsakiris, 2014; Tsakiris, 2010) and an interoceptively focused model (Seth, 2013), an FEP-inspired model of the bodily self is needed in which exteroceptive (tactile and visual) prediction errors are bound together with interoceptive prediction errors. Indeed, the renewed focus on the potential role of interoception for self-awareness, beyond emotional processing, resulted in new lines of research that attempted to study in parallel the integration of exteroceptive with interoceptive predictions errors, thereby adding the important interoceptive element of how "my body feels" to exteroceptive evidence (Aspell et al., 2013; Blefari, Martuzzi, Salomon et al., 2017; Filippetti & Tsakiris, 2017; Ronchi et al., 2015; Sel et al., 2017; Suzuki et al., 2013; Tsakiris, Jimenez, & Costantini, 2011).

Cardiac interoceptive signals and their cortical signatures have been related to bodily self-awareness in several recent studies. Inspired by classic bodily illusions, such as the RHI (Botvinick & Cohen, 1998), the Full-Body Illusion (Lenggenhager et al., 2007) and the Enfacement Illusion (Tsakiris, 2008) that rely on multisensory (e.g. visuo-tactile) stimulation to induce transient yet striking changes in body ownership, body identification, and self-face recognition, several studies have focused on the potential impact of cardiac interoceptive signals for these dimensions of self-awareness. Early studies focused on correlational designs to show that levels of explicit interoceptive accuracy were negatively correlated with the strength of the illusory experience of alterations in self-awareness such that individuals with lower interoceptive accuracy tend to experience a stronger RHI (Schauder et al., 2015; Tsakiris et al., 2011). These studies highlighted the dynamic balance between exteroceptive and interoceptive influences for self-awareness. The observation that participants with lower interoceptive accuracy experienced a stronger illusory sense of body ownership in the Rubber Hand Illusion suggested that in the absence of accurate interoceptive representations one's model of self is predominantly exteroceptive. Importantly, this finding suggested an antagonism between interoceptive and exteroceptive cues in bodily self-awareness. More recent studies have used cardiac signals as inducers of such changes in body ownership. In particular, the substitution of purely exteroceptive visuo-tactile stimulation by cardio-visual stimulation (i.e. a combination of interoceptive and exteroceptive signals) allowed researchers to probe a more active and potentially causal role of interoceptive signals for body-awareness. For example, Suzuki,

Garfinkel, Critchley, and colleagues (2013) showed that looking at a virtual hand that pulsates in synchrony with one's heartbeat can lead to the same changes in body ownership as the ones reported in the classic version of the Rubber Hand Illusion. Such findings were soon extended to the Full Body Illusion (Aspell et al., 2013) and the Enfacement Illusion (Sel, Azevedo, & Tsakiris, 2016). The effect of the synchronicity between cardiac and visual events that induce the illusory changes in self-awareness was also reflected in the attenuated amplitude of the neural response to heartbeats (i.e. Heartbeat Evoked Potentials; HEP), an effect that also correlated with explicit interoceptive accuracy. More excitingly, Park and colleagues confirmed the insula as the neural source of HEPs and demonstrated HEP modulations in the insula during self-identification using intracranial electroencephalography (EEG) (Park Bernasconi et al., 2017).

Taken together, these findings suggest that if exteroceptive influences highlight the malleability of body awareness, interoceptive signals seem to serve the stability of body awareness in response to exteroceptive stimulation, reflecting a psychological consequence of the biologically necessary function of homeostasis. Therefore, this attempt to unify the two sides of embodiment concerns equally the physiological and psychological basis of selfhood. At the physiological level, it is interoceptive autonomic signaling that ensures the stability (homeostasis) of the organism. At the psychological level, as visceral information can be in some sense described as inherently self-related (unlike exteroceptive sensations, which are externally caused), both predictive and non-predictive accounts suggest that the feed-forward integration of visceral with exteroceptive information provides some inherent selfhood and affect to conscious experiences. In other words, the high expected precision of visceral signals make them ideal for providing a continuous estimate of "self-stability."

2.4.2 The metacognitive self-model and visceral precision

The notion of a more global or emergent concept emphasizing the role of the hierarchical brain in iteratively predicting its own neural activity emerges naturally from considering the predictive brain as a whole, rather than as a single hierarchy or collection of hierarchies (auditory, visceral, etc.). Although cortical hierarchies are often depicted as a "pyramid," with one executive homunculus sitting atop relatively few inputs, recent advances in human tractography, functional connectivity, and monkey tracing studies challenge the plausibility of such a view. Instead, increasing evidence suggests that the global topology of brain connectivity is best described as a kind of centrifugal hierarchy (Figure 2.2).

From this global or bird's-eye view of the predictive brain, it is clear that a variety of models can be spun to explain how visceral sensations are propagated throughout the hierarchy. For example, in the model architecture depicted earlier, visceral sensations are treated as equal with other sensorimotor hierarchies. In this case "selfhood" emerges solely from the metacognitive nature of the deep hierarchy; that is, it is the global expectation of precision that embeds an inherently self-related notion in information processing. To put this another way, consider that the global self-model is essentially the

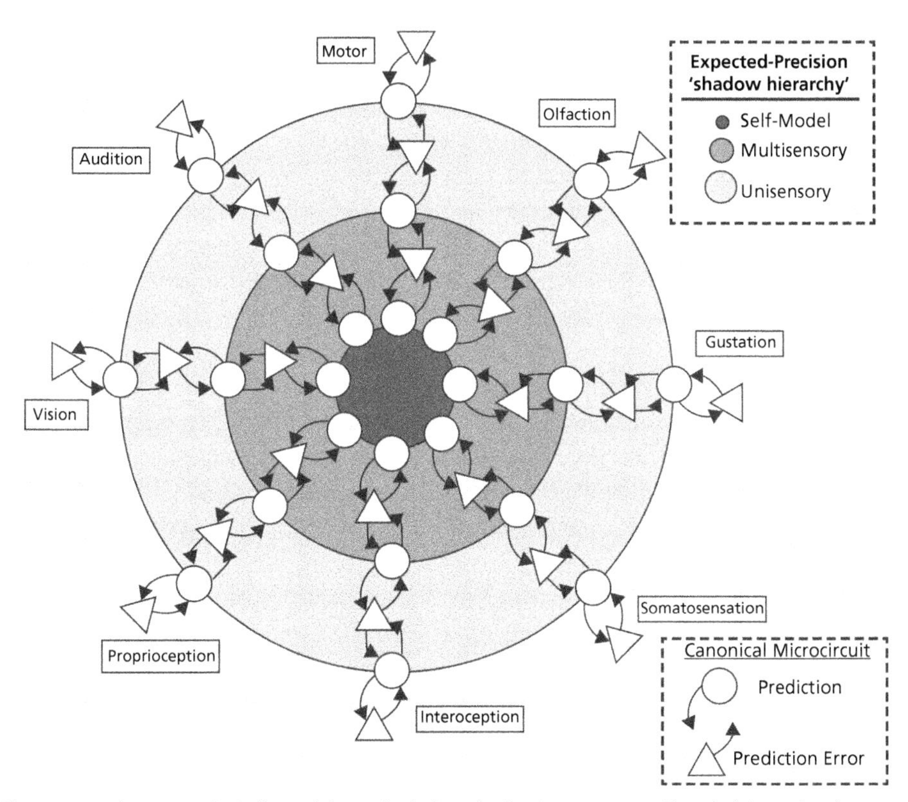

Figure 2.2 The Dynamic Self-Model. By depicting the brain as a "centrifugal" hierarchy, the self-model is revealed. At the "periphery" of the brain we find high-speed, sensory-motor hierarchies with a relatively high modularity and functional specialization. At the next level, multisensory cortices combine prediction errors from divergent sensory-viscero-motor hierarchies with descending "self-predictions" originating in the centermost layer. At the "center" of the hierarchy sits the "rich club," a network of hubs integrating multi-sensory prediction errors with global "self-predictions" oscillating at narrative timescales. The metastable interaction of these layers is further controlled by a neuromodulatory "shadow hierarchy" which estimates and optimizes expected precision from the most global (self-related) predictions down to the most local level of cortical processing.

brain's prediction of its own reliability. In this sense, global "experience predictions" (i.e. that I am this kind of agent, with these kinds of beliefs, who will experience some stimulus in a particular way) are inherently self-related and constrain lower-level brain dynamics.

However, there are numerous reasons to think that visceral sensations may enjoy some privileged status within the global hierarchy. Both neuroanatomically and functionally speaking, primary viscero-sensory and viscero-motor control centers such as the insular and cingulate cortices sit firmly within the "middle" integration layer and exhibit greater multisensory sensitivity than other "primary" sensory cortices. Further, these areas are rich in neuromodulatory neurons thought to encode expected precision, and visceral sensations themselves may have an a priori hyper-precision. Thus, rather than being a mere "arm" of the predictive hierarchy, the visceral brain may in fact form the backbone of the "shadow hierarchy" responsible for mediating perceptual and affective salience via precision optimization. In line with this hypothesis, recent studies have highlighted the far-reaching effects of the visceral brain on a global self-model by considering the role of visceral precision on metacognition.

The metacognitive ability to monitor our own experiences, actions, and beliefs and to form an accurate feeling of confidence is a crucial part of cognition in general and decision-making in particular. If our subjective beliefs become very divorced from reality, then poor decisions are sure to follow. Indeed, if perception itself is a kind of "Bayesian hallucination," then overly precise expectations may be doubly so; I may perceive friendly faces as hostile, or systematically undervalue my own competence, if my predictions are too precise. In general, there is an obvious overlap between the statistical notion of precision, and the metacognitive notion of confidence, but how do the two relate? Are we more confident when our brain is very precise? At what hierarchical level (i.e. self, integrative, or sensorimotor) does precision matter most for our subjective self-awareness? Most importantly for the current issue, how do visceral signals come into this picture?

Until now, these questions have been pursued primarily from the perspective of signal detection theory (SDT). Here, metacognition and confidence are presumed to arise from the feed-forward monitoring of decision-relevant information only. That is to say, according to the SDT model, all that really matters for subjective confidence is the (exteroceptive) evidence upon which my decision itself is based. Yet this view of the brain as a feed-forward device is clearly in contradiction to the predictive processing views explained in sections 2.2 and 2.3, where both feedback and multisensory integration are pervasive features of self-experience. Why then should our metacognition be so rationally secluded from the homeostatic visceral function of the body?

In contrast to this view, we argue that metacognition arises generally from the interaction of the global self-model, with more task- or performance-specific modules lower in the hierarchy. In this sense, global expectations of self-precision are a kind of metacognitive model of how accurate I expect to be on an upcoming trial, given both my visceral and exteroceptive precision. Put another way: if I expect to be very fatigued on an upcoming test, then I will also expect to be less confident on that material even if it is relatively easy. The metacognitive self-model thus emerges from the deepest levels of the cortical hierarchy, and enables the brain to both estimate and control its own self-efficacy in the face of an ever-changing environment. In this sense, descending expected precision signals are not only a crucial aspect of selfhood but also of our ability to monitor our performance and change our behavior when it is no longer adaptive.

In support of this view, it has recently been demonstrated that subjective exteroceptive confidence depends both on sensory precision, and on visceral surprise itself. To demonstrate this, Allen and colleagues utilized a novel task in which participants viewed moving dots on a screen and judged whether their average motion was to the left or right, and also rated their confidence (Allen et al., 2016). Unbeknownst to the participants, on every trial an unconscious neutral or disgust-related cue was presented using careful masking techniques. By carefully controlling the difficulty of the dot judgment, this study demonstrated that a sudden increase in interoceptive prediction error can reverse the impact of sensory precision, resulting in higher confidence for noisy trials and lower confidence for precise trials. In a complementary study, Hauser and colleagues (2017a) followed up on these results by administering the beta-blocking drug propranolol, which inhibits the activity of noradrenaline both in the central and autonomic nervous system, crucial for interoceptive arousal. Interestingly, this study found blocking noradrenaline actually improved the correspondence of perceptual accuracy and confidence, suggesting that blocking signals from the body renders metacognition "less embodied" and more concerned solely with exteroceptive evidence. In this sense, altering bodily signals is likely to influence a variety of biases in both health and disordered decision-making. This may have profound implications for how we understand and treat psychiatric disorders such as obsessive–compulsive disorder (OCD), anxiety, and psychosis, where aberrant visceral precision may result in overly precise (or imprecise) metacognitive self-model (Bliksted et al., 2017)), locking the patient into an unrealistically uncertain world.

Ultimately, the emerging understanding of a metacognitive self-model integrating interoceptive and exteroceptive sensations is still in its infancy. It remains to be seen, for example, the extent to which visceral signals influence perceptual or value-based decisions in a variety of different domains. Nevertheless, these sorts of findings are exactly what one would expect if visceral sensations are afforded higher a priori precision, and they suggest that in many domains our explicit, conscious self-awareness may be biased in subtle ways by the ongoing activity and predictability of the visceral body.

2.5 An after-thought: The ontogenetic origins of interoceptive precisions

In section 2.4, we described some key properties of domain-specific and more global self-models. In the future, it will be crucial to use a model-based approach in order to map how the varieties of self models (e.g. global, multisensory, metacognitive) interact with one another and to pit competing hypotheses about how visceral signals contribute to these models (e.g. by enhancing expected precision or prediction error) against one another. This will not only greatly accelerate the computational neuroscience of embodiment but also provide valuable tools to ask important questions, for instance, about the ontogenetic development of self-models the lifespan, as well as about the role of visceral signals for social awareness—the awareness of other people in relation to the self. It is precisely these ontogenetic and more social aspects of interoception that remain poorly understood. A large body of developmental research on the development of self-awareness (Lewis, 2001; Rochat, 2003) documents the importance of multisensory integration processes that will enable infants to match their mirror reflection with their own body and eventually to master delayed self-recognition, indicative of a more diachronic self-representation by the third year. In addition, an intersubjective approach suggests that infants learn self/other differentiation through social interactions of mutual attention (Reddy, 2003) where they detect the caregiver's contingent response to their emotion expression (see also the social-biofeedback model; Gergely & Watson, 1999). More recently, intersubjective approaches on the development of self-awareness have been extended to interoception (Fotopoulou & Tsakiris, 2017), whereby the development of the visceral and emotional circuit depends on a caregiver–infant relationship (Fox et al., 2007; Rinaman, 2009), often conceptualized as one of homeostatic regulation (Rinaman, 2009). Human infants are born immature, and they do not have the ability to perform by themselves the actions needed for addressing their internal sensations and needs. From eating and drinking to thermoregulation and even sleep, their bodily regulation depends largely on caregivers. Furthermore, the first months post-partum are characterized by relative instability of key cardiovascular variables (e.g. Heart Rate Variability (HRV), Vagal Tone) that become moderately stable by the end of the first year (Fox et al., 2007), due to physiological maturation (Fracasso et al., 1994). Importantly, their levels depend on caregiving (McLaughlin et al., 2015) such as parent–infant contingency during interaction (Feldman, 2007; Feldman et al., 2011), and are predictive of self-regulation abilities in three-year-old children (Fracasso et al., 1994).

From the point of view of interoceptive awareness, progress in this area has been hindered by the lack of appropriate experimental methods that would allow to measure interoceptive sensitivity in early infancy. Recently, Maister, Tang, and Tsakiris have tackled this issue by developing the iBEAT task, a non-verbal behavioral task that measures infants' sensitivity to their own heartbeat. During the task, five-month-old infants were shown an animated character that either moved in synchrony with their own heartbeat or out of synchrony with their heartbeat. Using this sequential looking time task, it was observed that infants spent longer more time looking at the character that was moving out of synchrony than the one moving in synchrony, suggesting that even at this early age infants are, at least implicitly, sensitive to their own interoceptive signals. Moreover, the infants' performance in the iBEAT task revealed interesting individual differences. Infants who displayed greater interoceptive sensitivity in the iBEAT task also had larger HEP amplitudes in a subsequent task when infants viewed short video clips of facial expressions, a finding that conforms to HEP measures in adults (Pollatos & Schandry, 2004). However, the question of what processes can account for such individual differences remains unanswered.

Methodological advances such as the development of the iBEAT task will enable the field to study the ontogenetic origins and longitudinal development of interoception as the infant enters an intersubjective world of carer–infant embodied and affective interactions. These interactions are thought to be critical for providing the means by which the infant will learn to relate specific homeostatic needs (e.g. pain) and their behavioral expression (e.g. crying) to contingent allostatic responses from the carer (e.g. soothing rather than feeding; see Fotopoulou & Tsakiris, 2017). If these coupled intersubjective embodied iterations turn out to be critical for developing a sense of one's self *inside* her body, as well as interoceptive inferences with higher precision and better metacognition, we will then be in a position to test empirically the causal and crucial role that interoception plays for development and its importance for mentalizing one's own bodily states and those of others (Fotopoulou & Tsakiris, 2017; Shah, Catmur, & Bird, 2017). In particular, this approach could be integrated with new methods for studying metacognitive processes in infants (Goupil & Kouider, 2016), revealing how changes in visceral sensitivity contribute to the emergence of accurate self-monitoring and advance our understanding of developmental disorders such as autism (Brewer et al., 2015; Quattrocki & Friston, 2014), eating (Badoud & Tsakiris, 2017; see also the Chapter 9 in the present volume) and affective disorders (see the Chapter 8 in the present volume).

2.6 Conclusion

One can distinguish among different kinds of "self models" within the predictive mind. The exteroceptive and interoceptive models, in a more feed-forward sense, integrate the action of a visceral hierarchy with ascending exteroceptive signals to provide the basic embodied context for the self. The second, by representing confidence itself, enforces systematic interactions between the different exteroceptive and interoceptive hierarchies (see also Garfinkel et al., 2015). Collectively, both are likely to contribute uniquely to our embodied self-experience. Considering the a priori high precision of interoception, in favour of which we argued in this chapter, the feed-forward multisensory integration of prediction errors may be a crucial mechanism for binding together conscious contents in an embodied way. The high priority of visceral sensations may provide a naturally reliable "anchor" on which to lodge a more permanent feeling of bodily self. However, these processes are themselves likely to be cognitive impenetrable, in the sense that they occur below the metacognitive self-inferences required for conscious access. Thus, the top-down representation of both visceral and exteroceptive confidence (or precision) is a likely precursor for explicit learning in these domains, and may be a critical target for ontogenetic and cultural development of social norms, expected behaviors, and ultimately our empathic understanding of other minds as embodied agents.

The hypothesis that interoception plays an important role in cognitive and emotional processes is well established in the fields of experimental psychology, cognitive neuroscience, and clinical psychology and psychiatry. The proposal we put forward about the psychological role of interoception, namely that interoception serves the stability of self-awareness, because of the primacy of a priori high precision of visceral channels, is in line with FEP-inspired models of self-awareness. This role is informed by the homeostatic principles that keep the organism within certain ranges of physiological function in adaptive response to external changes. At the same time, one should be aware of the long-lasting dichotomies in our disciplines that have fractionalized the self. FEP-inspired models of the bodily self can, in principle, go beyond such dichotomies to integrate the influential traditions that until now have been kept separate: the awareness of the self from the outside and from within. Rather than focusing on the apparent differences of these sources of information for the self, our field should consider their antagonism from a predictive coding perspective that can explain their integration, and how their relationship is reflected in the balance between stability and adaptation. In reference to classic embodied cognition approaches, which in certain ways depict a surface body, it was about time, as the growing body of evidence reviewed in this chapter shows, to ground the self to a non-hollow body with a dimension of visceral depth. This step may pave the way for new investigations that can fulfil a long-standing aim of psychology to link the physiological to the psychological self.

Acknowledgments

MA would like to thank Francesca Fardo and Matthew Apps for productive discussions on this work. MA was supported by a Wellcome grant 100227 (MA). The Wellcome Trust Centre for Neuroimaging is supported by core funding from Wellcome (091593/Z/10/Z). MT is supported by the European Research Council (ERC-2016-CoG- 724537) under the FP7 and the NOMIS Foundation Distinguished Scientist Award.

References

Ainley, V., **Apps, M. A. J.**, **Fotopoulou, A.**, and **Tsakiris, M.** (2016). "Bodily precision": A predictive coding account of individual differences in interoceptive accuracy. *Philosophical Transactions of the Royal Society B*, *371*, 20160003.

Allen, M., **Frank, D.**, **Schwarzkopf, D. S.**, **Fardo, F.**, **Winston, J. S.**, **Hauser, T. U.**, et al. (2016). Unexpected arousal modulates the influence of sensory noise on confidence. *eLife*, *5*, e18103.

Allen, M. and **Friston, K. J.** (2016). From cognitivism to autopoiesis: Towards a computational framework for the embodied mind. *Synthese*, 1–24.

Apps, M. A. J. and **Tsakiris, M.** (2014). The free-energy self: A predictive coding account of self-recognition. *Neuroscience and Biobehavioral Reviews*, *41*, 85–97.

Aspell, J. E., **Heydrich, L.**, **Marillier, G.**, **Lavanchy, T.**, **Herbelin, B.**, and **Blanke, O.** (2013). Turning body and self inside out: Visualized heartbeats alter bodily self-consciousness and tactile perception. *Psychological Science*, *24*, 2445–53.

Badoud, D. and **Tsakiris, M.** (2017). From the body's viscera to the body's image: Is there a link between interoception and body image concerns? *Neuroscience and Biobehavioral Reviews*, *77*, 237–46. <https://doi.org/10.1016/j.neubiorev.2017.03.017>

Barrett, L. F. and **Simmons, W. K.** (2015). Interoceptive predictions in the brain. *Nature Reviews Neuroscience*, *16*, 419–29.

Blefari, M. L., **Martuzzi, R.**, **Salomon, R.**, **Bello-Ruiz, J.**, **Herbelin, B.**, **Serino, A.**, et al. (2017). Bilateral Rolandic operculum processing underlying heartbeat awareness reflects changes in bodily self-consciousness. *European Journal of Neuroscience*, *45*(10), 1300–12. <https://doi.org/10.1111/ejn.13567>

Bliksted, V., **Samuelsen, E.**, **Sandberg, K.**, **Bibby, B. M.**, and **Overgaard, M. S.** (2017). Discriminating between first- and second-order cognition in first-episode paranoid schizophrenia. *Cognitive Neuropsychiatry*, **22**, 95–107.

Botvinick, M. and **Cohen, J.** (1998). Rubber hand feels touch that eyes see. *Nature*, *391*(February), 756. <https://doi.org/10.1038/35784>

Bruineberg, J., **Kiverstein, J.**, and **Rietveld, E.** (2016). The anticipating brain is not a scientist: The free-energy principle from an ecological-enactive perspective. *Synthese*, 1–28.

Brewer, R., Happé, F., Cook, R., and **Bird, G.** (2015). Commentary on "Autism, oxytocin and interoception": Alexithymia, not autism spectrum disorders, is the consequence of interoceptive failure. *Neuroscience and Biobehavioral Reviews, 56,* 348–53. <https://doi.org/10.1016/j.neubiorev.2015.07.006>

Bruineberg, J. and **Rietveld, E.** (2014). Self-organization, free energy minimization, and optimal grip on a field of affordances. *Frontiers in Human Neuroscience,* **8**, 599.

Bruineberg, J., Kiverstein, J., and **Rietveld, E.** (2016). The anticipating brain is not a scientist: The free-energy principle from an ecological-enactive perspective. *Synthese,* 1–28. <https://doi.org/10.1007/s11229-016-1239-1>

Clark, A. (2013). Whatever next? Predictive brains, situated agents, and the future of cognitive science. *Behavioral and Brain Sciences, 36,* 181–204.

Damasio, A. R. (1999). *The Feeling of What Happens: Body and Emotion in the Making of Consciousness.* New York, NY: Harcourt Brace.

Fardo, F., Auksztulewicz, R., Allen, M., Dietz, M. J., Roepstorff, A., and **Friston, K. J.** (2017). Expectation violation and attention to pain jointly modulate neural gain in somatosensory cortex. *NeuroImage,* **153**, 109–21.

Faull, O., Hayen, A., and **Pattinson, K.** (2017). Breathlessness and the body: Neuroimaging evidence for the inferential leap. bioRxiv:117408. <https://www.biorxiv.org/content/biorxiv/early/2017/03/24/117408.full.pdf>

Feldman, H. and **Friston, K. J.** (2010). Attention, uncertainty, and free-energy. *Frontiers in Human Neuroscience, 4,* 215

Feldman, R. (2007). Infant biological foundations synchrony and developmental outcomes. *Current Directions in Psychological Science, 16*(6), 340–5.

Feldman, R., Magori-Cohen, R., Galili, G., Singer, M., and **Louzoun, Y.** (2011). Mother and infant coordinate heart rhythms through episodes of interaction synchrony. *Infant Behavior and Development, 34*(4), 569–77

Filippetti, M. L. and **Tsakiris, M.** (2017). Heartfelt embodiment: Changes in body-ownership and self-identification produce distinct changes in interoceptive accuracy. *Cognition, 159,* 1–10.

Fotopoulou, A. (2013). Beyond the reward principle: Consciousness as precision seeking. *Neuropsychoanalysis, 15,* 33–8.

Fotopoulou, A. and **Tsakiris, M.** (2017). Mentalizing homeostasis: The social origins of interoceptive inference. *Neuropsychoanalysis, 19*(1), 3–28.

Fox, N. A., Schmidt, L. A., Henderson, H. A., and **Marshall, P. J.** (2007). Developmental psychophysiology: Conceptual and methodological issues. *Handbook of Psychophysiology,* (1995), 453–81.

Fracasso, M. P., Porges, S. W., Lamb, M. E., and **Rosenberg, A. A.** (1994). Cardiac activity in infancy: Reliability and stability of individual differences. *Infant Behavior & Development, 17*(3), 277–84.

Friston, K. (2005). A theory of cortical responses. *Philosophical Transactions of the Royal Society B, 360,* 815–36.

Friston, K. (2009). The free-energy principle: A rough guide to the brain? *Trends in Cognitive Sciences, 13,* 293–301.

Friston, K. (2010). The free-energy principle: A unified brain theory? *Nature Reviews Neuroscience, 11* 127–38.

Friston, K. (2013). Life as we know it. *Journal of the Royal Society Interface, 10,* 20130475.

Friston, K. and **Frith, C.** (2015). A duet for one. *Consciousness and Cognition, 36,* 390–405

Friston, K., Rigoli, F., Ognibene, D., Mathys, C., Fitzgerald, T., and **Pezzulo, G.** (2015). Active inference and epistemic value. *Cognitive Neuroscience, 6,* 187–214.

Gallagher, S. and **Zahavi, D.** (2013). *The Phenomenological Mind*. London: Routledge.

Gallagher, S. and **Allen, M.** (2016). Active inference, enactivism and the hermeneutics of social cognition. *Synthese*, 1–22.

Garfinkel, S. N., Seth, A. K., Barrett, A. B., Suzuki, K., and **Critchley, H. D.** (2015). Knowing your own heart: Distinguishing interoceptive accuracy from interoceptive awareness. *Biological Psychology*, *104*, 65–74.

Gergely, G. & Watson, J. S. (1999). Early social-emotional development: Contingency perception and the social biofeedback model. In: P. Rochat (ed.), *Early Social Cognition*. Hillsdale, NJ: Erlbaum, pp. 101–36.

Goupil, L. & Kouider, S. (2016). Behavioral and neural indices of metacognitive sensitivity in preverbal infants. *Current biology*, *26*(22), 3038–45.

Hauser, T. U., Fiore, V. G., Moutoussis, M., and **Dolan, R.J.** (2016). Computational psychiatry of ADHD: Neural gain impairments across marrian levels of analysis. *Trends in Neuroscience*, *39*, 63–73.

Hauser, T. U., Allen, M., Purg, N., Moutoussis, M., Rees, G., and **Dolan, R.J.** (2017a). Noradrenaline blockade specifically enhances metacognitive performance. *eLife*, *6*, e24901.

Hauser, T. U., Allen, M., Rees G, and **Dolan, R. J.** (2017b). Metacognitive impairments extend perceptual decision making weaknesses in compulsivity. *Scientific Reports*, *7*, 6614.

Heidegger, M. (1996). *Being and Time: A Translation of Sein und Zeit*. New York, NY: SUNY Press.

Hohwy, J. (2013). *The Predictive Mind*. Oxford: Oxford University Press.

Hohwy, J. (2014). The neural organ explains the mind. In: T. Metzinger and J. M. Windt (eds), *Open MIND*. Frankfurt am Main: MIND Group. <https://open-mind.net/papers/the-neural-organ-explains-the-mind>

Joffily, M. and **Coricelli, G.** (2013). Emotional valence and the free-energy principle. *PLoS Computational Biology*, *9*, e1003094.

Kanai, R., Komura, Y., Shipp, S., and **Friston, K.** (2015). Cerebral hierarchies: Predictive processing, precision and the pulvinar. *Philosophical Transactions of the Royal Society B*, *370*, 20140169.

Koster-Hale, J. and **Saxe, R.** (2013). Theory of mind: A neural prediction problem. *Neuron*, *79*, 836–48.

Lenggenhager, B., Tadi, T., Metzinger, T., and **Blanke, O.** (2007). Video ergo sum: Manipulating bodily self-consciousness. *Science*, *317*(5841), 1096–9. <https://doi.org/10.1126/science.1143439>

Lewis, M. (2011). The origins and uses of self-awareness or the mental representation of me. *Consciousness and Cognition*, *20*(1), 120–9.

McLaughlin, K. A., Sheridan, M. A., Tibu, F., Fox, N. A., Zeanah, C. H., and **Nelson, C. A.** (2015). Causal effects of the early caregiving environment on development of stress response systems in children. *Proceedings of the National Academy of Sciences of the USA*, *112*(18), 5637–42. <https://doi.org/10.1073/pnas.1423363112>

Meessen, J., Mainz, V., Gauggel, S., Volz-Sidiropoulou, E., Sütterlin, S., and **Forkmann, T.** (2016). The relationship between interoception and metacognition: A pilot study. *Journal of Psychophysiology*, *30*(2), 76–86.

Merleau-Ponty, M. (1996). *Phenomenology of Perception*. New Delhi: Motilal Banarsidass Publisher.

Miall, R. C. and **Wolpert, D. M.** (1996). Forward models for physiological motor control. *Neural Networks*, **9**, 1265–79.

Moran, R. J., Campo, P., Symmonds, M., Stephan, K. E., Dolan, R. J., and **Friston, K. J.** (2013). Free energy, precision and learning: The role of cholinergic neuromodulation. *Journal of Neuroscience*, *33*, 8227–36.

Park, H.-D., Bernasconi, F., Salomon, R., Tallon-Baudry, C., Spinelli, L., Seeck, M., et al. (2017). Neural sources and underlying mechanisms of neural responses to heartbeats, and their role in bodily self-consciousness: An intracranial EEG study. *Cerebral Cortex*, *116*, 1–14.

Pollatos, O. and **Schandry, R.** (2004). Accuracy of heartbeat perception is reflected in the amplitude of the heartbeat-evoked brain potential. *Psychophysiology*, *41*(3), 476–82.

Quattrocki, E. and **Friston, K.** (2014). Autism, oxytocin and interoception. *Neuroscience and Biobehavioral Reviews*, *47*, 410–30.

Razran, G. (1961). The observable and the inferable conscious in current Soviet psychophysiology: Interoceptive conditioning, semantic conditioning, and the orienting reflex. *Psychological Review*, *68*, 81–147.

Reddy, V. (2003). On being the object of attention: Implications for self–other consciousness. *Trends in Cognitive Sciences*, *7*(9), 397–402.

Rinaman, L. and **Koehnle, T. J. K.** (2009). The development of central visceral circuits. In: M. Blumberg, J. Freeman, and S. Robinson (eds), *Oxford Handbook of Developmental Behavioral Neuroscience*. Oxford: Oxford University Press, pp. 298–322.

Rochat, P. (2003). Five levels of self-awareness as they unfold early in life. *Consciousness and Cognition*, *12*(4), 717–31.

Ronchi, R., Bello-Ruiz, J., Lukowska, M., Herbelin, B., Cabrilo, I., Schaller, K., et al. (2015). Right insular damage decreases heartbeat awareness and alters cardio-visual effects on bodily self-consciousness. *Neuropsychologia*, *70*, 11–20.

Schauder, K. B., Mash, L. E., Bryant, L. K., and **Cascio, C. J.** (2015). Interoceptive ability and body awareness in autism spectrum disorder. *Journal of Experimental Child Psychology*, *131*, 193–200.

Sel, A., Azevedo, R. T., and **Tsakiris, M.** (2017). Heartfelt self: Cardio-visual integration affects self-face recognition and interoceptive cortical processing. *Cerebral Cortex*, *27*(11), 5144–55.

Seth, A. K., Suzuki, K., and **Critchley, H. D.** (2012). An interoceptive predictive coding model of conscious presence. *Frontiers in Psychology*, *2*, 395.

Seth, A. K. (2013). Interoceptive inference, emotion, and the embodied self. *Trends in Cognitive Sciences*, *17*, 565–73.

Shah, P., Catmur, C., and **Bird, G.** (2017). From heart to mind: Linking interoception, emotion, and theory of mind. *Cortex*, *93*, 220–3.

Sokolov, E. N. (1963). Higher nervous functions: The orienting reflex. *Annual Review of Physiology*, *25*, 545–80.

Stephan, K. E., Manjaly, Z. M., Mathys, C. D., Weber, L.A.E., Paliwal, S., Gard, T., et al. (2016). Allostatic self-efficacy: A metacognitive theory of dyshomeostasis-induced fatigue and depression. *Frontiers in Human Neuroscience*, *10*, 550.

Suzuki, K., Garfinkel, S. N., Critchley, H. D., and **Seth, A. K.** (2013). Multisensory integration across exteroceptive and interoceptive domains modulates self-experience in the rubber-hand illusion. *Neuropsychologia*, *51*, 2909–17.

Tsakiris, M. (2008). Looking for myself: Current multisensory input alters self-face recognition. *PLoS One*, *3*(12), e4040.

Tsakiris, M. (2010). My body in the brain: A neurocognitive model of body-ownership. *Neuropsychologia*, *48*(3), 703–12.

Tsakiris, M., Jimenez, A. T.-, and **Costantini, M.** (2011). Just a heartbeat away from one's body: Interoceptive sensitivity predicts malleability of body-representations. *Proceedings of the Royal Society B*, *278*(1717), 2470–6.

Chapter 3

Interoceptive signals, brain dynamics, and subjectivity

Mariana Babo-Rebelo and Catherine Tallon-Baudry

3.1 The embodied self: Visceral inputs as self-specifying signals

3.1.1 The self is rooted in the body

The question of the bodily basis of the self has long been debated by philosophers. Descartes (1641/1989) had a dualistic point of view, where the self is purely mental and thus detached from the body. However, his approach fails to explain the interaction between the mental and the physical domains. For instance, remembering a vivid, scary event from our past increases our heart rate. To solve this issue, Spinoza (1677/2005) proposed that mind and body form one unique entity so that any mental event is accompanied by bodily changes. Therefore, the self, as the subject of mental activity, has a bodily basis. William James (1890/1931) further elaborated the concept of self. He defined a hierarchy of the self where the bodily self is at the bottom and underlies more cognitive and higher-level forms of self, such as the social self or the spiritual self. For him, "our entire feeling of spiritual activity . . . is really a feeling of bodily activities" (Vol. 1, pp. 301–2, 1931). Every episode of our lives is accompanied by particular bodily feelings that remain associated with the memories we retain from those episodes. These bodily feelings give the memories the "warmth" necessary for memories to be felt as our own and a sense of continuity of the self along time as being one and the same.

More recently, the idea of the bodily basis of the self has been translated into biological terms, notably by Antonio Damasio (1994, 1999). Damasio defines the first level of self, the *proto-self*, as representing the unconscious monitoring of the moment by moment state of the body. This proto-self is non-conscious, and corresponds to a mechanism shared by all living organisms. When an object (a face, a melody, etc.) interacts with the organism, it modifies the organism's state, thereby modifying the proto-self. These new maps representing the interaction between the organism and the object can become conscious and generate the *core-self*. Because a multiplicity of objects is constantly interacting with the organism, the core-self is constantly generated and continuous in time. The *autobiographical self* is then composed of the collection of experiences of the core-self. The autobiographical self is extended in time and it places the subject at a given point in their personal history, with a past that constitutes their identity, and a perspective of the future. In this hierarchical model of the self, each level depends on the lower level, and therefore all depend on bodily mechanisms. For Damasio, the body ensures the stability of the self over time; that is, this feeling that we stay the same person throughout our lifetime. Because the range of internal bodily states compatible with life is actually limited, bodily representations are stable and so is the self.

While those proposals have been influential, they have also been met with criticism. In particular, on both James and Damasio's proposals, selfhood is rooted in *changes* in bodily states. For James, the "feeling of bodily activities" constitutes the core definition of the self, while for Damasio the proto-self is generated by the brain response to changes in the organism internal state. This is reminiscent of the James–Lange theory of emotions, where physiological changes generate the feeling of an emotion. This theory has been criticized on several grounds, but the most relevant point is that altering bodily states does not necessarily induce an emotion. Similarly, altering bodily states does not alter the self. For instance, the self is not deeply altered when stimulating the viscera by eating. The proposal we outline aims at overcoming this criticism. Briefly, we propose that organs endowed with pacemaker properties, such as the heart or the stomach, function as continuous sources of signals, sending the message to the central nervous system that a body is there—whatever the bodily state is. This information would then be used at the central level to generate an egocentric reference frame, from which first-person perspective can arise (Park & Tallon-Baudry, 2014; Tallon-Baudry et al., 2017). First-person perspective can be viewed as a basic building block necessary to all aspects of selfhood. First-person perspective is intrinsic to the simplest, pre-reflective aspect of the self that defines the subject who acts, perceives, or feels. In more complex aspects of the self, such as the autobiographical or social self, the self includes also a reflective component where the self is the object of introspection (Christoff et al., 2011; Gallagher, 2012; Legrand & Ruby, 2009; Zahavi, 2005).

In the first part of the chapter, we develop the idea that the neural monitoring of visceral signals could constitute the ground for selfhood. Then, we describe cardiac and gastric pacemaker properties as well as known anatomical pathways from the viscera to the central nervous system. In the third part of the chapter, we review the recent experimental evidence directly relating neural responses to heartbeats to different facets of the self—the bodily self, the self who thinks, and the self who perceives, and finally we discuss the hypothesis in light of these results.

3.1.2 The neural monitoring of visceral signals as the ground for the self

3.1.2.1 The importance of visceral electrical signals from the heart and gastrointestinal tract

In the search for a bodily basis of selfhood, emphasis has mostly been placed on the role of sensory and motor signals (from the skin, limbs, joints, vestibular system) in agency (Frith, Blakemore, & Wolpert, 2000) or bodily self-consciousness (Blanke & Metzinger,

2009) studies, leading to the proposal that the bodily self results from multi-sensory integration (Blanke, Slater, & Serino, 2015). While sensory and motor signals certainly play a role, they are mostly emitted *in response* to a particular stimulus or *as a feedback* from a motor action, whereas first-person perspective should be continuously defined. The case of locked-in patients, who are fully paralyzed but nevertheless conscious, also shows that the self can exist despite massive disruption of proprioceptive signals (Tononi & Koch, 2008). Conversely, asomatognosic patients cannot sense their somatosensory body but are aware of their visceral functions, such as breathing, the heart beating, or digestion. Such a patient described the strangeness of her bodily self but her first-person perspective remained intact; she was able to say "I" (Damasio, 1994). From this clinical case, Damasio hypothesized that "some body representations may be of greater value than others to ground the mind, namely, those that pertain to the organism's interior, specifically to the viscera and internal milieu" (2003, p. 193).

The heart and the gastrointestinal tract have a very distinctive property: they contain pacemaker cells that continuously and autonomously generate an electrical signal. This is well known for the heart, and results in cardiac contraction, at a rate of about one beat per second. The gastrointestinal tract is lined with a specific pacemaker cell type, the interstitial cells of Cajal (Sanders, Koh, & Ward, 2006), that intrinsically generate a slow electrical rhythm at rates varying between 3 cycles per minute in the stomach to 12 cycles per minute in the duodenum. This slow electrical rhythm controls the frequency of contraction of the gastrointestinal tract smooth muscle, but is generated at all times, even when fasting (Bozler, 1945). These signals, continuously emitted by the heart and gastrointestinal tract, are relayed up to the central nervous system, as will be detailed in section 3.2.1. The brain is constantly monitoring visceral signals which most of the time are processed implicitly and remain unnoticed. Visceral signals can sometimes become conscious to indicate a large deviation from homeostasis in order to trigger a protective behavior. However, such events remain quite rare, whereas the self is continuously present. It thus seems more likely that the self is rooted in the automatic, unconscious monitoring of visceral inputs, rather than in sparse, transient, conscious events.

3.1.2.2 Proposal for the biological implementation of the self

Our proposal is that the integration of the various visceral signals in the brain generates a body-centered reference frame (Park & Tallon-Baudry, 2014; Tallon-Baudry et al., 2017). Ascending visceral signals would be in this sense *self-specifying* because they define the self at the biological level. This reference frame would then be used by the brain to tag mental processes as being subjective or self-related.

One could argue that there is no need for a mechanism tagging my mental processes as being mine, since they happen in my brain and not someone else's. However, not all mental processes have "mineness." The vast literature on unconscious processing shows numerous examples where mental processes remain unconscious, without first-person perspective. Thus, not all neural processes are by default subjective or self-related, and a tagging mechanism might be useful to define "mineness" (Tallon-Baudry et al., 2017). In this view, first-person perspective would not be defined at the neural level by activity in specific brain regions but would be based on the neural monitoring of visceral afferents, which might take place in a quite extended network as detailed in the following.

3.2 Visceral signals: Pathways and mechanisms

3.2.1 Pathways from the viscera to the brain

Which neuronal pathways carry visceral sensory information? What is the nature of visceral information and how is it represented? Surprisingly, we know much less about visceroception than about other senses such as vision or audition. One reason is probably that it has attracted less attention than classical senses but it also seems that the organization of visceral pathways is more complex, with more parallel pathways and more cortical targets, than for exteroceptive senses. However, the existence of multiple pathways also speaks about the importance of visceral representations in the brain.

3.2.1.1 From the periphery to the brainstem

Information about heart contraction is transduced by baroreceptors, neurons sensing changes in pressure following blood ejection. This system is mostly dedicated to the regulation of arterial blood pressure. Baroreceptors are located in the heart walls, the aortic arch and the carotid bodies and, depending on their location, send ascending projections either through the vagus nerve or glossopharyngeal nerve and discharge at different moments of the cardiac cycle (Klabunde, 2012). Both vagal and glossopharyngeal pathways converge in the Nucleus Tractus Solitarius (NTS), where they also converge with spinal afferents (Nosaka et al., 1995). Neurons responding to the stimulation of baroreceptor afferents have been observed in the rat NTS (Nosaka et al., 1995). It is worth underlining that the baroreceptor route is not the only pathway that can be employed. Somatosensory receptors are likely to convey heartbeat-related information as well, although detailed mechanisms have not yet been elucidated. Indeed, the chest is innervated by somatosensory afferents that might respond to the impact of the heart on the chest, at each heartbeat (Khalsa et al., 2009). Finally, it has recently been shown that, at least *in vitro*, vascular events can alter directly firing rate (Kim et al., 2016), suggesting the possibility of a direct route from vessels to neurons that would bypass the peripheral mechanotransduction of cardiac contraction.

Regarding the stomach, the interstitial cells of Cajal, which generate the slow gastric basal rhythm, connect not only to smooth muscles but also to sensory neurons (Powley & Phillips, 2011). Sensory information from the gastrointestinal tract is, as cardiac information, relayed up to the NTS (Furness et al., 2013).

3.2.1.2 Central targets of visceral inputs

Visceral inputs reach a number of cortical targets. The insular cortex receives vagal inputs in a number of mammalian species (Saper, 2002) and appears viscerotopically organized, with cardiopulmonary inputs targeting the posterior (granular) insula (Cechetto & Saper, 1987). While the insula is sometimes presented as *the* primary visceral cortex, visceral information is also mapped in a number of other regions, that should not be neglected: the ventral anterior cingulate cortex (Vogt, Pandya, & Rosene, 1987) and somatosensory cortices SI and SII (Kern et al., 2013; Korn, Wendt, & Albe-Fessard, 1966; Newman, 1962). More recently, Dum, Levinthal, and Strick (Dum et al., 2009) showed that motor cingulate regions receive inputs from the spinothalamic tract.

While anatomical tracing or stimulation studies show the existence of multiple cortical targets of visceral inputs, much emphasis has been placed on the role of the insula, following the proposal by Craig (Craig, 2002, 2009). In his view, interoceptive information would be represented in the posterior insula, and then integrated with other sensory and cognitive processes in a gradient progressing toward the anterior insula, thereby generating self-awareness. Following this influential theory, a number of brain imaging studies used a region-of-interest approach targeting the insula, but did not test other candidate regions. There is no doubt that the right anterior insula is important to explicitly report interoceptive feelings, as elegantly demonstrated by (Critchley et al., 2004). However, as will be detailed in section 3.3.4, the role of the insula appears more limited in the absence of heartbeat-related tasks (Babo-Rebelo, Richter, & Tallon-Baudry, 2016a; Babo-Rebelo et al., 2016b; Park et al., 2016; Park et al., 2014).

3.2.1.3 An impact of visceral inputs on brain dynamics?

Visceral information can reach a number of different cortical targets but does it have an impact on brain dynamics? Evidence accumulates to suggest a strong cross-talk between brain dynamics and physiological signals, such as skin conductance levels (Fan et al., 2012; James, Henderson, & Macefield, 2013; Nagai et al., 2004), respiration fluctuations (Yuan et al., 2013), or heart rate (de Munck et al., 2008). Classically, physiological measures have been considered as reflecting brain outputs. The most well-known case is fluctuations in pupil diameter, which are thought to be directly reflecting noradrenergic release by the locus coeruleus (Aston-Jones & Cohen, 2005; Joshi et al., 2016), or electrodermal activity, reflecting sympathetic output (Beissner et al., 2013). More generally, there is a strong bias to think that physiological measures reflect mostly top-down autonomic control, from the brain to the peripheral organs. In human brain imaging, physiological signals are mostly considered as a source of noise that needs to be regressed out of the data (Birn, 2012; Glover, Li, & Ress, 2000; Shmueli et al., 2007).

The importance of a bottom-up influence of visceral inputs on brain dynamics should nonetheless be considered. Indeed, up to 80% of the fibers of the vagus nerve are ascending (Agostoni et al., 1957), suggesting that the bottom-up transfer of information is prioritized relative to top-down transfer of information. Besides, while there is no doubt that pupil diameter is under strong central control, other organs generate their own activity. As mentioned earlier, the stomach intrinsically generates a slow (~0.05 Hz) electrical wave, known as the gastric basal rhythm (Sanders et al., 2006). A recent study investigated a potential link between the gastric basal rhythm with resting-state brain dynamics (Richter et al., 2017). There it was shown that the phase of the gastric basal rhythm constrains the amplitude of alpha oscillations in the right anterior insula and occipito-parietal regions, with the gastric slow rhythm accounting for 8% of the variance of alpha rhythm amplitude fluctuations. Importantly, the coupling was mostly due to an *ascending* influence from the stomach on the brain. So-called intrinsic brain activity might thus be—at least partly—constrained by visceral pacemakers.

3.2.2 Neural responses to heartbeats

To demonstrate a link between the self and ascending visceral information, one needs a measure of visceral processing. We will thus focus here on the heart for which such a measure is available: the heartbeat-evoked response.

Neural responses to heartbeats are computed by averaging brain activity, recorded with electroencephalography (EEG) or magnetoencephalography (MEG), locked to heartbeats (Figure 3.1). Heartbeat-evoked responses (HERs) were firstly explored in the 1980s by the group of Schandry (Schandry, Sparrer, & Weitkunat, 1986).

HERs appear to be generated in an impressive range of brain areas. Initial source localization (Pollatos, Kirsch, & Schandry, 2005) found dipole locations compatible with the anterior cingulate cortex, the medial frontal gyrus, the right insula, and the left somatosensory cortex. A more recent EEG study found sources in posterior cingulate cortex/supplementary motor area (Park et al., 2016). MEG recordings, which have a better spatial resolution than EEG, have shown the involvement of the right inferior parietal lobule, ventral posterior cingulate cortex, and ventromedial prefrontal cortex in the generation of HERs (Babo-Rebelo et al., 2016a; Park et al., 2014). HERs were also found in the insula, using a region of interest analysis of high-density EEG (Couto et al., 2015) or MEG data (Babo-Rebelo et al., 2016a), as well as in intracranial EEG (Babo-Rebelo et al., 2016b; Park et al., 2017). Intracranial electro-corticographic (EcoG) grid recordings also revealed prominent HERs in the primary somatosensory cortex (Kern et al., 2013). Many studies reported different effect latencies, ranging from 200–650 ms after the R-peak (Kern et al. 2013, for a review), potentially reflecting the different latencies at which baroreceptors can fire in a cardiac cycle, or the existence of different cortical relays.

3.3 Neural responses to heartbeats encode the self

Neural responses to heartbeats are a measure of the neural monitoring of cardiac activity. We now review recent evidence showing a link between these responses and three facets of the self: bodily awareness, the self in spontaneous thoughts, and the self as the subject of visual perception.

3.3.1 Neural responses to heartbeats and bodily awareness

Direct evidence for a link between HERs and bodily awareness comes from a study on full-body illusions (Park et al., 2016), induced by stroking the participant's back (Lenggenhager et al., 2007) in synchrony with the strokes applied to a virtual body displayed in front of the participant. If the stroking is asynchronous, participants do not experience the

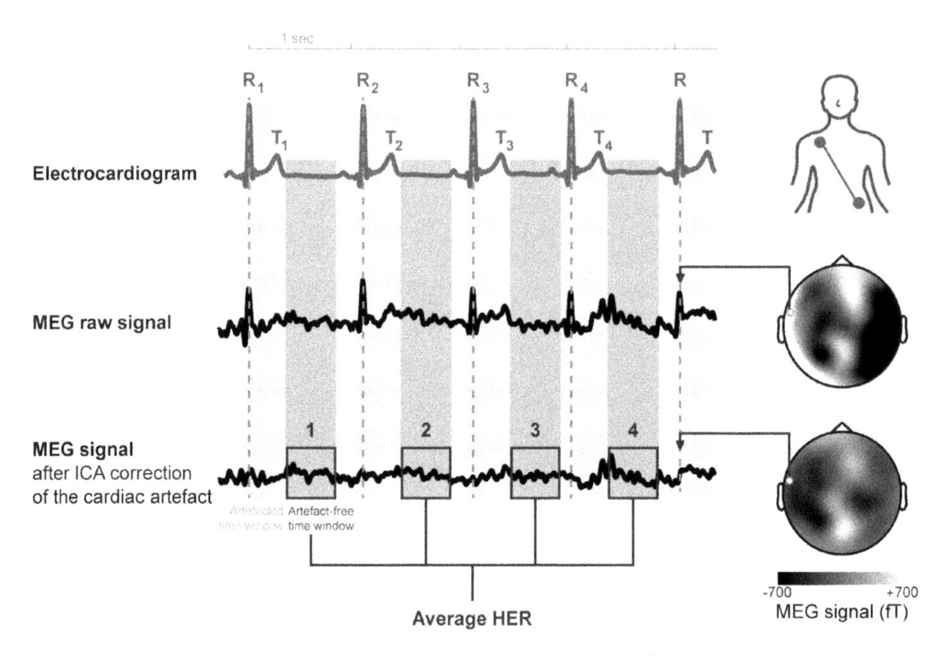

Figure 3.1 What is a Heartbeat-Evoked Response (HER)? Example from real data. Example of raw data in a single participant, with an electrocardiogram (ECG, top row), recorded here between the right clavicle and left abdomen, magnetoencephalographic (MEG) raw data (middle raw), and after correction of the cardiac field artefact (bottom row), from the MEG sensor highlighted in white on the topographical maps. The ECG shows major deflections or R-waves (corresponding to ventricular depolarization and the beginning of myocardial contraction), followed by T-waves (corresponding to ventricular repolarization). The interval between R peaks is quite variable in healthy participants. The R and T waves are also detected on MEG raw data, a phenomenon called the cardiac-field artefact (light-grey shaded areas). One thus has to be cautious when searching for brain responses to heartbeats: MEG (or EEG) data includes cardiac signals. The cardiac field artefact typically affects sensors located in temporal regions, as shown on the topographic map. We combine two solutions to avoid including the cardiac field artefact in our analysis. First, we analyze only the portion of MEG data corresponding to an electrical "silence" of the heart, when the heart relaxes and refills, after the end of the T wave (dark-grey shaded area). We also correct the MEG data from the cardiac-field artefact (bottom row), using independent component analysis (ICA). The heartbeat-evoked response (HER) is then computed as the average of the data segments in the dark-grey shaded area.

illusion. HER amplitude was found to differ depending on whether the stroking was synchronous or asynchronous and correlated with the strength of the experienced illusion (Park et al., 2016). This effect was associated with the posterior cingulate cortex/supplementary motor area (PCC-SMA) (Figure 3.2a). Similar findings were obtained with a modified version of the enfacement illusion (Sel, Azevedo, & Tsakiris, 2016). Participants watched a morphed face which decreased in luminance synchronously or asynchronously with their heartbeats. This manipulation induced a bias in a subsequent self-recognition task where the other person's face was included to a greater extent in the representation of

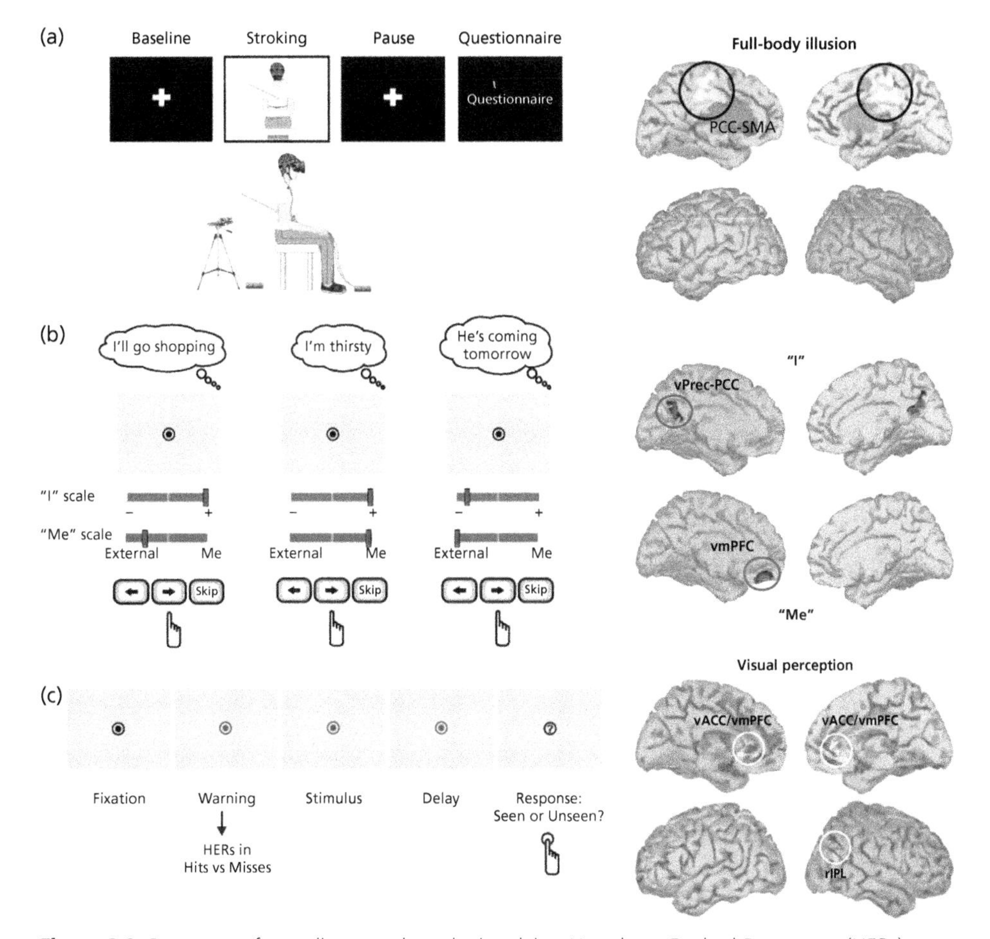

Figure 3.2 Summary of paradigms and results involving Heartbeat-Evoked Responses (HERs). (a)—HERs covary with the bodily self (Park et al., 2016). Participants were stroked on the back, while visualizing their own back being stroked in front of them, in a virtual reality setting. When the stroking was synchronous with the visual input, participants may experience the illusion of being located closer to the virtual body. The amplitude of HERs recorded during the stroking phase varied with illusion strength. This effect was located in the posterior cingulate cortex-supplementary motor area (PCC-SMA). (b)—HERs encode the self-relatedness of spontaneous thoughts (Babo-Rebelo et al., 2016a; Babo-Rebelo et al., 2016b). Participants had to mind-wander while fixating. They were interrupted at random intervals and had to evaluate the self-relatedness of the interrupted thought on the "I" scale (how much were they involved as the subject or agent in the thought) and on the "Me" scale (was the thought referring to themselves, the "Me," or to something external). Participants could skip the answer if they did not know how to rate the thought. HERs in the ventral precuneus-posterior cingulate cortex (vPrec-PCC) encoded the involvement of the "I" in the thought, while HERs in the ventromedial prefrontal cortex (vmPFC) independently encoded the "Me" dimension. (c)—HERs predict conscious visual perception (Park et al., 2014). Participants fixated a central point and were presented with a faint visual stimulus (annulus grating at threshold of visibility). They had to report if they had seen the stimulus or not. The amplitude of HERs before stimulus onset predicted whether the stimulus was going to be subsequently seen or not. This effect was located in the ventral anterior cingulate cortex/ventromedial prefrontal cortex (vACC/vmPFC) and in the right inferior parietal lobule (rIPL). Note that differential neural responses to heartbeats were observed in the default network during fixation (spontaneous thoughts, panel b; perception at threshold before stimulus onset, panel c) while in the virtual body experiment (panel a), differential responses to heartbeats are maximal in premotor regions.

one's own face after synchronous stimulation. HER amplitude differed between synchronous and asynchronous conditions, in centro-parietal electrodes (Sel et al., 2016).

Changes in bodily awareness are thus associated with changes in HER amplitude. Those results speak in favor of the hypothesis that the neural monitoring of visceral signals is linked to self-awareness. Still, it remains to be determined whether neural responses to heartbeats are related to other facets of the self, beyond bodily awareness.

3.3.2 **Neural responses to heartbeats and the self in spontaneous thoughts**

The most basic level of self is the self as the *subject* who acts, feels, and perceives from a first-person perspective. Actions, feelings, and perceptions can then be reflected upon. This corresponds to a second level of self, where the self is the *object* of introspection. This distinction between the self as the subject and the self as the object is reminiscent of phenomenological theories distinguishing a pre-reflective from a reflective form of self (Christoff et al., 2011; Gallagher, 2012; Legrand and Ruby, 2009; Zahavi, 2005). This idea can be operationalized in spontaneous thoughts, by distinguishing the "I" from the "Me." The "I" is always present, but can be more or less engaged. The "I" is engaged when one is the agent, the first-person subject of the thought, for example in a thought like "I will go to the supermarket," as opposed to "It's raining" or "He has to go to the supermarket." In contrast, the "Me" corresponds to a reflective dimension of thoughts, when one is thinking about oneself, about one's feelings or bodily state for instance, as in "I am tired" (Babo-Rebelo et al., 2016a; Babo-Rebelo et al., 2016b). Could HERs correspond to the biological implementation of the "I", of the "Me", or both?

This question was assessed in a thought-sampling paradigm, where participants were asked to mind-wander while fixating on a screen (Babo-Rebelo et al., 2016a). They were interrupted at random intervals and had to report whether they were engaged as the "I" and as the "Me" during the interrupted thought. HER amplitude was shown to correlate with the self-relatedness of thoughts, but in different regions for the "I" and the "Me." The amplitude of HERs in the ventral precuneus and posterior cingulate regions (vPrc-PCC) co-varied with the engagement of the "I" in the ongoing thought (Figure 3.2b). The "Me" dimension was associated with HERs in the ventromedial prefrontal cortex (vmPFC) (Figure 3.2b). Although the "I" and the "Me" were often combined in a given thought, we could demonstrate that the association between the "I" and HERs in vPrc-PCC was orthogonal to the association between the "Me" and HERs in vmPFC.

These MEG results were then replicated with intracranial recordings, by showing a trial-by-trial parametrical modulation of HERs along with the level of involvement of each self-dimension in each sampled thought (Babo-Rebelo et al., 2016b). The main effects were found in midline regions of the default-network, but a region of interest analysis additionally revealed that HERs in the right anterior insula were modulated by the degree of engagement of the "I" in thoughts. HERs thus encode the self-relatedness of thoughts, along both the "I" and the "Me" self-dimensions, but in distinct regions.

3.3.3 Neural responses to heartbeats and the self as the subject of visual perception

The existence of a first-person subject underlying any conscious perception has been overlooked in cognitive neuroscience (Tallon-Baudry et al., 2017). Indeed, the hallmark of conscious vision is that the participant reports his/her perception: for conscious perception to exist, there must be a *subject* of experience (Park and Tallon-Baudry, 2014; Tallon-Baudry et al., 2017). In the experiment by Park and colleagues (Park et al., 2014), participants had to report the presence or absence of near-threshold gratings. HER amplitude in the ventral anterior cingulate/ventromedial prefrontal cortex (vACC/vmPFC) and the right posterior inferior parietal lobule (rIPL), before stimulus presentation, predicted whether the visual stimulus was going to be consciously perceived or not (Figure 3.2c) (Park et al., 2014). This effect corresponded to changes in visual sensitivity (d') and not to changes in the criterion of response, suggesting that information carried by neural responses to heartbeats is used as sensory evidence in the seen/unseen decision.

Differential HERs predicting conscious vision can here be interpreted as corresponding to fluctuations in the engagement of the self as the experiencing subject, the one who wonders whether or not he/she has seen the stimulus. Note that only weak, subthreshold differences in HERs could be detected in the right insula.

3.3.4 Reconsidering the role of the insula

In the three experiments mentioned above (Babo-Rebelo et al., 2016a; Babo-Rebelo et al., 2016b; Park et al., 2016, 2014) that directly relate interoceptive processing with the "I," the "Me," or the bodily self, the insula did not appear to be the key player. This raises questions about the "hypothesis that the anterior insula engenders human awareness" (Craig, 2009).

There is no doubt that the insula is involved in cardiac processing, and indeed neural responses to heartbeats were observed in the posterior (Park et al., 2017) and anterior (Babo-Rebelo et al., 2016b) insula using iEEG. fMRI studies further suggest that (a) the insula is involved in cardiac-visual integration (Blefari et al., 2017; Ronchi et al., 2015; Salomon et al., 2016), (b) the insula is activated when explicitly paying attention to interoceptive signals (Critchley et al., 2004; Farb, Segal, & Anderson, 2013), and (c) the anterior insula is involved in self-related bodily processing (Blanke et al., 2014; Brass & Haggard, 2010; Heydrich & Blanke, 2013; Karnath & Baier, 2010). When combined, these three sets of results could suggest a link between cardiac processing and the interoceptive/bodily self in the insula.

However, there are several reasons why the role of the insula might have been overestimated. First, it is not clear whether there is a true anatomical overlap between interoception and self-related processes. This is all the more important that the insula is an extended structure, with numerous subdivisions (Deen, Pitskel, & Pelphrey, 2011). Second, even if there were an overlap between self-related activations and interoception, it does not necessarily follow that there is a true interaction between interoception and the self. For instance, it could be that paying attention to interoceptive signals and paying attention to some aspects of the self both require saliency estimation, a process implemented in the insula for a variety of tasks, independently from the self or interoceptive processing (Menon & Uddin, 2010). Last, the reverse inference suggesting that insular activity is a signature of interoceptive processing might be flawed, as any reverse inference (Poldrack, 2011). The insula is activated by a wealth of different processes, not necessarily related to the self nor to interoception (Chang et al., 2013; Duncan & Owen, 2000).

3.3.5 **Changes in neural responses to heartbeats in the absence of physiological changes**

Theories rooting the self in the body have focused on the role of *bodily* changes (see section 3.1.1). Importantly, none of the results reported earlier were associated with differences in cardiorespiratory parameters (heart rate, heart rate variability, peripheral blood pressure, respiratory patterns), suggesting that cardio-respiratory state did not change. This is in line with the hypothesis that bodily information exists and impacts neural processing even in the absence of bodily changes. In addition, several arousal measures, such as the pupil diameter, interbeat interval, heart rate variability, electrodermal activity, or alpha power did not differ between conditions, ruling out the possibility that HER differences reflected distinct global arousal states. Altogether, this suggests that the amplitude changes of HERs encoding the self are related to neural, rather than bodily, fluctuations, as further discussed in section 3.4. A heartbeat could be considered as a physically constant stimulus generating neural responses whose amplitude varies from one stimulus to the next, a phenomenon which is well known for exteroception. For instance, the repeated presentation of a physically identical visual stimulus can elicit brain responses of different amplitudes, depending on neural and cognitive parameters.

The fact that neural responses to heartbeats can vary independently from changes in cardiac parameters seems incompatible with interoceptive prediction error accounts of selfhood (Seth, 2013; Seth & Friston, 2016). In this framework, cardiac inputs should vary and deviate from the corresponding homeostatic prediction, thereby generating prediction error signals at the origin of a sense of self.

3.4 **Towards a biological implementation of the self?**

We have presented evidence that neural responses to heartbeats encode changes in bodily awareness, encode self-relatedness in spontaneous thoughts, and predict the seen or unseen fate of a visual stimulus. Such results are in line with the hypothesis that neural responses to heartbeats constitute a marker of the first-person perspective inherent to self-consciousness, bodily consciousness, and perceptual consciousness. However, the results show a *correlation* between HER amplitude and the self, while the hypothesis that neural responses to heartbeats play a causal role in the generation of first-person perspective remains to be directly tested. It is thus worth examining the different interpretations of the correlations between HER amplitude and the self.

A first interpretation of the changes in amplitude of HERs is that HERs are a nonspecific marker of enhanced brain activity. Any region being particularly active at a given moment would then show changes in HER amplitude. In this view, if two conditions induce different levels of activity in a given region, responses to heartbeats in this region differ as well. The fact that differential HERs are found in regions which are expected to be differently activated, such as default-network regions during the resting state or passive fixation (Babo-Rebelo et al., 2016a; Babo-Rebelo et al., 2016b; Park et al., 2014), or bodily/motor regions during full-body illusions (Park et al., 2016), could support this interpretation. However, in the aforementioned three experiments, HER differences could not be trivially explained by different levels of neural activity (e.g. alpha power, slow fluctuations) differing between conditions. Still, not all features of brain activity (e.g. high-frequency bands) were investigated. Ruling out definitively the hypothesis that neural responses to heartbeats are a non-specific marker of cortical reactivity will prove difficult, since it implies measuring all aspects of cortical reactivity and demonstrating the absence of a difference, which is a notoriously difficult task.

A second hypothesis is that ascending visceral signals themselves differ between conditions, leading in turn to differential neural responses to heartbeats. In this hypothesis, information about the self can be found directly in cardiac data. For instance, cardiac afferent signals would determine whether or not a stimulus is likely to be seen, or whether a spontaneous thought is self-related. However, there were no differences in the measured cardiac parameters (electrocardiogram, heart rate, heart rate variability, and blood pressure), but more subtle differences may have gone unnoticed. Other parameters, such as volume of blood ejected at each heartbeat, were not measured and might vary.

The third hypothesis is that self-related information is present in brain responses to ascending visceral signals, not in the visceral signals themselves. Cardiac or gastric ascending signals would function as constant sources of signal, indicating that a body is there but not necessarily conveying more specific information. Note that other organs or systems might also contribute, but the pacemaker properties of the heart and the gastrointestinal tract make them particularly relevant. These ascending signals could interact with ongoing brain activity, anchoring some aspects of brain activity in a body-centered reference frame and hence implementing first-person perspective. The mechanisms underlying this interaction remain to be investigated. Cardiac signals would contribute to a body-centered reference frame, which would be used by the brain to anchor thoughts or percepts to the self (Park & Tallon-Baudry, 2014). The amplitude of these neural responses would then be a marker of the self-relatedness of neural activity in this region. Note that given that visceral signals target a large number of cortical areas, this mechanism could take place in many different brain regions, wherever a self versus non-self distinction is relevant for the task at play.

3.5 Conclusion

Building on a long tradition relating the self to bodily signals, we have proposed to revise this hypothesis and to focus on visceral inputs. Such signals display interesting characteristics, notably the fact that they are continuously emitted, in the absence of bodily movement but also in the absence of bodily state changes. Visceral inputs would indicate to the brain the mere presence of a body, and could thus act as continuous self-specifying signals. Neural responses to heartbeats, which can be measured non-invasively in humans, offer a valuable tool to experimentally probe the link between the neural monitoring of visceral inputs and the self. Recent results show correlations between neural responses to heartbeats and the self, not only, as initially hypothesized, when the self is implicit (the self as the agent, the self experiencing a visual input) but also in situations where the self is explicit or reflective (bodily awareness, thinking about oneself). These results are compatible with our proposal that the integration of visceral signals generates a subject-centered reference frame underlying the different facets of the self. However, the results so far are only correlational, and moving to causation will prove an important, but difficult, step. In addition, some questions remain open, for instance how neural responses to heartbeats interact with stimulus or thought content.

References

Agostoni, E., **Chinnock, J. E.**, **Daly, M. D. B.**, and **Murray, J. G.** (1957). Functional and histological studies of the vagus nerve and its branches to the heart, lungs and abdominal viscera in the cat. *Journal of Physiology*, *135*(1), 182–205. <https://doi.org/10.1113/jphysiol.1957.sp005703>

Aston-Jones, G. and **Cohen, J. D.** (2005). An integrative theory of locus coeruleus-norepinephrine function: Adaptive gain and optimal performance. *Annual Review of Neuroscience*, *28*(1), 403–50. <https://doi.org/10.1146/annurev.neuro.28.061604.135709>

Babo-Rebelo, M., **Richter, C.**, and **Tallon-Baudry, C.** (2016a). Neural responses to heartbeats in the default network encode the self in spontaneous thoughts. *Journal of Neuroscience*, *36*(30), 7829–40. <https://doi.org/https://doi.org/10.1523/JNEUROSCI.0262-16.2016>

Babo-Rebelo, M., **Wolpert, N.**, **Adam, C.**, **Hasboun, D.**, and **Tallon-Baudry, C.** (2016b). Is the cardiac monitoring function related to the self in both the default network and right anterior insula? *Philosophical Transactions of the Royal Society B*, *371*(1708), 1–13. <https://doi.org/10.1098/rstb.2016.0004>

Beissner, F., **Meissner, K.**, **Bär, K.-J.**, and **Napadow, V.** (2013). The autonomic brain: An activation likelihood estimation meta-analysis for central processing of autonomic function. *Journal of Neuroscience*, *33*(25), 10503–11. <https://doi.org/10.1523/JNEUROSCI.1103-13.2013>

Birn, R. M. (2012). The role of physiological noise in resting-state functional connectivity. *NeuroImage*, *62*(2), 864–70. <https://doi.org/10.1016/j.neuroimage.2012.01.016>

Blanke, O. and **Metzinger, T.** (2009). Full-body illusions and minimal phenomenal selfhood. *Trends in Cognitive Sciences*, *13*(1), 7–13. <https://doi.org/10.1016/j.tics.2008.10.003>

Blanke, O., **Pozeg, P.**, **Hara, M.**, **Heydrich, L.**, **Serino, A.**, **Yamamoto, A.**, et al. (2014). Neurological and robot-controlled induction of an apparition. *Current Biology*, *24*, 2681–6. <https://doi.org/10.1016/j.cub.2014.09.049>

Blanke, O., **Slater, M.**, and **Serino, A.** (2015). Behavioral, neural, and computational principles of bodily self-consciousness. *Neuron*, *88*(1), 145–66. <https://doi.org/10.1016/j.neuron.2015.09.029>

Blefari, M. L., **Martuzzi, R.**, **Salomon, R.**, **Bello-Ruiz, J.**, **Herbelin, B.**, **Serino, A.**, et al. (2017). Bilateral rolandic operculum processing underlying heartbeat awareness reflects changes in bodily self-consciousness. *European Journal of Neuroscience*, *45*, 1300–12. <https://doi.org/10.1111/ijlh.12426>

Bozler, E. (1945). The action potentials of the stomach. *American Journal of Physiology*, *144*, 693–700. <http://ajplegacy.physiology.org/content/144/5/693.article-info>

Brass, M. and **Haggard, P.** (2010). The hidden side of intentional action: The role of the anterior insular cortex. *Brain Structure and Function*, *214*, 603–10. <https://doi.org/10.1007/s00429-010-0269-6>

Cechetto, D. F. and **Saper, C. B.** (1987). Evidence for a viscerotopic sensory representation in the cortex and thalamus in the rat. *Journal of Comparative Neurology*, *262*(1), 27–45. <https://doi.org/10.1002/cne.902620104>

Chang, L. J., **Yarkoni, T.**, **Khaw, M. W.**, and **Sanfey, A. G.** (2013). Decoding the role of the insula in human cognition: Functional parcellation and large-scale reverse inference. *Cerebral Cortex*, *23*(3), 739–49. <https://doi.org/10.1093/cercor/bhs065>

Christoff, K., **Cosmelli, D.**, **Legrand, D.**, and **Thompson, E.** (2011). Specifying the self for cognitive neuroscience. *Trends in Cognitive Sciences*, *15*(3), 104–12. <https://doi.org/10.1016/j.tics.2011.01.001>

Couto, B., **Adolfi, F.**, **Velasquez, M.**, **Mesow, M.**, **Feinstein, J.**, **Canales-Johnson, A.**, et al. (2015). Heart evoked potential triggers brain responses to natural affective scenes: A preliminary study. *Autonomic Neuroscience: Basic and Clinical*, *193*, 132–7. <https://doi.org/10.1016/j.autneu.2015.06.006>

Craig, A. D. (2002). How do you feel? Interoception: The sense of the physiological condition of the body. *Nature Reviews Neuroscience*, *3*(8), 655–66. <https://doi.org/10.1038/nrn894>

Craig, A. D. (2009). How do you feel—now? The anterior insula and human awareness. *Nature Reviews Neuroscience*, *10*(1), 59–70. <https://doi.org/10.1038/nrn2555>

Critchley, H. D., **Wiens, S.**, **Rotshtein, P.**, **Ohman, A.**, and **Dolan, R. J.** (2004). Neural systems supporting interoceptive awareness. *Nature Neuroscience*, *7*(2), 189–95. <https://doi.org/10.1038/nn1176>

Damasio, A. R. (1994). *Descartes' Error. Emotion, Reason, and the Human Brain*. New York, NY: Avon Books.

Damasio, A. R. (1999). *The Feeling of what Happens: Body, Emotion and the Making of Consciousness*. New York, NY: Harcourt.

Damasio, A. R. (2003). *Looking for Spinoza. Joy, Sorrow, and the Feeling Brain*. New York, NY: Harcourt.

de Munck, J. C., **Gonçalves, S. I.**, **Faes, T. J. C.**, **Kuijer, J. P. A.**, **Pouwels, P. J. W.**, **Heethaar, R. M.**, et al. (2008). A study of the brain's resting state based on alpha band power, heart rate and fMRI. *NeuroImage*, *42*(1), 112–21. <https://doi.org/10.1016/j.neuroimage.2008.04.244>

Deen, B., **Pitskel, N. B.**, and **Pelphrey, K. a.** (2011). Three systems of insular functional connectivity identified with cluster analysis. *Cerebral Cortex*, *21*(7), 1498–506. <https://doi.org/10.1093/cercor/bhq186>

Descartes, R. (1989, orig. pub. 1641). *Discourse on Method and Meditations*. (trans. J. Veitch). New York, NY: Amherst.

Dum, R. P., **Levinthal, D. J.**, and **Strick, P. L.** (2009). The spinothalamic system targets motor and sensory areas in the cerebral cortex of monkeys. *Journal of Neuroscience*, *29*(45), 14223–35. <https://doi.org/10.1523/JNEUROSCI.3398-09.2009>

Duncan, J. and **Owen, A. M.** (2000). Common regions of the human frontal lobe recruited by diverse cognitive demands. *Trends in Neurosciences*, *23*(10), 475–83. <https://doi.org/10.1016/S0166-2236(00)01633-7>

Fan, J., **Xu, P.**, **Van Dam, N. T.**, **Eilam-Stock, T.**, **Gu, X.**, **Luo, Y.**, et al. (2012). Spontaneous brain activity relates to autonomic arousal. *Journal of Neuroscience*, *32*(33), 11176–86. <https://doi.org/10.1523/JNEUROSCI.1172-12.2012>

Farb, N. a S., **Segal, Z. V**, and **Anderson, A. K.** (2013). Mindfulness meditation training alters cortical representations of interoceptive attention. *Social Cognitive and Affective Neuroscience*, *8*(1), 15–26. <https://doi.org/10.1093/scan/nss066>

Frith, C. D., **Blakemore, S. J.**, and **Wolpert, D. M.** (2000). Abnormalities in the awareness and control of action. *Philosophical Transactions of the Royal Society of London B*, *355*(1404), 1771–88. <https://doi.org/10.1098/rstb.2000.0734>

Furness, J. B., **Rivera, L. R.**, **Cho, H.-J.**, **Bravo, D. M.**, and **Callaghan, B.** (2013). The gut as a sensory organ. *Nature Reviews Gastroenterology & Hepatology*, *10*, 729–40. <https://doi.org/10.1038/nrgastro.2013.180>

Gallagher, S. (2012). *Phenomenology*. London: Palgrave Macmillan.

Glover, G. H., **Li, T. Q.**, and **Ress, D.** (2000). Image-based method for retrospective correction of physiological motion effects in fMRI: RETROICOR. *Magnetic Resonance in Medicine*, *44*(1), 162–7. <https://doi.org/10.1002/1522-2594(200007)44:1<162::AID-MRM23>3.0.CO;2-E>

Heydrich, L. and **Blanke, O.** (2013). Distinct illusory own-body perceptions caused by damage to posterior insula and extrastriate cortex. *Brain*, *136*, 790–803. <https://doi.org/10.1093/brain/aws364>

James, C., **Henderson, L.**, and **Macefield, V. G.** (2013). Real-time imaging of brain areas involved in the generation of spontaneous skin sympathetic nerve activity at rest. *NeuroImage*, *74*, 188–94. <https://doi.org/10.1016/j.neuroimage.2013.02.030>

James, W. (1931, orig. pub. 1890). *The Principles of Psychology*. New York, NY: Henry Holt and Company. <https://doi.org/10.1037/11059-000

Joshi, S., **Li, Y.**, **Kalwani, R. M.**, and **Gold, J. I.** (2016). Relationships between pupil diameter and neuronal activity in the locus coeruleus, colliculi, and cingulate cortex. *Neuron*, *89*(1), 221–34. <https://doi.org/10.1016/j.neuron.2015.11.028>

Karnath, H. O. and **Baier, B.** (2010). Right insula for our sense of limb ownership and self-awareness of actions. *Brain Structure and Function*, *214*, 411–17. <https://doi.org/10.1007/s00429-010-0250-4>

Kern, M., **Aertsen, A.**, **Schulze-Bonhage, A.**, and **Ball, T.** (2013). Heart cycle-related effects on event-related potentials, spectral power changes, and connectivity patterns in the human ECoG. *NeuroImage*, *81*, 178–90. <https://doi.org/10.1016/j.neuroimage.2013.05.042>

Khalsa, S. S., **Rudrauf, D.**, **Feinstein, J. S.**, and **Tranel, D.** (2009). The pathways of interoceptive awareness. *Nature Neuroscience*, *12*(12), 1494–6. <https://doi.org/10.1038/nn.2411>

Kim, K. J., **Diaz, J. R.**, **Iddings, J. A.**, and **Filosa, J. A.** (2016). Vasculo-neuronal coupling: Retrograde vascular communication to brain neurons. *Journal of Neuroscience*, *36*(50), 12624–39. <https://doi.org/10.1523/JNEUROSCI.1300-16.2016>

Klabunde, R. E. (2012). *Cardiovascular Physiology Concepts*. Philadelphia, PA: Lippincott, Williams & Wilkins.

Korn, H., **Wendt, R.**, and **Albe-Fessard, D.** (1966). Somatic projection to the orbital cortex of the cat. *Electroencephalography and Clinical Neurophysiology*, *21*(3), 209–26. <https://doi.org/10.1016/0013-4694(66)90071-X>

Legrand, D. and **Ruby, P.** (2009). What is self-specific? Theoretical investigation and critical review of neuroimaging results. *Psychological Review*, *116*(1), 252–82. <https://doi.org/10.1037/a0014172>

Lenggenhager, B., **Tadi, T.**, **Metzinger, T.**, and **Blanke, O.** (2007). Video ergo sum: Manipulating bodily self-consciousness. *Science*, *317*(5841), 1096–9. <https://doi.org/10.1126/science.1143439>

Menon, V. and **Uddin, L. Q.** (2010). Saliency, switching, attention and control: A network model of insula function. *Brain Structure and Function*, *214*(5–6), 655–67. <https://doi.org/10.1007/s00429-010-0262-0>

Nagai, Y., **Critchley, H. D.**, **Featherstone, E.**, **Trimble, M. R.**, and **Dolan, R. J.** (2004). Activity in ventromedial prefrontal cortex covaries with sympathetic skin conductance level: A physiological account of a "default mode" of brain function. *NeuroImage*, *22*(1), 243–51. <https://doi.org/10.1016/j.neuroimage.2004.01.019>

Newman, P. P. (1962). Single unit activity in the viscero-sensory areas of the cerebral cortex. *Journal of Physiology*, *160*(2), 284–97. <https://doi.org/10.1113/jphysiol.1962.sp006846>

Nosaka, S., **Murase, S.**, **Murata, K.**, and **Inui, K.** (1995). "Aortic baroreceptor" neurons in the nucleus tractus solitarius in rats: Convergence of cardiovascular inputs as revealed by heartbeat-locked activity. *Journal of the Autonomic Nervous System*, *55*(1–2), 69–80. <http://www.ncbi.nlm.nih.gov/entrez/query.fcgi?cmd=Retrieve&db=PubMed&dopt=Citation&list_uids=8690854>

Park, H.-D. and **Tallon-Baudry, C.** (2014). The neural subjective frame: From bodily signals to perceptual consciousness. *Philosophical Transactions of the Royal Society of London B*, *369*(1641), 20130208. <https://doi.org/10.1098/rstb.2013.0208>

Park, H.-D., **Correia, S.**, **Ducorps, A.**, and **Tallon-Baudry, C.** (2014). Spontaneous fluctuations in neural responses to heartbeats predict visual detection. *Nature Neuroscience*, *17*(4), 612–18. <https://doi.org/10.1038/nn.3671>

Park, H.-D., **Bernasconi, F.**, **Bello-Ruiz, J.**, **Pfeiffer, C.**, **Salomon, R.**, and **Blanke, O.** (2016). Transient modulations of neural responses to heartbeats covary with bodily self-consciousness. *Journal of Neuroscience*, *36*(32), 8453–60. <https://doi.org/10.1523/JNEUROSCI.0311-16.2016>

Park, H.-D., **Bernasconi, F.**, **Salomon, R.**, **Tallon-Baudry, C.**, **Spinelli, L.**, **Seeck, M.**, et al. (2017). Neural sources and underlying mechanisms of neural responses to heartbeats, and their role in bodily self-consciousness: An intracranial EEG study. *Cerebral Cortex*, 1–14. <https://doi.org/10.1093/cercor/bhx136>

Poldrack, R. A. (2011). Inferring mental states from neuroimaging data: From reverse inference to large-scale decoding. *Neuron*, *72*(5), 692–7. <https://doi.org/10.1016/j.neuron.2011.11.001>

Pollatos, O., **Kirsch, W.**, and **Schandry, R.** (2005). Brain structures involved in interoceptive awareness and cardioafferent signal processing: A dipole source localization study. *Human Brain Mapping*, *26*(1), 54–64. <https://doi.org/10.1002/hbm.20121>

Powley, T. L. and **Phillips, R. J.** (2011). Vagal intramuscular array afferents form complexes with interstitial cells of Cajal in gastrointestinal smooth muscle: Analogues of muscle spindle organs? *Neuroscience*, *186*, 188–200. <https://doi.org/10.1016/j.neuroscience.2011.04.036>

Richter, C. G., **Babo-Rebelo, M.**, **Schwartz, D.**, and **Tallon-Baudry, C.** (2017). Phase-amplitude coupling at the organism level: The amplitude of spontaneous alpha rhythm fluctuations varies with the phase of the infra-slow gastric basal rhythm. *NeuroImage*, *146*, 951–8. <https://doi.org/10.1016/j.neuroimage.2016.08.043>

Ronchi, R., **Bello-Ruiz, J.**, **Lukowska, M.**, **Herbelin, B.**, **Cabrilo, I.**, **Schaller, K.**, et al. (2015). Right insular damage decreases heartbeat awareness and alters cardio-visual effects on bodily self-consciousness. *Neuropsychologia*, *70*, 11–20. <https://doi.org/10.1016/j.neuropsychologia.2015.02.010>

Salomon, R., **Ronchi, R.**, **Donz, J.**, **Bello-Ruiz, J.**, **Herbelin, B.**, **Martet, R.**, et al. (2016). The insula mediates access to awareness of visual stimuli presented synchronously to the heartbeat. *Journal of Neuroscience*, *36*(18), 5115–27. <https://doi.org/10.1523/JNEUROSCI.4262-15.2016>

Sanders, K. M., **Koh, S. D.**, and **Ward, S. M.** (2006). Interstitial cells of Cajal as pacemakers in the gastrointestinal tract. *Annual Review of Physiology*, *68*(1), 307–43. <https://doi.org/10.1146/annurev.physiol.68.040504.094718>

Saper, C. B. (2002). The central autonomic nervous system: Conscious visceral perception and autonomic pattern generation. *Annual Review of Neuroscience*, *25*, 433–69. <https://doi.org/10.1146/annurev.neuro.25.032502.111311>

Schandry, R., **Sparrer, B.**, and **Weitkunat, R.** (1986). From the heart to the brain: A study of heartbeat contingent scalp potentials. *International Journal of Neuroscience*, *30*(4), 261–75. <https://doi.org/10.3109/00207458608985677>

Sel, A., **Azevedo, R. T.**, and **Tsakiris, M.** (2016). Heartfelt self: Cardio-visual integration affects self-face recognition and interoceptive cortical processing. *Cerebral Cortex*, 1–12. <https://doi.org/10.1093/cercor/bhw296>

Seth, A. K. (2013). Interoceptive inference, emotion, and the embodied self. *Trends in Cognitive Sciences*, *17*(11), 565–73. <https://doi.org/10.1016/j.tics.2013.09.007>

Seth, A. K. and **Friston, K. J.** (2016). Active interoceptive inference and the emotional brain. *Philosophical Transactions of the Royal Society B, 371*(20160007). <https://doi.org/10.1098/rstb.2016.0007>

Shmueli, K., van Gelderen, P., de Zwart, J. A., Horovitz, S. G., Fukunaga, M., Jansma, J. M., et al. (2007). Low-frequency fluctuations in the cardiac rate as a source of variance in the resting-state fMRI BOLD signal. *NeuroImage, 38*(2), 306–20. <https://doi.org/https://doi.org/10.1016/j.neuroimage.2007.07.037>

Spinoza, B. de. (2005, orig. pub. 1677). *Ethics* (trans. E. Curley). London: Penguin Classics.

Tallon-Baudry, C., Campana, F., Park, H.-D., and **Babo-Rebelo, M.** (2017). The neural monitoring of visceral inputs, rather than attention, accounts for first-person perspective in conscious vision. *Cortex,* 1–11. <https://doi.org/10.1016/j.cortex.2017.05.019>

Tononi, G. and **Koch, C.** (2008). The neural correlates of consciousness: An update. *Annals of the New York Academy of Sciences, 1124,* 239–61. <https://doi.org/10.1196/annals.1440.004>

Vogt, B. A., Pandya, D. N., and **Rosene, D. L.** (1987). Cingulate cortex of the rhesus monkey: I. Cytoarchitecture and thalamic afferents. *Journal of Comparative Neurology, 262*(2), 256–70. <https://doi.org/10.1002/cne.902620207>

Yuan, H., Zotev, V., Phillips, R., and **Bodurka, J.** (2013). Correlated slow fluctuations in respiration, EEG, and BOLD fMRI. *NeuroImage, 79,* 81–93. <https://doi.org/10.1016/j.neuroimage.2013.04.068>

Zahavi, D. (2005). *Subjectivity and Selfhood: Investigating the First-Person Perspective.* Cambridge, MA: MIT Press.

Chapter 4

The embodiment of time: How interoception shapes the perception of time

Marc Wittmann and Karin Meissner

4.1 Introduction: From phenomenology to neuroscience

Conscious awareness and subjective time are intricately connected. In phenomenological analyses, self-consciousness and time consciousness cannot be separated. In a phenomenal description, consciousness can be seen as a world that is present, as an island of presence in the continuous flow of time. This "window of presence" is concerned with what is happening right now (Metzinger, 2004; Revonsuo, 2006). This description complements the analysis of time experience by Edmund Husserl (1928) and William James (1890), both of whom also discerned two complementary aspects of temporality. Subjective time is described as (a) a continuous flow and (b) the feeling of a present moment. The flow constitutes itself through the experience of passage created by the sequence of (a) an expectation of what is going to happen, (b) the actual experience of what is happening right now, and (c) memory of what has happened. Besides the flow of time, the unity of the present moment (or the feeling of "nowness") is a basic property of consciousness, which comprises the qualitative character of subjective experience. Felt presence is not a duration-less instant in time but is temporally extended and for which neural correlates are assumed and investigated (Pöppel, 1997; Varela, 1999; Lloyd, 2012; Northoff, 2016).

Conscious experience has a first-person mode of "givenness." Conscious states are inherently given to me as the experiencer, or phenomenal experience is mine (Nagel, 1974; Metzinger, 2008; Kiverstein, 2009). This quality of "mineness" thus includes a minimal sense of self within experience. The act of conscious perception includes a basic form of self-consciousness (Zahavi, 2005). Moreover, the self as part of present experience is extended. This temporal extension of the presence stems from temporal properties, past moments, present awareness, and expectations, all being interwoven in present experience. Husserl (1928) termed these facets of present awareness as retention, impression, and protention, respectively, forming the implicit temporal structure of any conscious experience. The phenomenological connection between "time" and the "self" can, therefore, be expressed as follows: I become aware of what is happening now *to me* through what just happened *to me* and expectations of what might happen *to me*. The realization of a self (what happens to me) is created through this tripartite structure of consciousness (Kiverstein, 2009). According to this conceptualization, time consciousness and self-consciousness are manifestations of the same underlying process.

The last connection needed in this short phenomenological introduction to our neuroscientific inquiry on subjective time is the concept of embodiment, the notion that subjective time emerges through bodily processes. According to the enactive/embodied cognition models of subjectivity (Varela, Thompson, & Rosch, 1991/2016), the phenomenal first-person perspective depends on the physical self. In other words, the mental self is created by the continuous visceral and proprioceptive input from the body. The physical self is the functional (bodily) anchor of subjective experience (Metzinger, 2008). Subjective time emerges only through the existence of the self across time as an enduring and embodied entity. In his phenomenological analysis, Maurice Merleau-Ponty (1945) was most explicit when he declared that every mental act is based on a bodily function. Accordingly, one has to understand time as subject and the subject as time ("*Il faut comprendre le temps comme sujet et le sujet comme temps*," Merleau-Ponty, 1945, p. 483); the physical self and subjective time are inseparable.

4.2 Neural models of time perception

The dimension of time is undoubtedly essential for human cognitive functioning. There are many temporal levels of organization in perception and action, ranging from the processing of milliseconds of duration up to daily rhythms and beyond (Buhusi & Meck, 2005; Wittmann, 2016). Specifically, the feeling of time passing and the estimation of duration in the seconds and minutes range are fundamental for orientation in the world and for decision-making. The neural underpinnings of subjective time are, however, poorly understood; there is no consensus on *how* and *where* time is processed in the brain (Wittmann & van Wassenhove, 2009).

Regarding functional principles, regardless of questions of neural implementation, there are several conceptualizations concerning time perception which are summarized here. For one, memory decay has repeatedly been suggested to govern the experience of duration (Staddon, 2005). The underlying idea is that memory capacity decreases over time; therefore, memory decay could function as a clock. An alternative model of time perception encompassing a memory sub-function is the *dual klepsydra model* (Wackermann & Ehm, 2006), where subjective time is represented by the states of lossy accumulators. The accumulator receives inflow during the presentation of a stimulus to be timed (producing the representation of duration), but, at the same time, a continuous outflow reflects the loss of representation over time. In further conceptualizations, energy expenditure has been proposed to underlie subjective duration (Mach, 1911; Marchetti, 2009). It has been shown that a greater demand on mental activity while analyzing more complex or novel situations expands subjective duration. In contrast, experienced repetition leads to higher coding efficiency and to shorter duration estimates (Eagleman &

Pariyadath, 2009). Accordingly, the experience of duration would be a function of the amount of energy expended during the timed interval.

The most influential cognitive model is based on the idea of a pacemaker-accumulator clock. A pacemaker would produce a series of pulses like the ticks of a clock, and the number of pulses recorded during an interval would lead to experienced duration (Treisman, 2013; Gibbon, Church, & Meck, 1984). In a variant of that model, an attentional gate is assumed to open only when attention is directed to time. Time units then enter the accumulator. Accordingly, the more attention is paid to the passage of time, the longer duration is experienced (Zakay & Block, 1997; Wearden, 2016). This notion fits well with everyday experience. Time expands when we become aware of it, like in a waiting situation. Its strong heuristic value probably explains why this model is predominantly used in psychology to account for empirical results.

Regarding the neuroanatomy and neurophysiology of time perception, several models have been brought forward to provide an answer on which brain areas and which neural mechanisms underlie duration judgments. The following summary is by no means exhaustive, but provides a rough sketch of the most prominent ideas. Related to the timing of events ranging from the milliseconds to a few seconds at most, a general mechanism for different magnitudes, such as time, space, and number, has been proposed in the right posterior parietal cortex (Bueti & Walsh, 2009), as well as mechanisms related to neural-delay conduction pathways in the cerebellum (Ivry et al., 2002). Alternatively, it has been suggested that many neural networks have intrinsic temporal-processing properties. Accordingly, duration estimation for very brief events lasting less than half a second are related to time-dependent neural changes, such as short-term synaptic plasticity (Buonomano, Bramen, & Khodadadifar, 2009). Subjective duration is thus an emergent property (or processed at a later stage) stemming from modality-related processes in the brain (van Wassenhove, 2009). One of the most prominent recent neural models is the striatal beat-frequency model, which assumes coincidence detection mechanisms involving oscillatory signals with various frequencies in cortico-striatal circuits (Matell & Meck, 2004). Phases of different cortical oscillators are read out by neurons located in the striatum and give rise to a unique activation pattern over time that distinguishes different durations. Neural oscillations of various frequencies have been shown to be associated with mechanisms, such as coincidence detection (neural phase timing), as well as related to different cognitive functions, including interval timing: the synchronous timing of events and temporal expectation (van Wassenhove, 2016). Therefore, an oscillatory model favouring synchronization and coincidence detection seems a promising avenue for future research (Kononowicz & van Wassenhove, 2016). Although a specific model employing oscillatory mechanisms has not received unanimous empirical support, EEG data show the involvement of neural oscillations in time perception, at least with intervals of up to a few seconds' duration (Kononowicz & van Rijn, 2015).

The dopaminergic system plays a key role regarding the involvement of neurotransmitters in the perception of time. Many studies in animals and humans have shown that dopamine-receptor agonists and antagonists provoke a relative overestimation and underestimation of duration, respectively (Rammsayer, 2009; Coull, Cheng, & Meck, 2011). Complementing these findings, carriers of genotypic variants modulating D2 receptor density in the striatum were associated with duration-discrimination variability (but not accuracy) in a timing task with a stimulus duration of around 500 ms (Wiener, Lohoff, & Coslett, 2011). In contrast, duration-discrimination variability with visual stimuli lasting around two seconds was associated with a polymorphism related to an enzyme modulating synaptic dopaminergic metabolism in the prefrontal cortex. These outcomes clearly show how different durations are processed by different neural systems. Other transmitter systems also influence subjective time. One study using sub-second visual stimuli showed that resting-state GABA concentration correlated with timing accuracy in humans (Terhune et al., 2014). The neuromodulator oxytocin induces a subjective time dilation for happy female faces and a time compression for happy male faces in heterosexual male viewers (Colonnello, Domes, & Heinrichs, 2016), showing how transient physiological states influence duration estimates. Other studies have revealed the involvement of the serotonergic (5-HT) transmitter system in the estimation of longer time intervals. For example, intake of sub-threshold doses of psilocybin, a hallucinogenic substance and 5-HT 2A/1A receptor agonist, interfered with a duration-reproduction task with intervals up to 5 seconds (Wackermann et al., 2008). Even though participants did not notice any changes in their states of consciousness, duration reproduction was less accurate compared to a placebo condition. Gene polymorphisms associated with the serotonin system, but not the dopamine system, were associated with duration discrimination of intervals lasting between 3.2 and 6.4 seconds (Sysoeva, Tonevitsky, & Wackermann, 2010).

Complementing these findings on the duration-dependent involvement of transmitter systems, meta-analyses of neuroimaging data point to at least two distinct neural timing systems. A timing system for sub-second intervals is more strongly governed by subcortical systems in the brain, and a more cognitively controlled system of supra-second timing is more strongly related to cortical areas in the brain (Lewis & Miall, 2003; Wiener, Turkeltaub, & Coslett, 2010). Further neuroimaging evidence supports a dual system separating intervals below and above two seconds (Morillon, Kell, & Giraud, 2009). Several systems probably function in coordination with each other, and individual systems become dominant, depending on the time range involved (Petter et al., 2016). Almost all of these models of human time perception are based on empirical findings with intervals ranging from milliseconds to a few seconds. These time intervals are definitely important for the understanding of individual sensorimotor processing required when performing sports, playing music, driving a car, or even for our survival as *homo sapiens* in interpersonal communication and when hunting and gathering (Wittmann & Pöppel, 1999). Brain-based models of human time perception rarely encompass empirical data from longer time intervals in the multiple-second range. The few existing neuroimaging studies employing multiple-second intervals show that a multitude of areas in the brain are activated including the basal ganglia and several cortical areas (Hinton & Meck, 2004; Wittmann et al., 2010). Subjective time as an experience and as related to everyday decision-making is crucially dependent upon the perception of the passage of time and duration in the multiple-second range (Wittmann & Paulus, 2009). The feeling of boredom, when time drags on and duration expands, or of time pressure, when there does not seem to be enough time to finish something, are commonly encountered in everyday experience and strongly influence our decisions (Zakay, 2014). These perceptions of time are related to the feeling of time passing and most likely cannot be explained by mechanisms dealing with sensorimotor processes lasting between a fraction of a second and up to three seconds.

4.3 **Body time: Attention, affect, and interoception**

A considerable body of evidence indicates an intricate interplay between affective states and subjective time. Subjects overestimate the duration of emotionally arousing pictures or short audio files with emotional content presented from several hundred milliseconds to a few seconds (Droit-Volet, Brunot, & Niedenthal, 2004; Noulhiane et al., 2007; Wackermann et al., 2014). This relative overestimation of duration is typically explained by the above-mentioned cognitive model of prospective time perception, the pacemaker-accumulator model (Zakay & Block, 1997; Wearden, 2016). Accordingly, increased physiological arousal leads to a higher pacemaker rate which, in turn, leads to a larger accumulation of temporal units over a given time interval (Droit-Volet & Meck, 2007; Wittmann & Paulus, 2008). Temporal dilation effects of emotionally arousing stimuli seem to be related to the embodiment of emotions, at least when judging the duration of presented photos with emotional faces. Participants relatively overestimated the duration of presented faces when they were free to spontaneously imitate perceived emotions (Effron et al., 2006). When subjects had a pen in their mouths that prevented the mimicking of emotions, the duration of faces was judged to be relatively shorter. The effects of emotions on duration estimation are also observed with longer time intervals. In a retrospective duration-judgment task with three video clips lasting 45 seconds each, a fear-inducing horror video led to a relative overestimation compared to a serious documentary and a funny cartoon, the latter being estimated as having lasted the shortest time (Pollatos, Laubrock, & Wittmann, 2014). In other words, the highly arousing horror video elicited time dilation, whereas the cartoon was experienced as "time flies when you are having fun." These relative over- and underestimations were boosted when subjects were instructed to pay attention to their bodily reactions to the film clips. In a further condition, when subjects were instructed to focus on physical sensations (interoceptive focus), they over- and underestimated the two emotional films even more strongly compared to the neutral documentary.

The notion that feelings and emotions depend on visceral and somatosensory feedback from the peripheral nervous system goes back at least to the theories of James and Lange in the late nineteenth century. Related modern theories postulate that body signals are integrated with perceptual, motivational, social, and cognitive information, leading to the awareness of complex emotional states (Damasio, 1999; Singer, Critchley, & Preuschoff, 2009). For example, one empirical study showed how those individuals who were more sensitive in perceiving their heartbeat also felt more aroused while judging photos with emotional content (Pollatos et al., 2007). The timing of the heartbeat is decisive for generating affective experience. It was shown that fearful faces were detected more accurately and were judged as more arousing when photos were presented at the cardiac systole compared to when they were presented at the diastole. This behavior and experience corresponded with fMRI-recorded higher amygdala responses (Garfinkel et al., 2014). Conscious emotional experiences are directly felt in the body, and people can draw emotion-specific activation maps of physical sensations (Nummenmaa et al., 2014). It is argued that perception of these emotion-triggered and topologically specific body changes generates consciously felt emotions.

A direct link between the perception of time and physical processes was proposed by Craig (2009, 2015). Craig suggested that the experience of time is related to emotional and visceral processes because they share a common underlying neural system, the interoceptive system, including the insular cortex. Through integrating the ascending somatic signals, the insula would be involved in creating a series of conscious emotional moments in time. As a consequence, the sense of duration would be created by these successive moments of self-realization, essentially formed by information originating within the body. In this context, it is important to note that the underlying computational cognitive architecture regarding discrete or continuous processing over time is still debated (Madl et al., 2016). The aforementioned phenomenological insight of the dual embodiment of self and time corresponds to a recent conceptualization of time-awareness in neuroscience (Wittmann, 2016). Thus, everyday experience becomes understandable. In situations such as when waiting, where one easily gets frustrated, one attends to time and is comparably aroused, one is strongly aware of his/her own emotional and body feelings, and, as a consequence, subjective duration expands. The insular cortex is an integral part of the saliency network involved in cognitive control and attentional processes (Menon & Uddin, 2010). The same brain network is also involved in the functions of body awareness, attentional control and the sense of time. In combining these three functions, one can argue that "attending to time" is equivalent to "attending to bodily signals." This at least is the strong hypothesis.

An fMRI study by Critchley, Wiens, Rotshtein, and Dolan (2004) was probably the first to link the insular cortex anatomy and activity, interoception, attention, and explicit timing abilities. Participants took part in an interoceptive task where they had to judge the timing of their own heartbeats in relation to a series of presented tones. Activation in the right anterior insula predicted accuracy in the heartbeat-detection task; that is, whether the tones were synchronous with the own heartbeat or not. Grey-matter volume in that specific region was also correlated with interoceptive timing accuracy, as well as with subjective ratings of heartbeat awareness. The striking novel information this influential research report provided is that the right anterior insula is involved in temporally fine-tuned conscious sensing of bodily processes. Empirical findings now identify the role of the insular cortex in temporally integrating the heartbeat with exteroceptive signals (Salomon et al., 2016). The awareness of visual stimuli depends on when they appear in relation to the heartbeat. When stimuli occur close to the heartbeat, detection of external stimuli is less accurate. More empirical research is now confirming the notion that visual conscious experience is dependent upon neural events locked to the heartbeats (Park et al., 2014). A recent line of research using fMRI technology and psychophysiological measurements complements these findings on the timing of sub-second events: insular-cortex activation and direct physiological responses, such as the heart rate and skin conductance levels, are also related to the estimation of duration in the multiple-second range (Wittmann et al., 2010; Meissner & Wittmann, 2011).

4.4 **Body time: Climbing activation**

The initial motivation to use longer time intervals in our research stems from an applied research agenda. Trait-like impulsivity, such as that found in many psychiatric disorders such as borderline personality disorder or drug dependence, is associated with an over-estimation of duration in the multiple-second to minute range (Berlin & Rolls, 2004; Wittmann et al., 2007). In accordance with our embodiment concept of subjective time, impulsivity can be understood as a strongly felt urge for immediate gratification, which is generated through the interoceptive system, including insular-cortex functioning (Turel & Bechara, 2016). To test individuals later with higher levels of impulsivity, we began to test healthy young students with a duration-reproduction task while recording activation via functional neuroimaging (fMRI) technology. The computerized duration-reproduction task became the standard experimental timing task for the following investigations reported here (for details on the methods used, see Wittmann et al., 2010, 2011; Wittmann & Meissner, 2011; Otten et al., 2015). In the duration-reproduction task, participants were instructed to reproduce the duration of tones with intervals of 3, 9, and 18 seconds. In each trial a 1.2 kHz tone was presented for one of the three durations (encoding phase), followed by a variable pause after which a second, 2 kHz tone was presented. After the second tone had started (reproduction phase), subjects had to stop the tone by pressing a key when they estimated that the duration of the first tone had elapsed. Although subjects were requested not to count, to prevent any such tendency the participants had to complete a secondary working-memory task. At the beginning of each trial, four numbers between zero and nine were presented to be memorized. After the second tone had been switched off by the subject, one number appeared, and the subjects had to respond by pressing one of two buttons for "yes" and "no" whether the presented number was one of the four from the beginning of the trial.

In the first of two fMRI studies (Wittmann et al., 2010), several areas of activation in sub-cortical and cortical areas were detected for the contrasts between the encoding and reproduction phases and, very similarly, for the two timing phases contrasted with a control reaction-time task. In the control task, subjects had to wait the same duration (3, 9, 18 seconds), but had to press a button as fast as possible at the end of the tone. Because we employed comparably long intervals, we were able to analyze activation patterns in the identified areas of activation over time. Time-activity curves showed an increasing (climbing) activation pattern over time in the left and right posterior insula during the

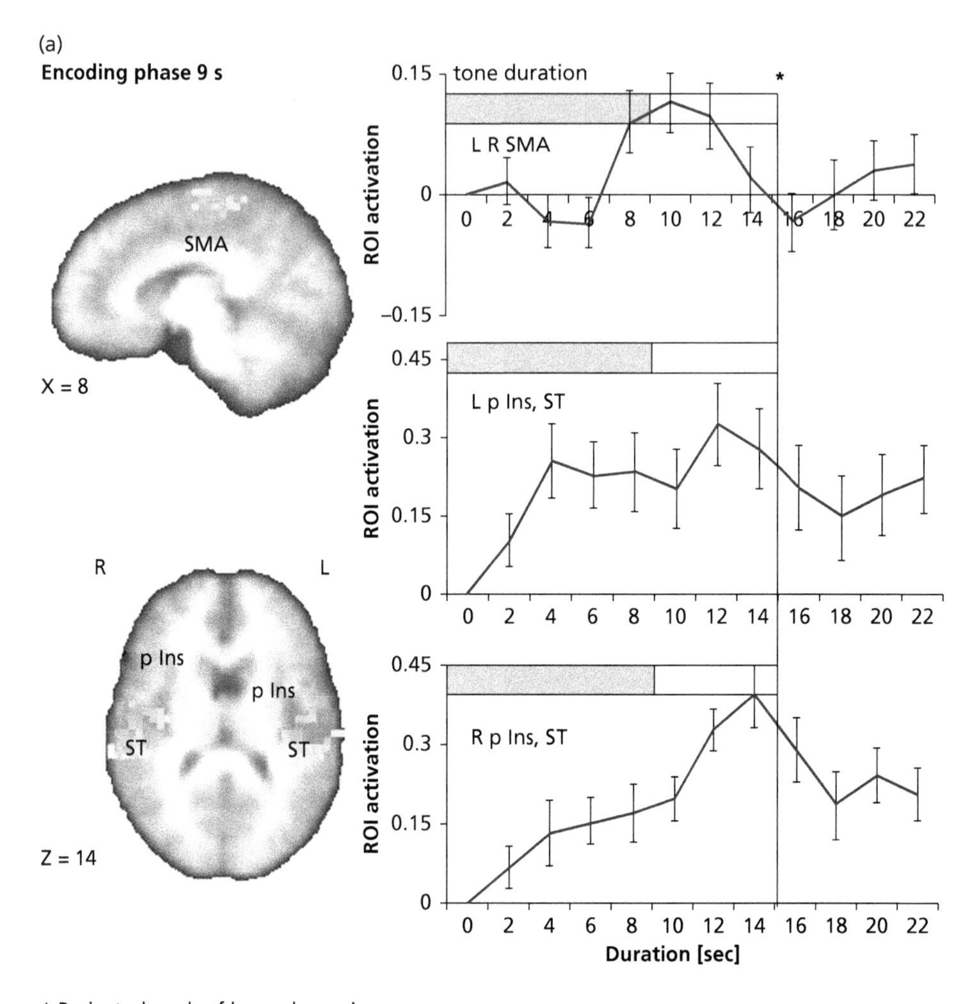

* Projected peak of hemodynamic response

Figure 4.1 Brain activity during the 9-s (4.1a) and 18-s (4.1b) encoding phase. A sagittal (x = 8) and an axial slice (z = 14) show significant brain activity ($p < 0.01$, corrected) in three regions encompassing a bilateral medial frontal area (SMA), left and right posterior insula (p Ins) as well as superior temporal cortex (ST) as related to the encoding versus control contrast in the 9- and 18-s conditions. Individual time activity curves (set to zero at the onset of the stimulus) show an inverted u-shape function in the SMA and climbing brain activity that peaks at the end of the stimulus (with a delay of around 6 s reflecting the hemodynamic response function) for left (L) and right (R) p Ins, ST.

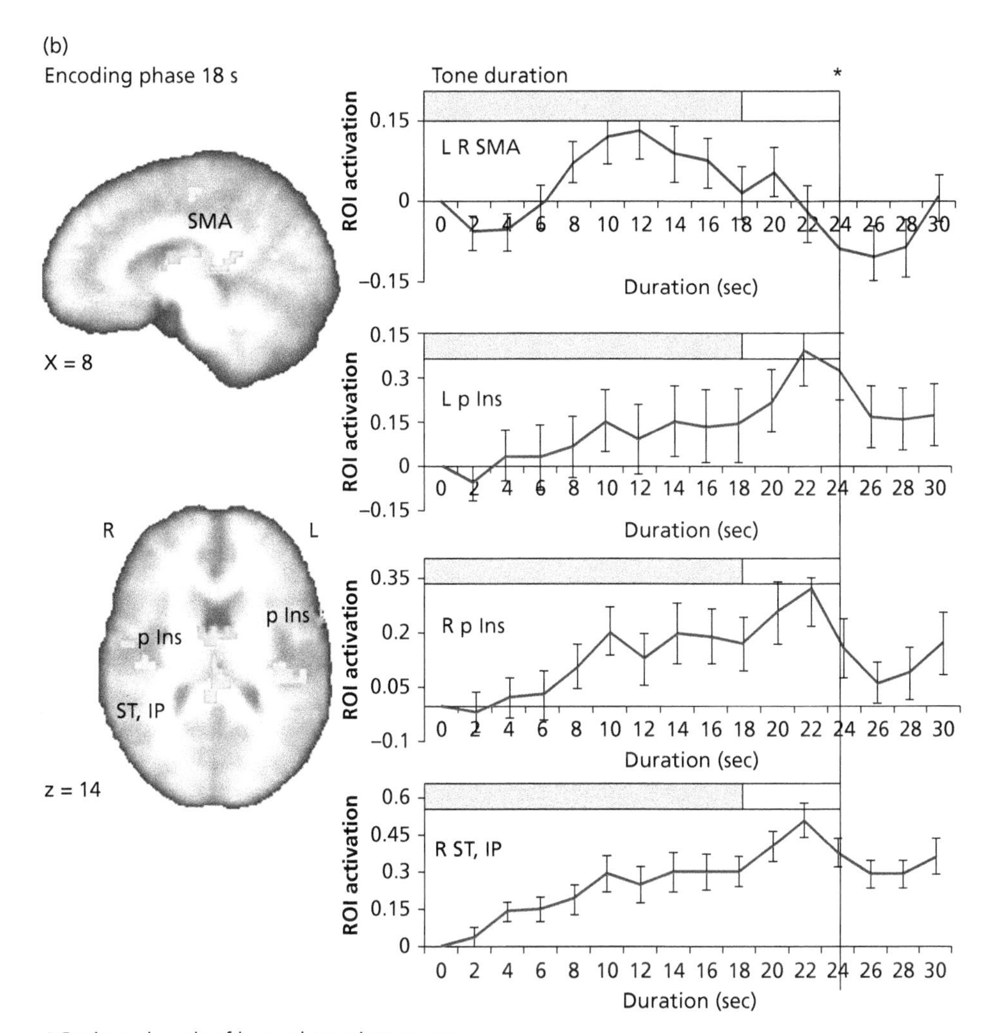

* Projected peak of hemodynamic response

Figure 4.1 Continued

encoding phase (Figure 4.1). Most notably, this region of activation encompassed the dorsal posterior insula, which is the primary interoceptive area (Craig, 2015). This neural signature was interpreted as being related to the accumulation of subjective duration. Time-activity curves in the reproduction phase revealed similar climbing activation which peaked shortly before the motor response in the left and right anterior insula, the inferior frontal cortex, and the pre-SMA. These results were interpreted as an indication that the anterior insula and related areas are involved in the comparison of the two presented intervals (encoding, reproduction phase). In a following fMRI study assessing time perception with students covering a range of self-reported impulsivity levels, we were able to replicate the main findings of time-activity curves in the posterior and anterior insula (Wittmann et al., 2011).

Following the fMRI results of insular cortex activation, we next investigated whether performance in the duration-reproduction task was related to individual interoceptive awareness and with measurable changes in autonomic activity during the task (Meissner & Wittmann, 2011). Healthy volunteers participated in two tasks: (a) the heartbeat-perception task conducted before the timing task as a measure of interoceptive sensitivity and (b) the auditory duration-reproduction task. Temporal intervals of 8-, 14- and 20-second duration were used while skin-conductance levels and cardiac and respiratory periods were recorded. First of all, a relationship was found between the accuracy in perceiving one's resting-state heartbeat and performance in the following timing task. The heartbeat-perception task was used as suggested originally by Schandry (1981). Subjects are asked to count their own heartbeats and report the number at the end of a designated interval. Participants who had higher interoceptive accuracy (they deviated less from the true number of heartbeats) performed more accurately (with less deviation) in the duration-reproduction task (for a discussion of different interoceptive dimensions, see Garfinkel et al., 2015). This indicated that a generally better access to visceral signals—ascending signals from the heart—enables a more accurate representation of duration. Regarding psychophysiological indices during the duration-reproduction task, cardiac periods increased (the heart rate slowed down) and skin-conductance levels decreased (a sign of relaxation) progressively and almost linearly during the encoding of the 8-, 14-, and 20-second intervals (Figure 4.2). These analyses point to a possible relationship between changes in physiological signals from the body and time-perception accuracy. It is important to emphasize that it is not the mean heart rate during a target interval that is predictive of timing behavior, as was assessed by Schwarz and colleagues (2013), but the changing (or increase) in cardiac periods over time.

The findings of linearly increasing cardiac periods and decreasing skin-conductance levels during the auditory duration-estimation task were replicated in a follow-up study where we compared the behavior of meditators to non-meditators (Otten et al., 2015). Moreover, these physiological changes over time were also observed during an additional visual duration-reproduction task. Results thus strongly support the modality independence of mechanisms. One finding from the initial study (Meissner & Wittmann, 2011) was not replicated: the heartbeat perception scores in the Schandry task (1981) were not associated with timing performance in the auditory and visual duration-estimation tasks. The accuracy index of interoception was, therefore, not predictive of time-perception accuracy in the following duration-reproduction tasks. A visible ceiling effect—individuals were overall better aware of their heartbeats than in the former study—could potentially explain the lack of replication. Methodological considerations also have to be discussed, such as the use of more objective psychophysiological tasks when assessing interoceptive accuracy (Garfinkel et al. 2015). One association with the interoception task used was that heartbeat-perception scores were positively related to correct answers in a divided-attention test (Otten et al., 2015). This result confirms a previously found correlation between the Schandry task and divided-attention performance, adding evidence for the embodiment conception of mental functioning (Matthias et al., 2009).

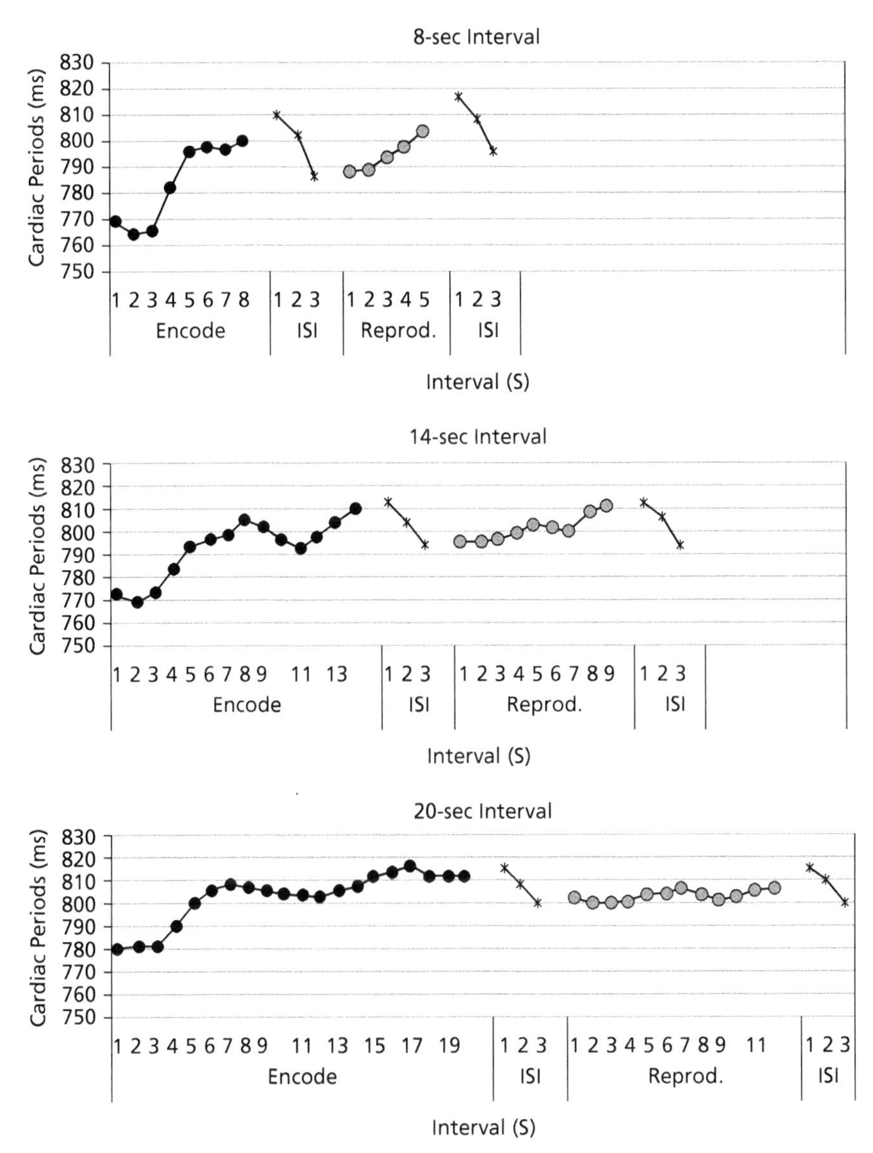

Figure 4.2 Mean second-to-second changes of cardiac periods (s) during the encoding interval, the reproduction interval, and the first 3 s of the subsequent inter-stimulus intervals (ISI) for tones of 8-s, 14-s, and 20-s duration. Due to individual differences in the length of the reproduced intervals, the reproduction intervals were restricted to the initial seconds that were available for all subjects, namely the first 5 s, 9 s, and 12 s of the 8-s, 14-s, and 20-s intervals, respectively.

Another potential component of the heartbeat related to time-estimation behavior has recently been proposed: heart rate variability as an indicator of vagal control was measured during a baseline resting period. Using different indices of heart rate variability, a positive correlation was found between duration-reproduction accuracy of multiple-second intervals and the root mean square of successive differences (RMSSD) of inter-beat intervals (Pollatos et al., 2014). A positive correlation was also reported between cardiac vagal tone (HF) and errors in a millisecond timing task: the greater the variability, the better the temporal judgment (Cellini et al., 2015). These results fit with the model of neuro-visceral integration, where a greater vagal tone (stronger parasympathetic activation) is associated with more efficient attentional regulation and response flexibility (Thayer & Brosschot, 2005). A higher general vagal tone as measured in the resting-state condition could thereby facilitate the allocation of attention involved in time perception and lead to more accurate duration judgment. However, these first study results have to be followed up by studies that clarify the role of autonomic cardiac regulation in relation to respiratory rate for performance in time perception tasks.

4.6 Applied research on embodied time

The upsurge of studies on meditation techniques is relevant for conceptual issues of the conscious self and subjective time. In mindfulness meditation, functional aspects of self-consciousness are modulated by specific processes during meditation induction, that is by increased attentional focus on body states and emotion regulation (Hölzel et al., 2011). An important aspect that is noticed by novices during a meditation session and by experienced individuals at least at the beginning of a session is that subjective time slows down considerably as the physical self becomes the focus of attention (Kabat-Zinn, 2005). This phenomenon is understandable within the conceptualization of insular cortex function underlying the subjective passage of time. fMRI studies show how the instruction to focus on "being in the present—here and now" and on breathing sensations results in an increase in neural activation in the insular cortex in experienced meditators (Farb et al., 2007, Farb, Segal, & Anderson, 2012).

An interoceptive view on subjective time might also be fruitful for an understanding of psychiatric and neurologic syndromes related to distorted notions of the physical and mental self, emotional states, and time perception (Hartocollis, 1983). Schizophrenia can even be seen as a disturbance of the embodied self (de Haan & Fuchs, 2010; Seth, 2013). Disturbances in time perception are reported by individual patients as the feeling of being "stuck in time" (Vogeley & Kupke, 2007; Giersch & Mishara, 2017). Collected reports show that for some of those patients, time is not passing and that the experienced presence feels expanded: "What is the future? One cannot reach it. . . Time stands still . . . This is boring, stretched time without an end." (Fischer, 1929). Recent experimental approaches show impairments in the consciously felt passage of time, as well as in implicit measures of time continuity (Giersch et al., 2009; Lalanne et al., 2012). Similar distortions can also be seen in individual patients with schizotypal disorders, such as the depersonalization syndrome, which are accompanied by depressive symptoms. These patients experience a detachment from their own bodies and, in case studies, exhibit disturbances in the subjective sense of time that are complemented by impairments in objective timing tasks (D'Allonnes, 1905; Zaytseva et al., 2015). These empirical findings correspond with the notion that the underlying self and time disturbances are related to disruptions in embodied perceptual experience.

The passage of time can also be studied in patients who suffer from physical symptoms. Wittmann and colleagues (2006) showed that patients with a life-threatening illness who had a lower health-related quality of life and higher anxiety levels reported time to pass more slowly. This finding suggests that the burden of symptoms slows down the passage of time. This corresponds with preliminary results from an experimental study in which nausea was experimentally induced by optokinetic stimulation: Participants with higher nausea levels at the end of the 20-minute nausea-stimulation period reported time to have passed more slowly than participants with lower nausea levels ($n = 69$, Spearman's rho = −0.31, $p < 0.01$) (Meissner et al., in preparation). Although the specific mediators of the association between symptom severity and the passage of time have yet to be identified, these findings indicate the close relationship between the affective bodily self and subjective time.

To sum up our analysis of the literature, a variety of time-perception models exist simultaneously. Recent research presented here has added the idea of an "embodiment of subjective time" implying the relationship between emotional physical states and the processing of time duration. The classification of human time perception into different time ranges indicates that different neural mechanisms are involved, depending on the length of the processed time interval. To find consensus on this issue, research on the neural basis of time perception has to test more systematically for duration-dependent effects by expanding the range of tested intervals within one study.

References

Berlin, H. A. and **Rolls, E. T.** (2004). Time perception, impulsivity, emotionality, and personality in self-harming borderline personality disorder patients. *Journal of Personality Disorders, 18*, 358–78.

Bueti, D. and **Walsh, V.** (2009). The parietal cortex and the representation of time, space, number and other magnitudes. *Philosophical Transactions of the Royal Society B, 364*, 1831–40.

Buhusi, C. V. and **Meck, W. H.** (2005). What makes us tick? Functional and neural mechanisms of interval timing. *Nature Reviews Neuroscience, 6*, 755–65.

Buonomano, D. V., Bramen, J., and **Khodadadifar, M.** (2009). Influence of the interstimulus interval on temporal processing and learning: Testing the state-dependent network model. *Philosophical Transactions of the Royal Society B, 364*(1525), 1865–73.

Cellini, N., Mioni, G., Levorato, I., Grondin, S., Stablum, F., and **Sarlo, M.** (2015). Heart rate variability helps tracking time more accurately. *Brain and Cognition, 101*, 57–63.

Colonnello, V., Domes, G., and **Heinrichs, M.** (2016). As time goes by: Oxytocin influences the subjective perception of time in a social context. *Psychoneuroendocrinology, 68*, 69–73.

Coull, J. T., Cheng, R.-K., and **Meck W. H.** (2011). Neuroanatomical and neurochemical substrates of timing. *Neuropsychopharmacology Review, 36*, 3–25.

Craig, A. D. (2009). Emotional moments across time: A possible neural basis for time perception in the anterior insula. *Philosophical Transactions of the Royal Society B*, **364**, 1933–42.

Craig, A. D. (2015). *How Do You Feel? An Interoceptive Moment with your Neurobiological Self.* Princeton, NJ: Princeton University Press.

Critchley, H. D., Wiens, S., Rotshtein, P., and **Dolan, R. J.** (2004). Neural systems supporting interoceptive awareness. *Nature Neuroscience, 7*, 189–95.

Damasio, A. (1999). *The feeling of What Happens: Body and Emotion in the Making of Consciousness.* San Diego, CA: Harcourt Inc.

D'Allonnes, G.-R. (1905). Rôle des sensations internes dans les émotions et dans la perception de la durée. *Revue Philosophique de la France et de l'Étranger, 60*, 592–623.

de Haan, S. and **Fuchs, T.** (2010). The ghost in the machine: Disembodiment in schizophrenia—two case studies. *Psychopathology, 43*, 327–33.

Droit-Volet, S., Brunot, S., and **Niedenthal, P. M.** (2004). Perception of the duration of emotional events. *Cognition and Emotion, 18*, 849–58.

Droit-Volet, S. and **Meck, W. H.** (2007). How emotions colour our perception of time. *Trends in Cognitive Sciences, 11*, 504–13.

Eagleman, D. and **Pariyadath, V.** (2009). Is subjective duration a signature for coding efficiency? *Philosophical Transactions of the Royal Society B, 364*, 1841–52.

Effron, D. A., Niedenthal, P. M., Gil, S., and **Droit-Volet, S.** (2006). Embodied temporal perception of emotion. *Emotion, 6*, 1–9.

Farb, N. A., Segal, Z. V., Mayberg, H., Bean, J., McKeon, D., Fatima, Z., et al. (2007). Attending to the present: Mindfulness meditation reveals distinct neural modes of self- reference. *Social Cognitive and Affective Neuroscience, 2*, 313–22.

Farb, N. A., Segal, Z. V., and **Anderson, A. K.** (2012). Mindfulness meditation training alters cortical representations of interoceptive attention. *Social Cognitive and Affective Neuroscience, 8*, 15–26.

Fischer, F. (1929). Zeitstruktur und Schizophrenie. *Zeitschrift für die gesamte Neurologie und Psychiatrie, 121*, 544–74.

Garfinkel, S. N., Minati, L., Gray, M. A., Seth, A. K., Dolan, R. J., and **Critchley, H. D.** (2014). Fear from the heart: Sensitivity to fear stimuli depends on individual heartbeats. *Journal of Neuroscience, 34*, 6573–82.

Garfinkel, S. N., Seth, A. K., Barrett, A. B., Suzuki, K., and **Critchley, H. D.** (2015). Knowing your own heart: Distinguishing interoceptive accuracy from interoceptive awareness. *Biological Psychology, 104*, 65–74.

Gibbon, J., Church, R. M., and **Meck, W. H.** (1984). Scalar timing in memory. In J. Gibbon and L. Allan (eds), *Annals of the New York Academy of Sciences: Vol. 423. Timing and Time Perception*. New York, NY: New York Academy of Sciences, pp. 52–77.

Giersch, A., Lalanne, L., Corves, C., Seubert, J., Shi, Z., Foucher, J., et al. (2009). Extended visual simultaneity thresholds in patients with schizophrenia. *Schizophrenia Bulletin, 35*, 816–25.

Giersch, A. and **Mishara, A.** (2017). Disrupted continuity of subjective time in the milliseconds range in the self-disturbances of schizophrenia: Convergence of experimental, phenomenological, and predictive coding accounts. *Journal of Consciousness Studies, 24*, 62–87.

Hartocollis, P. (1983). *Time and Timelessness, Or, The Varieties of Temporal Experience (A Psychoanalytic Inquiry)*. New York, NY: International Universities Press.

Hinton, S. C. and **Meck, W. H.** (2004). Frontal–striatal circuitry activated by human peak-interval timing in the supra-seconds range. *Cognitive Brain Research, 21*, 171–82.

Hölzel, B. K., Lazar, S. W., Gard, T., Schuman-Olivier, Z., Vago, D. R., and **Ott, U.** (2011). How does mindfulness work? Proposing mechanisms of action from a conceptual and neural perspective. *Perspectives on Psychological Science, 6*, 537–59.

Husserl, E. (1928). *Vorlesungen zur Phänomenologie des inneren Zeitbewußtseins.* Halle: Max Niemeyer Verlag.

Ivry, R. B., Spencer, R. M., Zelaznik, H. N., and **Diedrichsen, J.** (2002). The cerebellum and event timing. *Annals of the New York Academy of Sciences, 978,* 302–17.

James, W. (1890). *The Principles of Psychology.* London: MacMillan.

Kabat-Zinn, J. (2005). *Coming to Our Senses.* New York, NY: Hyperion.

Kiverstein, J. (2009). The minimal sense of self, temporality and the brain. *Psyche, 15,* 59–74.

Kononowicz, T.W. and **van Rijn, H.** (2015). Single trial beta oscillations index time estimation. *Neuropsychologia, 75,* 381–9.

Kononowicz, T.W. and **van Wassenhove, V.** (2016). In search of oscillatory traces of the internal clock. *Frontiers in Psychology, 7*(224), 1–5.

Lalanne, L., van Assche, M., Wang, W., and **Giersch, A.** (2012). Looking forward: An impaired ability in patients with schizophrenia? *Neuropsychologia, 50,* 2736–44.

Lewis, P. A. and **Miall, R. C.** (2003). Distinct systems for automatic and cognitively controlled time measurement: Evidence from neuroimaging. *Current Opinion in Neurobiology, 13,* 250–5.

Lloyd, D. (2012). Neural correlates of temporality: Default mode variability and temporal awareness. *Consciousness and Cognition, 21,* 695–703.

Mach, E. (1911). *Die Analyse der Empfindungen und das Verhältnis des Physischen zum Psychischen.* Jena: Verlag von Gustav Fischer.

Madl, T., Franklin, S., Snaider, J., and **Faghihi, U.** (2016). Continuity and the flow of time: A cognitive science perspective. In: B. Mölder, V. Arstila, and P. Øhrstrøm (eds), *Philosophy and Psychology of Time.* Cham: Springer International Publishing, pp. 135–60.

Marchetti, G. (2009). Studies on time: A proposal on how to get out of circularity. *Cognitive Processes, 10,* 7–40.

Matell, M. S. and **Meck, W. H.** (2004). Cortico-striatal circuits and interval timing: Coincidence detection of oscillatory processes. *Cognitive Brain Research, 21,* 139–70.

Matthias, E., Schandry, R., Duschek, S., and **Pollatos, O.** (2009). On the relationship between interoceptive awareness and the attentional processing of visual stimuli. *International Journal of Psychophysiology, 72,* 154–9.

Meissner, K. and **Wittmann, M.** (2011). Body signals, cardiac awareness, and the perception of time. *Biological Psychology, 86,* 289–97.

Menon, V. and **Uddin, L.Q.** (2010). Saliency, switching, attention and control: A network model of insula function. *Brain Structure and Function, 214,* 655–67.

Merleau-Ponty, M. (1945). *Phénoménologie de la perception.* Paris: La Librairie Gallimard.

Metzinger, T. (2004). *Being No One. The Self-Model Theory of Subjectivity.* Cambridge MA: MIT Press.

Metzinger, T. (2008). Empirical perspectives from the self-model theory of subjectivity: A brief summary with examples. In: R. Banerjee and B. K. Chakrabarti (eds), *Progress in Brain Research, 168.* Amsterdam: Elsevier, pp. 215–45.

Morillon, B., Kell, C. A., and **Giraud, A. L.** (2009). Three stages and four neural systems in time estimation. *Journal of Neuroscience, 29,* 14803–11.

Nagel, T. (1974). What it is like to be a bat? *The Philosophical Review, 83,* 435–50.

Northoff, G. (2016). Slow cortical potentials and "inner time consciousness"—A neuro-phenomenal hypothesis about the "width of present". *International Journal of Psychophysiology, 103,* 174–84.

Noulhiane, M., Mella, N., Samson, S., Ragot, R., and **Pouthas, V.** (2007). How emotional auditory stimuli modulate time perception. *Emotion, 7,* 697–704.

Nummenmaa, L., Glerean, E., Hari, R., and **Hietanen, J.K.** (2014) Bodily maps of emotions. *Proceedings of the National Academy of Sciences of the USA, 111,* 646–51.

Otten, S., Schötz, E., Wittmann, M., Kohls, N., Schmidt, S., and **Meissner, K.** (2015). Psychophysiology of duration estimation in experienced mindfulness meditators and matched controls. *Frontiers in Psychology, 6,* 1215.

Park, H. D., Correia, S., Ducorps, A., and **Tallon-Baudry, C.** (2014). Spontaneous fluctuations in neural responses to heartbeats predict visual detection. *Nature Neuroscience, 17,* 612–18.

Petter, E. A., Lusk, N. A., Hesslow, G., and **Meck, W. H.** (2016). Interactive roles of the cerebellum and striatum in sub-second and supra-second timing: Support for an initiation, continuation, adjustment, and termination (ICAT) model of temporal processing. *Neuroscience & Biobehavioral Reviews, 71,* 739–55.

Pöppel, E. (1997). A hierarchical model of temporal perception. *Trends in Cognitive Sciences, 1,* 56–61.

Pollatos, O., Herbert, B. M., Matthias, E., and **Schandry, R.** (2007). Heart rate response after emotional picture presentation is modulated by interoceptive awareness. *International Journal of Psychophysiology, 63,* 117–24.

Pollatos, O., Laubrock, J., and **Wittmann, M.** (2014). Interoceptive focus shapes the experience of time. *PloS One, 9,* e86934.

Pollatos, O., Yeldesbay, A., Pikovsky, A., and **Rosenblum, M.** (2014). How much time has passed? Ask your heart. *Frontiers in Neurorobotics, 8,* 15.

Rammsayer, T. (2009). Effects of pharmacological induced dopamine-receptor stimulation on human temporal information processing. *NeuroQuantology, 7,* 103–13.

Revonsuo, A. (2006). *Inner Presence. Consciousness as a Biological Phenomenon.* Cambridge, MA: MIT Press.

Salomon, R., Ronchi, R., Dönz, **J., Bello-Ruiz, J., Herbelin, B., Martet, R.,** et al. (2016). The insula mediates access to awareness of visual stimuli presented synchronously to the heartbeat. *Journal of Neuroscience, 36,* 5115–27.

Schandry, R. (1981). Heart beat perception and emotional experience. *Psychophysiology, 18,* 483–8.

Schwarz, M. A., Winkler, I., and **Sedlmeier, P.** (2013). The heart beat does not make us tick: The impacts of heart rate and arousal on time perception. *Attention, Perception & Psychophysics, 75,* 182–93.

Seth, A. K. (2013). Interoceptive inference, emotion, and the embodied self. *Trends in Cognitive Sciences, 17,* 565–73.

Singer, T., Critchley, H. D., and **Preuschoff, K.** (2009). A common role of insula in feelings, empathy and uncertainty. *Trends in Cognitive Sciences, 13,* 334–40.

Staddon, J. E. R. (2005). Interval timing: Memory, not a clock. *Trends in Cognitive Sciences, 9,* 312–14.

Sysoeva, O. V., Tonevitsky, A., and **Wackermann, J.** (2010). Genetic determinants of time perception mediated by the serotonergic system. *PLoS One 5,* e12650.

Thayer, J. F. and **Brosschot, J. F.** (2005). Psychosomatics and psychopathology: Looking up and down from the brain. *Psychoneuroendocrinology, 30,* 1050–8.

Terhune, D. B., Russo, S., Near, J., Stagg, C. J., and **Kadosh, R. C.** (2014). GABA predicts time perception. *Journal of Neuroscience, 34,* 4364–70.

Treisman, M. (2013). The information-processing model of timing (Treisman, 1963): Its sources and further development. *Timing & Time Perception, 1,* 131–58.

Turel, O. and **Bechara, A.** (2016) A triadic reflective-impulsive-interoceptive awareness model of general and impulsive information system use: Behavioral tests of neuro-cognitive theory. *Frontiers in Psychology, 7,* 601.

van Wassenhove, V. (2009). Minding time in an amodal representational space. Philosophical *Transactions of the Royal Society of London B,* **364**, 1815–30.

Wittmann, M., Vollmer, T., Schweiger, C., and **Hiddemann, W.** (2006). The relation between the experience of time and psychological distress in patients with hematological malignancies. *Palliative & Supportive Care, 4,* 357–63.

van Wassenhove, V. (2016). Temporal cognition and neural oscillations. *Current Opinion in Behavioral Sciences, 8*, 124–30.

Varela, F. J., Thompson, E., and **Rosch, E.** (1991/2016). *The Embodied Mind: Cognitive Science and Human Experience*. Cambridge, MA: MIT Press.

Varela, F. J. (1999). Present-time consciousness. *Journal of Consciousness Studies, 6*, 111–40.

Vogeley, K. and **Kupke, C.** (2007). Disturbances of time consciousness from a phenomenological and a neuroscientific perspective. *Schizophrenia Bulletin, 33*, 157–65.

Wackermann, J. and **Ehm, W.** (2006). The dual klepsydra model of internal time representation and time reproduction. *Journal of Theoretical Biology, 239*, 482–93.

Wackermann, J., Wittmann, M., Hasler, F., and **Vollenweider, F. X.** (2008). Effects of varied doses of psilocybin on time interval reproduction in human subjects. *Neuroscience Letters, 435*, 51–5.

Wackermann, J., Meissner, K., Tankersley, D., and **Wittmann, M.** (2014). Effects of emotional valence and arousal on acoustic duration reproduction assessed via the "dual klepsydra model". *Frontiers in Neurorobotics, 8*, 11.

Wearden, J. (2016). *Psychology of Time Perception*. London: Palgrave Macmillan.

Wiener, M., Turkeltaub, P., and **Coslett, H. B.** (2010). The image of time: A voxel-wise meta-analysis. *NeuroImage, 49*, 1728–40.

Wiener, M., Lohoff, F. W., and **Coslett, H. B.** (2011). Double dissociation of dopamine genes and timing in humans. *Journal of Cognitive Neuroscience, 23*, 2811–21.

Wittmann, M. and **Pöppel, E.** (1999). Temporal mechanisms of the brain as fundamentals of communication—with special reference to music perception and performance. *Musicae Scientiae, 3* (Suppl.), 13–28.

Wittmann, M., Leland, D. S., Churan, J., and **Paulus, M. P.** (2007). Impaired time perception and motor timing in stimulant-dependent subjects. *Drug and Alcohol Dependence, 90*, 183–192.

Wittmann, M. and **Paulus, M. P.** (2008). Decision making, impulsivity and time perception. *Trends in Cognitive Sciences, 12*, 7–12.

Wittmann, M. and **Paulus, M. P.** (2009). Temporal horizons in decision making. *Journal of Neuroscience, Psychology, and Economics, 2*, 1–11.

Wittmann, M. and **van Wassenhove, V.** (2009). The experience of time: Neural mechanisms and the interplay of emotion, cognition and embodiment. *Philosophical Transactions of the Royal Society B, 364*, 1809–13.

Wittmann, M., Simmons, A. N., Aron, J. L., and **Paulus, M. P.** (2010). Accumulation of neural activity in the posterior insula encodes the passage of time. *Neuropsychologia, 48*, 3110–20.

Wittmann, M., Simmons, A. N., Flagan, T., Lane, S. D., Wackermann, J., and **Paulus, M. P.** (2011). Neural substrates of time perception and impulsivity. *Brain Research, 1406*, 43–58.

Wittmann, M. (2016). *Felt Time. The Science of How We Experience Time*. Cambridge MA: MIT Press.

Zahavi, D. (2005). *Subjectivity and Selfhood: Investigating the First-Person Perspective*. Cambridge, MA: MIT Press.

Zakay, D. and **Block, R. A.** (1997). Temporal cognition. *Current Directions in Psychological Science*, 6(1), 12–16.

Zakay, D. (2014). Psychological time as information: The case of boredom. *Frontiers in Psychology*, 5, 917.

Zaytseva, Y., Szymanski, C., Gutyrchik, E., Pechenkova, E., Vlasova, R., and **Wittmann, M.** (2015). A disembodied man: A case of somatopsychic depersonalization in schizotypal disorder. *PsyCh Journal*, 4, 186–98.

Chapter 5

The neurobiology of gut feelings

Qasim Aziz and James K. Ruffle

5.1 Introduction

Interoception is defined as a "sensitivity to stimuli arising inside of the body," in contrast to exteroception which can be defined as a "sensitivity to stimuli arising outside of the body." There are a myriad of "gut feelings" which, taken together, form the construct of gastrointestinal (GI) interoception. The GI tract is the second most innervated bodily organ, second only to the brain, and specific modalities span from interoceptive awareness percepts including visceral sensation and pain signalling, hunger, or nausea, but also those outside of conscious perception including the interoceptive impact of sub-threshold sensory stimuli. These modalities are processed by means of neuroanatomical pathways ascending to the level of the brainstem, subcortical and cortical brain regions which may invoke a cognitive or bodily response. Additionally, humoral mechanisms play a critical role in visceral interoception, as does the autonomic nervous system (ANS). Moreover, these intricate signals are influenced by various individual factors, including core physiology such as gender or genetics and ANS tone, but also complex psyche components such as personality traits. In fact, some research suggests that the intestinal bacterial flora composition may even influence how we "feel."

Visceral interoceptive information reaches the brain through an array of neural, humoral, and immune pathways, amalgamating in an abundance of ascending signalling data which ensures homeostasis within the GI tract, many of which do not reach conscious awareness of interoceptive signals, for example in regulating GI motility and secretion. However, those that engender conscious perception include sensations of hunger, satiety, nausea, the urge to defecate, and, probably the most studied interoceptive signal in GI physiology, pain (Derbyshire, 2003).

To begin, the neuroanatomical pathways of sensory signalling in the GI tract will be described. Since the core emphasis in visceral interoception research has consisted of understanding the sensory spectrum of the gut, with a vast research body investigating pain, this therefore will form a key aspect in this chapter. When describing the neurobiology and neuroanatomy of visceral sensory signalling this chapter will, for clarity, use visceral pain as the sensory example. Additional conscious GI interoceptive signals will be discussed later throughout the chapter, including that of hunger and nausea. Sequentially, the humoral pathways underpinning the neurobiology of gut feelings will be described, including the brain–gut axis, and tie in how inter-individual factors hold an influential role in the regulation of these interoceptive signals.

5.2 Interoceptive signalling pathways

5.2.1 Ascending sensory pathways of visceral pain

Following a visceral insult that would instigate pain, nociceptive GI afferents localized in the visceral tissue are activated. The ascending neural pathways from the GI tract are encompassed in two main afferent routes: (a) the spinal pathway and (b) the tenth cranial nerve (CNX), the vagus nerve (Coen, Hobson, & Aziz, 2012). These two afferent types converge at multiple supra-spinal levels, with the vagus projecting to the nucleus tractus solitarii (NTS), a group of brainstem nuclei that receives numerous inputs including that originating from baroreceptors, GI and pulmonary afferents (Altschuler et al., 1989). For lamina I neurons, these relay principally to the parabrachial nucleus, before subsequently ascending to higher centers, whilst spinothalamic tract fibers may project directly to thalamic regions (Craig, 2003).

Both spinal and vagal afferents also indirectly project to subcortical and cortical areas, including the thalamus (ventral posterior lateral, medial dorsal, and ventral medial posterior nuclei), insula, amygdala, prefrontal cortex (PFC), primary somatosensory cortex (SI), secondary somatosensory cortex (SII), and the anterior cingulate cortex (ACC). By large these regions are thought to exhibit a degree of "viscerotopic" organization, meaning that specific anatomical parts of the nuclei correspond to different visceral components (Altschuler et al., 1989; Aziz et al., 2000). That being said, some exceptions do exist, with the ventral posterior lateral aspect of the thalamus as an example of a region that does not display viscerotopic organization (Coen et al., 2012). Overall, by these elaborate nuclei interconnections, a visceral sensory "neuromatrix" exists both for innocuous and nociceptive (painful) stimuli (Melzack & Wall, 1965).

5.2.2 Humoral signalling

In addition to the vagal and spinal homeostatic afferent pathways, an intricate humoral pathway also aids in homeostatic regulation of visceral interoceptive signalling, reaching the central nervous system by circulating substances. There are at least three disparate humoral pathways permitting information transfer. First, the ventricular humoral pathway (also known as the classical pathway) detects changes in substances at the level of the third and fourth ventricle, engaging the adjacent circumventricular organs including the area postrema, organum vasculosum of lamina terminalis, and subfornical organ (Figure 5.1) (Ceunen, Vlaeyen, & Van Diest, 2016). In turn, processed humoral information projects to the NTS, hypothalamus, PB nucleus, dorsal motor nucleus, nucleus ambiguous, insula, ACC, sympathetic medullary nuclei, and midline thalamic regions.

Second, the blood–brain humoral pathway (also known as the non-classical pathway) detects changes in substances passing the blood–brain barrier. This pathway, which invokes processing at the NTS, hypothalamus, amygdala, and monoamine systems, aims

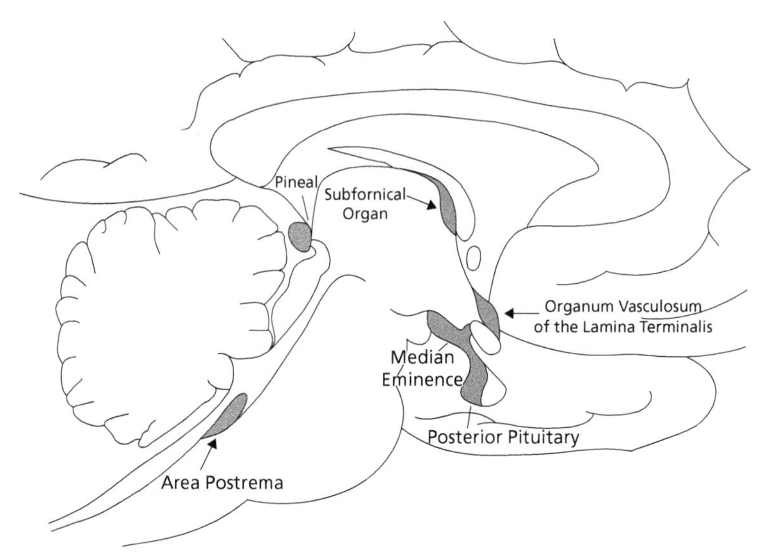

Figure 5.1 Location of circumventricular organs in the rat brain. AP = area postrema, ME = median eminence, OVLT = organum vasculosum of the lamina terminalis, P = pineal gland, PP = posterior pituitary, SFO = subfornical organ. (Lechan & Toni, 2016).

to influence information relay between insula, cingulate cortices, and ventral striatum. Third, the microglial humoral pathway (also known as the extraneuronal pathway) refers to the response engendered by residing microglia within circumventricular organs, leptomeninges, and choroid plexus in the presence of both pathogen and/or inflammation.

There exists a complex intercommunication between interoceptive signalling modalities. Whilst for comprehensibility academic literature will describe neural, humoral, and indeed immune interoceptive signalling mechanisms in a reductionist and disparate fashion, there exists significant interconnection and influence from one modality to the next, which convolutes further with the influence of inter-individual variability. As an example highlighted by (Browning & Travagli, 2011), the visceral feeling state of dyspepsia can be influenced by both psychological factors such as stress but also food indigestion. With both stress and indigestion, glucagon-like peptide 1 (GLP-1), cholecystokinin (CCK), and corticotrophin releasing factor (CRF) are released, which cause increase in cyclic AMP levels at brainstem regions. By these humoral factors increasing a localized increase in cAMP at vago-vagal neurocircuitry, the dampening effect of GABAergic synapses is decreased. Therefore, signals from normally innoxious events such as meal ingestion are processed inappropriately and gastric function disrupted (Browning & Travagli, 2011; Tack, Bisschops, & Sarnelli, 2004).

5.3 The "brain–gut axis"

The "brain–gut axis" refers to the bi-directional signalling processes between the brain and the gut (Aziz and Thompson, 1998). Although physiological axes such as the "hypothalamic pituitary axis" (HPA) have been historically described for some time, the construct of physiological data transfer between the brain and the gut has become a rapidly developing area of interoceptive research particularly in the last few decades (Aziz and Thompson, 1998). A variety of research disciplines, albeit with a particular emphasis on functional neuroimaging, have provided a wealth of evidence to support the proposal of a brain–gut axis such that it has become an adopted term and central component to contemporaneous research in visceral sensation (Omran and Aziz, 2014). By large, a "visceral sensory neuromatrix" has been largely determined, including not only aforementioned sensory neural components but also the autonomic nervous system (ANS), neuroendocrine HPA, and neuroimmune systems (Van Oudenhove, Coen, & Aziz, 2007).

The brain–gut axis has served as an answer to the proposal that an intricate communication system between the GI tract and the brain *must* exist in order to permit interoception, but also to regulate GI function by means of brain to gut signalling. In addition, the physiological, anatomical, and psychological factors that influence this bi-directional signalling pathway have become an intriguing area of brain–gut axis research, not least about how its function may be perturbed in various disorders, a poignant example being irritable bowel syndrome (IBS) (Farmer & Ruffle, 2015).

5.4 The autonomic nervous system

The autonomic nervous system (ANS) is a key aspect of the bi-directional nature of the brain–gut axis. Comprised of two largely opposing arms, the sympathetic (SNS) and parasympathetic nervous system (PNS), its function is to integrate changes in the external environment with the internal self so as to maintain homeostasis. The functions of the ANS are numerous and essential throughout the body, including regulation of metabolism and critical components of the cardiorespiratory system. Importantly, it also plays a key role in visceral interoception, including pain processing via the vagal nerve, the main branch of the PNS (Ruffle et al., 2018; Ruffle et al., 2017a). Whilst the vagal nerve is largely comprised of afferent fibers, the efferent arm is posited to have a key role in modulation of visceral nociceptive signals (Botha et al., 2015), GI motility (Frokjaer et al., 2016), cardiorespiratory regulation, and inflammation (Bonaz et al., 2013).

5.5 Brain processing of gastrointestinal sensory signalling

5.5.1 Visceral pain processing

Although research in visceral sensory representation in the brain is continually evolving, the brain regions arguably best implicated thus far in pain processing are those of the SI, SII, cingulate cortex, insula, PFC, thalamus, and amygdala (Aziz et al., 1997; Coen et al., 2007; Derbyshire, 2003; Van Oudenhove et al., 2007). These regions have been elucidated by means of stimulation of multiple visceral sites including the esophagus, stomach, and rectum, but also varying stimulation methods such as mechanical, electrical, or acid-induced stimulation.

Neuroanatomical and behavioral studies suggest that pain processing in the brain is divided into medial and lateral pain systems. The somatosensory cortices, SI and SII, act to encode the intensity and localization of the painful stimulus, referred to as the "lateral pain system" (Aziz et al., 2000; Van Oudenhove et al., 2007). The multifaceted region of the cingulate, including the ACC and PFC, as well as interconnection to the anterior insula, amygdala, hippocampus, PAG, and brainstem, forms the "medial pain system," which plays an important role in in both the affective-motivational (experience of pain unpleasantness and related anxiety) and cognitive-evaluative (both anticipation of and attention to pain) (Gregory et al., 2003; Kulkarni et al., 2005).

The insula cortex holds a key role in interoception (Craig, 2002). Indeed, for visceral sensation, the right anterior insula has been regarded by some groups as the "interoceptive cortex," playing a key role in the awareness of the bodily self as a feeling entity (Craig, 2002). Although multimodal in its role, the insula is thought to have roles in processing the affective dimension of pain whereby it may integrate the experience of pain with emotional information (Ploner et al., 2011). The insula additionally has efferent outputs to other key brain regions including the amygdala, hypothalamus, and periaqueductal gray (PAG), which have additional roles in the processing of visceral pain (Carrive & Bandler, 1991; Gregory et al., 2003). The amygdala has an important role in the affective dimension of pain, and is regarded as the brain's "fear center" (Stein et al., 2007). Additionally, both the amygdala and PAG play key roles in the descending modulation of pain (Tracey et al., 2002).

The PFC is understood to aid in the cognitive influence on visceral pain (Apkarian et al., 2005). The PFC is a cluster of various sub-regions, of which the orbitofrontal cortex (OFC) processes visceral sensory information and encodes the affective, motivational, and hedonic aspects (Kringelbach, 2005). Furthermore, the OFC assists in the decisions pertaining to the autonomic and behavioral response to the stimulus, including the intricate interaction between cognition (e.g. anticipation to pain) and emotion to pain (Bantick et al., 2002). The dorsolateral PFC (dlPFC) is another important sub-region, which is involved in cognition, specifically the attention and anticipation of visceral pain (Aziz et al., 2000).

The thalamus is an important subcortical cluster of nuclei located in the center of the brain. Its many roles include pain processing. Specifically, it transfers information between cortical regions via the relay nuclei, but it also has projections to higher cortical regions. It is implicated in both pain sensation and the arousal response, yielding connectivity to the aforementioned insula cortex, SI, and PFC (Aziz et al., 1997; Craig et al., 1994). In the context of neuroimaging however, its activation is not *always* reported in the context of visceral pain, compared to somatosensory where it appears to be more consistently activated (Coen et al., 2012).

5.5.2 Brain networks in visceral sensation

Advances in functional neuroimaging over the last decade has permitted the ability to determine proposed brain networks for visceral sensory and pain processing (Labus et al.,

Table 5.1 Networks of visceral sensation

Homeostatic Afferent	Emotional Arousal	Cognitive-Modulatory
Thalamus	Amygdala	ACC
Insula	LC	Amygdala
OFC	ACC	Insula
Dorsal ACC		OFC

Three key networks for visceral sensation. Abbreviations: ACC, anterior cingulate cortex; LC, locus coeruleus; OFC, orbitofrontal cortex.

From Omran & Aziz, 2014

2008; Tillisch & Labus, 2011). These networks are determined by means of correlating brain activity during functional neuroimaging of a painful visceral stimulus, thus inferring the interaction or "networking" between several brain regions. At present, it has been suggested that three main brain networks may be key in the visceral pain matrix, as follows: (a) the homeostatic-afferent network, comprising the thalamus, insula, OFC, and dorsal ACC; (b) the emotional arousal network, comprising the amygdala, LC, and ACC sub-regions; and (c) the cortical-modulatory network, comprising the ACC, amygdala, insula, and medial aspect of the OFC (Table 5.1, Figure 5.2) (Labus et al., 2008; Stein et al., 2007; Tillisch & Labus, 2011).

The roles of these networks in processing a complex visceral interoceptive signal such as pain differ. The homeostatic-afferent network is understood to be responsible for the processing of the interoceptive physiological input via the PB nucleus, whilst the emotional arousal network is responsible for how the brain would interpret and perceive the stimulus (Pezawas et al., 2005; Tillisch & Labus, 2011). Lastly, the cortical-modulatory network aids in the modulation of the pain experience, tying in to the aforementioned process of descending analgesia (Coen et al., 2012).

5.6 Descending analgesia in visceral pain

A key mantra of the brain–gut axis is the bi-directionality of neural signalling. Signals transmit caudally from brain to gut, and one such example is that of "descending analgesia," a phenomenon that permits the brain to modulate the sensation of visceral pain (Melzack & Wall, 1965). Most central brain structures that receive a visceral sensory input, whether noxious or innocuous, additionally relay information caudally as a means to modulate the sensory transmission of visceral afferents, in particular to the dorsal horn of the spinal cord. One key region in descending analgesia is the ACC which, prior to further caudal transmission, projects to the amygdala and PAG which may allow both affective and cognitive factors to modulate the visceral pain experience (Dunckley et al., 2005; Tracey et al., 2002). The amygdala and PAG caudally project to the locus coeruleus (LC), and onwards to the dorsal horn of the spinal cord. It should be noted that the construct of descending analgesia is not specific to visceral pain but engenders

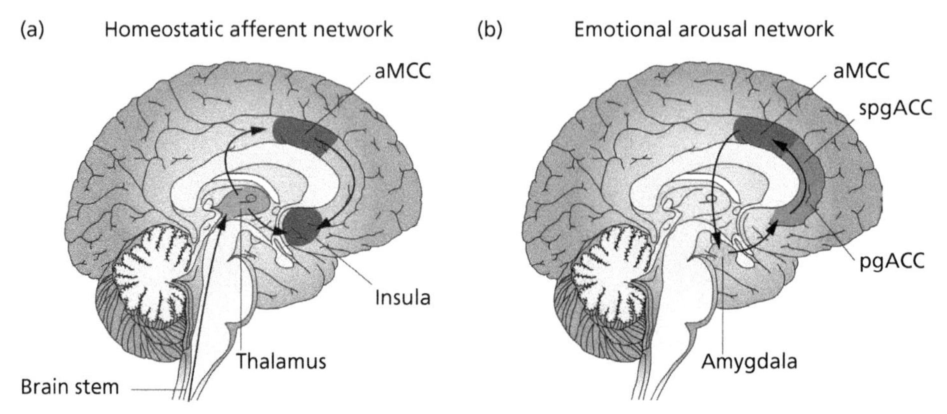

Figure 5.2 Networks of brain activation in visceral stimulation studies. (a) The homeostatic–afferent network encompasses areas that are thought to resemble those of pain when stimulated in visceral pain studies both in participants with a FGID and in participants who are otherwise healthy. The core regions are shown.(b) The emotional arousal network is depicted. Cognitive (e.g. expectation and anticipation), emotional (e.g. sadness), and psychological aspects have all been shown to be involved in visceral perceptions and this progress has established what is known as the "emotional arousal network." The central components of this network are the amygdala and parts of the ACC. Abbreviations: ACC, anterior cingulate cortex; aMCC, anterior midcingulate cortex; FGID, functional gastrointestinal disorder; pgACC, perigenual ACC; sgACC, subgenual ACC.

Reprinted by permission from *Nature Reviews Gastroenterology & Hepatology*, 11 (9), Functional brain imaging in gastroenterology: to new beginnings, Yasser Al Omran and Qasim Aziz, pp. 565–76, Figure 1, doi:10.1038/nrgastro.2014.89, Copyright © 2014, Springer Nature.

somatosensory nociception also, overall referred to famously as Melzack and Wall's pain "gate control theory" (see Melzack & Wall, 1965). Interestingly however, this has formed an important area of visceral pain research regarding how individual factors such as the psyche, including personality or anxiety, also influence descending analgesia (Farmer et al., 2014a; Farmer et al., 2013; Tracey, 2011). Such roles for individual factors will be further described later.

5.7 Additional interoceptive modalities

Visceral states include numerous modalities other than core sensory and pain pathways. These range from sensations under the umbrella of conscious interoceptive awareness, such as nausea and hunger, to far more complex visceral states such as anticipation of a visceral threat, or sub-threshold sensation to reach conscious awareness. These differing modalities will be discussed in the following sections.

5.7.1 Nausea

Nausea is a common and distressing symptom, often preceding vomiting. Numerous evidence has purported that the bi-directional interactions between brain–gut axis, in addition to both autonomic and endocrine systems (in particular arginine vasopressin, ghrelin, and cortisol), play important roles in the experience of nausea. Indeed, the sensory experience of nausea is often accompanied by numerous physiological changes, including pallor, sweating, and gastric dysrhythmia (Sanger & Andrews, 2006).

The neurobiology of nausea has been implicated the ANS, in particular the vagal pathway to cortical brain regions. Through mechanism similar to that of pain as described earlier, abdominal vagal afferent fibers reach the NTS and area postrema which are thought to play a major role in integrating both the emetic and nausea response. Our understanding of the neurobiology of nausea is further complicated by studies illustrating that abdominal vagal afferents are *not* essential for its sensation, given that humans with bilateral abdominal vagotomy can still experience nausea (Sanger & Andrews, 2006). It is important to note, however, the difference between emesis, the act of vomiting, and nausea, the physiological sense of feeling sick. Whilst the two often occur together, they are not equivalent. Because there are no clear animal models of nausea (whilst there are for emesis), the neurobiology of emesis has been clearly demonstrated, with a particular emphasis at the brainstem level, given that decerebrate animal models still can exhibit emetic behavior (Miller, Nonaka, & Jakus, 1994).

Functional neuroimaging studies suggest that "higher" cortical regions and the vestibular system are particularly important in the genesis of nausea. In a recent functional magnetic resonance imaging (fMRI) study, it has been shown that nausea (induced by visual stimulus) is associated with decreased plasma ghrelin and vasopressin, with increased ACC, inferior frontal, and middle occipital gyri activity (Farmer et al., 2015). Meanwhile, cerebellar areas showed decreased activity, including the declive nucleus and parahippocampal gyrus (Farmer et al., 2015).

5.7.2 Hunger

Hunger or appetite is an additional visceral interoceptive state. Comprising interconnections between behavior and core physiology, it has been purported that four main brain areas play key role in the control of appetitive behavior. These are as follows: (a) amygdala/hippocampus, (b) insula, (c) OFC, and (d) striatum, together formulating a complex interoceptive phenomena of learning about reward (food), allocation of attention and resource/effort (to food), and the integration between bodily homeostasis regarding energy stores, GI contents, and extrinsic signals such as food availability (Figure 5.3) (Dagher, 2009).

Homeostatic and GI information is largely relayed by circulating gut peptide hormones and nutrients, which act at the hypothalamus. Additional brain structures are also involved, as is the vagal nerve, in regulating appetite and the behaviors as described earlier, which are perturbed if their interconnections are disrupted. For example, one study has shown that lesion-induced disruption of the amygdala–OFC interconnection abolishes sensory-specific satiety—that is, a normal response whereby food fed to satiety loses its incentive properties (Holland & Gallagher, 2004). The PFC additionally adds cognitive influence over the apparent brain network of appetite regulation.

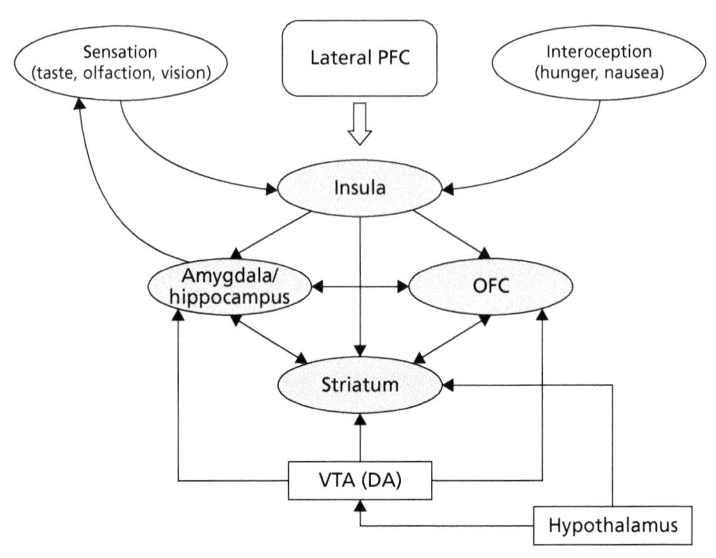

Figure 5.3 A brain network for appetitive behavior. (Not all connections are depicted)
PFC, prefrontal cortex; OFC, orbitofrontal cortex; VTA, ventral tegmental area; DA, dopamine.
Reprinted by permission from *International Journal of Obesity*, 33 (S2), The neurobiology of appetite: hunger as addiction, A. Dagher, pp. S30–S33, Figure 1, doi: 10.1038/ijo.2009.69, Copyright © 2009, Springer Nature.

5.7.3 **Interoceptive awareness of sensory signals**

Under normal physiological conditions, stimulation of intestinal afferents does not typically reach conscious awareness. However, these neural signals likely still reach the brainstem in order to subsequently trigger GI reflexes to maintain bodily homeostasis, and thus permit interoceptive awareness (Kern & Shaker, 2002). Without this process, there would be no feedback loop to maintain the internal GI milieu. Until relatively recently, it was also unknown whether viscerosensory signals of interoceptive awareness even reach higher cortical regions.

In an early study, by means of rectal distension to a threshold below conscious perception in healthy volunteers, it was shown that these afferent signals, whilst not strong enough to reach conscious perception, are still registered in the cortex, and are detectable by functional neuroimaging. However, the degree of magnitude of activity of these cortical areas was much smaller than a visceral interoception sensory afferent signal that would reach the level of conscious perception (Kern & Shaker, 2002). The areas activated following stimulation that was not consciously perceived were fourfold: sensorimotor, parietal-occipital, ACC, and insula (Kern & Shaker, 2002). The group posited that these areas of activation came as a consequence of vagal or spinal afferents as discussed earlier in this chapter. Additionally, given that sensorimotor cortical regions are supplied by spinal afferents alone, it was suggested that visceral interoception sensory signals that do not reach conscious perception may be relayed to the cortex by spinal afferents, whilst the vagal nerve be more implicated in conscious sensation or pain *proper* (Kern & Shaker, 2002). In follow-up studies from the same group, the effect of esophageal acid stimulation to below-conscious perception thresholds were additionally explored, revealing similar findings of activity in the cingulate, insula and sensorimotor regions (Kern, Chai, & Lawal, 2009). Indeed, more recent studies have also shown how the functional connectivity of interoceptive regions such as the insula are modulated by esophageal acid stimulation below a threshold of conscious perception (Babaei et al., 2013).

5.7.4 Anticipation of visceral threat

An additional visceral interocept that has gained attention over the last decade is that of anticipation to a bodily threat. Largely achieved by means of the threat of pain (e.g. to be told one would soon receive visceral pain), it has been shown that anticipation is processed at the brain level quite differently to that of pain *proper.* When expecting a threat which merits emotional arousal, one's anticipation modulates the sequential cognitive response to that stimuli, such as the stress and anxiety that might accompany it.

Numerous groups have studied pain anticipation in an effort to characterize brain regions implicated, and perhaps even that an anticipatory brain network should such exist. One frequently proposed brain region in anticipation is the anterior insula, given its well-described roles in conscious interoceptive awareness. However, additionally proposed regions include the ACC, PAG, PFC, medial frontal lobe, amygdala, and OFC. These regions are implicated in the processing of visceral pain also, and thus their documented activation prior to actual pain *proper* is interesting in the context of modulation, certainly warranting further study (Bishop et al., 2004; Coen et al., 2011; Fairhurst et al., 2007; Ploghaus et al., 2001; Ruffle et al., 2015b). In the context of disease, anticipation of pain in IBS is different from healthy controls as they inactivate certain brain regions, including the ACC and amygdala, to a lesser degree than IBS patients, possibly representing a maladaptive coping strategy to pain in IBS patients (Berman et al., 2008).

5.8 Inter-individual factors in visceral interoception

A major focus into advancing our understanding to the "neurobiology of gut feelings" has been to characterize the factors of an individual which influence visceral interoceptive processing, referred to as the "inter-individual factors." In gastroenterology, furthermore, the Rome working collaborative group has previously highlighted how lack of understanding of these factors at present significantly limits advancements in the field (Drossman & Hasler, 2016). To date, there are an array of factors which have been discovered, and span genetics, physiology, neuroanatomy, and psychophysiology. Taking this a step further, some groups have suggested the concept of visceral pain "endophenotypes" (Farmer & Aziz, 2014; Ruffle et al., 2017b; Tracey, 2011). In understanding the neurobiology of visceral interoception, it is important to take these factors into account, and thus will be discussed later in this chapter.

5.8.1 Gender

One frequently studied difference in visceral interoception is that of gender. It has been often documented that women demonstrate both higher pain sensitivity and greater prevalence of chronic visceral pain conditions than the male counterparts (Kano et al., 2013), IBS being an example discussed in section 5.9.2. In fact, some contemporaneous studies have even moved to studying *only* males *or* females, so as to eliminate the possibility of a gender confound in their results. These gender differences have been and continue to be investigated with the ever-advancing tools in neuroimaging. As one example, a previous study utilizing acute esophageal pain, by mechanical distension, showed that female subjects display greater brain activity in the mid-cingulate cortex, anterior insula, and premotor cortex regions well associated with the emotional arousal constituent of visceral pain processing which led the group to suggest that females may attribute greater emotional importance to an acute visceral pain stimulus than males (Kano et al., 2013). These findings of increased activity in emotional arousal brain regions have also been reported by other groups using connectivity analysis (Labus et al., 2008).

5.8.2 **Genetic**

Genetic differences have additionally been investigated in the brain processing of visceral signals. For example, polymorphisms in the 5-hydroxytryptamine (5-HT) signalling system have been shown to play a role in processing of interoceptive signals, the subsequent stress response a signal may invoke and furthermore the emotional regulation that accompanies it (Kilpatrick et al., 2015). Specific to visceral pain, the 5-HT (serotonin) transporter gene-linked polymorphic region (5-HTTLPR) has been shown to affect the brain response. In a neuroimaging study of brain connectivity in healthy males exposed to painful mechanical rectal distension, the *S/S* genotype of 5-HTTLPR was associated with significantly greater hippocampal-amygdala strength, an important central processing component of the stress response and emotion regulation, compared to alternative genotypic carriers (Kilpatrick et al., 2015). Indeed, additional studies have also suggested that the 5-HTTLPR genotype is associated with a differing extent of emotional regulation in visceral pain, whereby the *S/S* genotype has been shown to correspond to greater cerebral blood flow (as a surrogate to brain activity) in the ACC, hippocampus, and OFC in one study (Fukudo & Kanazawa, 2011; Fukudo et al., 2009), while to the insula, inferior frontal gyrus, supplementary motor area, and precentral gyrus in another (Schaub et al., 2013). Furthermore, it has been suggested that the functional gene polymorphism may predict the efficacy of a selective serotonin re-uptake inhibitor (SSRI) in the use of visceral pain, a finding particular poignant in current GI practice where SSRIs have been investigated for their utility in relieving IBS symptoms (Farmer & Ruffle, 2015; Tack et al., 2006).

5.8.3 **Autonomic physiology**

Abnormalities in the activity of the ANS are apparent in numerous GI disorders, many of which are associated with perturbation in visceral interoception processes (frequently pain). These clinical disorders specific to the GI tract include functional chest pain, IBS, inflammatory bowel disease, and Ehlers–Danlos syndrome (Bonaz et al.,

2013; De Wandele et al., 2014; Hoff et al., 2016; Ruffle et al., 2015a; Ruffle et al., 2018; Spaziani et al., 2008). Over the last decade, accumulating evidence has suggested an anti-nociceptive role for the PNS whereby many of these aforementioned disorders exhibit a paucity of baseline vagal tone when compared to healthy controls (Botha et al., 2015; Farmer et al., 2014a). The exact mechanism by which abnormal function of the vagus may lead to anti-nociception is not yet known, although it has been proposed to have an anti-nociceptive and anti-inflammatory function (Farmer et al., 2016; Ruffle et al., 2017a).

Baseline autonomic function is an additional important variable to account for in understanding the brain processing of visceral interoceptive stimuli. With structural neuroimaging, it has been shown that cortical thickness of the mid-cingulate cortex correlates with degree of resting parasympathetic activity, quantified by heart rate variability (HRV) (Winkelmann et al., 2016). Meanwhile, using fMRI it has additionally been shown that activity in the ACC and cerebellum correlates with vagal tone (Kano et al., 2014). Using vertex analysis, it has recently been reported that the shapes of subcortical nuclei are influenced by both the resting SNS and PNS tone of an individual (Ruffle et al., 2018). Specifically, SNS was positively correlated to outward shape changes of the brainstem, nucleus accumbens, amygdala, and pallidum, whilst PNS vagal tone was negatively correlated to inward shape changes of the amygdala and pallidum. Furthermore, vagal tone was correlated to total volume of the brainstem and the putamen. Needless to say, it is clear that baseline autonomic function in an individual influences their processing of visceral neural signals.

5.8.4 **Psychophysiological**

The emotional and affective dimension of a visceral signal, especially a threat such as pain, is a key aspect to its cognitive interpretation. Psychophysiological factors such as personality traits have historically been thought highly important in the cognitive processes underpinning processing a threat such as pain (Harkins, Price, & Braith, 1989). However, in the context of the viscera, the influence of personality has only relatively recently been studied. Using mechanical esophageal distension in induce visceral pain, it has been shown with fMRI that personality, anxiety, negative emotion, and sociability influence central brain processing of anticipation and actual visceral pain (Coen et al., 2008; Coen et al., 2011; Kumari et al., 2007; Paine et al., 2009a; Paine et al., 2009b; Ruffle et al., 2015b).

During a study by Coen and colleagues, in anticipation to visceral pain, higher neuroticism scores were associated with greater activity in the thalamus, parahippocampal gyrus, and ACC, but these regions had lower activity during visceral pain *proper*. These regions are previously attributed to the emotional and cognitive appraisal of pain, but it is thought that these findings may reflect the neurotic individual's tendency to a heightened arousal during pain anticipation yet an avoidance coping response during pain (Coen et al., 2011). Notably, neuroticism has strong ties to IBS also and is a risk factor for unexplained chronic abdominal pain in the disorder (Hazlett-Stevens et al., 2003). Referring to extraversion, in a follow-up study it was shown that during both pain anticipation and visceral pain, a higher degree of extraversion was associated with greater activity to the right insula, which may link to the sympathetic-predominant response to threat which higher extraversion individuals display (Ruffle et al., 2015b).

5.8.5 Microbiota

The human microbiota is a diverse and dynamic ecosystem within the GI tract, which has evolved to be symbiotic to the host. An estimated 10^{14} microorganisms populate the adult gut (Ley, Peterson, & Gordon, 2006). Whilst sterile prenatally, inoculation occurs vertically during birth, and over the course of the first year of life it is fully established. Throughout an individual's life, this ecosystem is determined by genetics, diet, and environment (Dominguez-Bello et al., 2011). The microbiota protects the body from external pathogens, aids in digestion and metabolism, and additionally acts as a source for neurochemicals in numerous bodily processes, including neural transmission. As an example, the microbiota is responsible for 95% of bodily serotonin (Sommer & Backhed, 2013).

The microbiota has formed an interesting area of GI research in recent years, culminating in the suggestion that it forms an aspect in bi-directional brain–gut axis communication; the brain influences the microbiota, and the microbiota influences the brain (Figure 5.4) (De Vadder et al., 2014). The central nervous system can influence the GI microbiota composition (a) directly, for example by means of neurotransmitter release (e.g. serotonin) from enterochromaffin cells, neurones, and immune cells, or (b) indirectly, by fluctuations in GI motility and secretions by autonomic tone (this subsequently affecting blood flow and nutrient availability for said microbiota) (Rhee, Pothoulakis, & Mayer, 2009).

To investigate the effect of microbiota on the brain, studies have largely relied on the premise of sterility in prenatal animals and maintenance in sterile environments postnatally (see Cryan & Dinan, 2012; Cryan & O'Mahony, 2011). Using these methods, groups have shown that the microbiota affect the central nervous system by affecting behavioral traits in animals, accompanied by changes in neurotrophic factors such as brain-derived neurotrophic factor (BDNF) in regions such as the hippocampus (Bercik et al., 2011). Numerous animal examples are apparent (Cryan & Dinan, 2012; Cryan & O'Mahony, 2011; Farmer, Randall, & Aziz, 2014b).

In GI disease, it is also thought that changes to the gut microbiota may play an important role. The frequent comorbidity of mood disorders in GI disorders, including both IBS and coeliac disease, has been proposed in part due to changes in the microbiota. Furthermore, microbiota may perturb the brain–gut axis, one poignant example being that of post-infection IBS (Spiller & Lam, 2012). The concept of the microbiota influencing the neurobiology of gut feelings is an exciting and developing field expected to reveal significant developments for our understanding of the GI microbiota and its impact on interoception (Farmer et al., 2014b; Rhee et al., 2009).

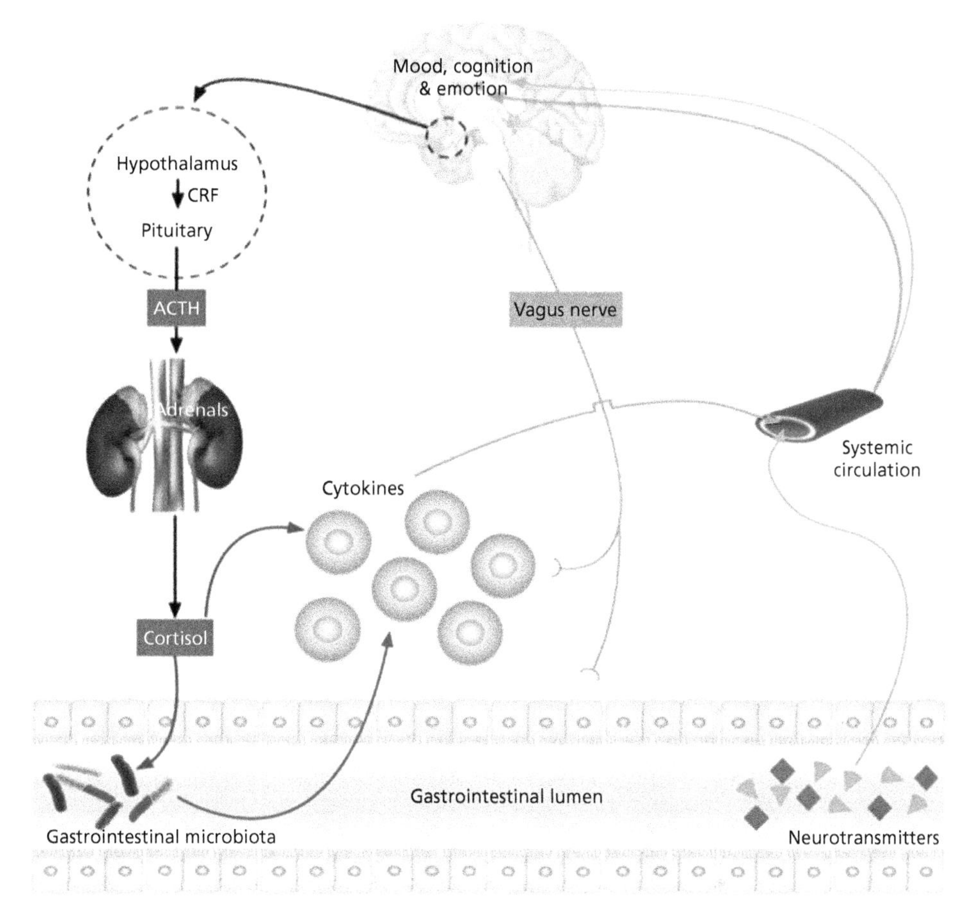

Figure 5.4 Bidirectional brain–gut–microbiota pathways. Multiple pathways, including but not limited to neural, endocrine, and immune, exist in which the gastrointestinal microbiota may modulate the brain. Abbreviations: ACTH, adrenocorticotrophic hormone; CRF, corticotrophin releasing hormone.

5.8.6 **Combining factors to form complex endophenotypes**

One future direction of this research area is the possibility of combining these factors to form visceral "endophenotypes" as a form of statistical dimension reduction of multiple data arrays into a simpler construct (Tracey, 2011). Endophenotypes are measurable components of a disease/condition, which may include neuroanatomical or cognitive characteristics that have simpler ties to underpinning factors such as genetics. Clustering individuals into endophenotypes has been suggested as a means to aid identification of patients at risk for developing chronic pain.

Using a group of healthy controls, it has been previously shown that more pain-sensitive and pain-resistant phenotypes do indeed exist, using arrays of physiological, psychophysiological, and genetic data (Farmer et al., 2014a; Farmer et al., 2013). With data coalesced into two main clusters, individual's in pain cluster 1, at baseline, show higher neuroticism and anxiety, a preponderance for the *SS/LS* 5-HTTLPR genotype, higher baseline sympathetic tone, lower parasympathetic tone, and higher serum cortisol. During pain however, this group tolerated it less, habituated less to the stimulus, showed a greater parasympathetic nervous system activation, a sympathetic nervous system withdrawal, and had an elevated serum cortisol. In contrast, pain cluster 2 at baseline showed higher extraversion but lower anxiety, a preponderance for the *L/L* genotype, lower serum cortisol, a higher parasympathetic tone with low sympathetic tone. During pain however, the group tolerated the pain stimulus to a greater extent, displayed a greater habituation effect and a parasympathetic withdrawal coupled to a sympathetic activation. Using fMRI, individuals with high extraversion and low anxiety have been shown preferentially to activate the frontal cortex, insula, and left thalamus during pain in comparison to cluster 1 individuals, see (Farmer et al., 2014a; Farmer et al., 2013). In a follow-up study of this cohort, it has also recently been shown that visceral pain endophenotypes can be accurately predicted using machine learning with whole-brain connectivity data with over 85% accuracy (Ruffle et al., 2017b).

5.9 **Comparing gut feelings in health and disease**

5.9.1 **Chronic pain**

Acute and chronic pain both have a distinct neurobiology, and indeed visceral pain is no exception. Some authorities have even called for chronic pain to be considered an individual disease entity (Tracey & Bushnell, 2009). Herein two common causes of chronic visceral pain will be discussed, IBS and inflammatory bowel disease (IBD). Both IBS and IBD are associated with altered interoception, and thus these conditions also demonstrate altered brain processing of acute visceral painful compared to healthy controls.

5.9.2 **Irritable bowel syndrome**

IBS is one of the most often studied "functional" GI disorders with regards to neuroimaging of visceral interoception in disease, in part attributable to its incomplete understanding and high prevalence of between 5% and 20% (Farmer & Ruffle, 2015). IBS is more prevalent in women, and is associated with a significant socioeconomic burden by means of a reduction in health-related quality of life, not least large healthcare costs from recurrent consultation and over-investigation. It has been described as one of the most common persistent "pain syndromes," where dysregulation of the aforementioned brain–gut axis is a core aspect of the underpinning disorder. This in turn leads to the development of a visceral hypersensitivity state. Denoted by the Rome working group criteria, now in its fourth iteration, IBS patients by definition experience recurrent abdominal pain which improves with defecation (Drossman & Hasler, 2016).

As discussed earlier in the chapter, there are three key networks in the processing of a visceral pain, the homeostatic-afferent, the emotional arousal, and the cortical-modulatory. In IBS, a disorder for which the presence of recurrent visceral pain is part of its very definition, the homeostatic-afferent and emotional arousal networks demonstrate increased engagement (Tillisch & Labus, 2011). Because the pathophysiology of IBS has been difficult to understand, multiple groups have turned to neuroimaging as a means to investigate it. These studies have demonstrated that the majority of the visceral pain neuromatrix is activated as described earlier (Mayer et al., 2005), however, differences from healthy controls *are* apparent. A meta-analysis has shown that patients with IBS display more consistent brain activation in emotional arousal network regions, including the pregenual ACC and amygdala, as well as brainstem regions implicated in the cortical-modulatory aspects of descending analgesia (Tillisch, Mayer, & Labus, 2011). Structural brain differences in IBS patients and controls have also been studied, revealing that IBS patients exhibit a *decreased* grey matter density (GMD) in many regions involved in visceral pain processing, including the thalamus, PFC, posterior parietal cortex, and ventral striatum, but an *increase* in GMD in the ACC and OFC, areas involved in the cognitive and attentional aspects of visceral pain (Seminowicz et al., 2010). Additionally, it is possible that increased anxiety in the IBS group also affects these findings (Seminowicz et al., 2010), not least the change in baseline autonomic tone (Ruffle et al., 2015a; Ruffle et al., 2018). It is possible that duration of disease (Blankstein et al., 2010) or indeed important inter-individual factors influence such results. Further research is certainly warranted.

It is also possible to investigate white matter tract differences between chronic visceral pain conditions and healthy controls, by means of diffusion tensor imaging. Using probalistic tractography, a reduced structural connectivity was demonstrated in IBS patients between the amygdala and the dorsolateral PFC, possibly related to a decreased or insufficient inhibition of emotional arousal circuitry leading to amplification of the visceral pain experience (Labus et al., 2010). Notably, healthy control studies investigating brain white matter have shown a complex neural network for visceral pain including the insula, thalamus, ACC, PFC, SI, and SII (Moisset et al., 2010). However, the degree of white matter connectivity between these regions has been shown to be highly variable, most likely due to inter-individual variability factors (Moisset et al., 2010). Lastly, the influence of genetic factors on the processing of visceral interoceptive signals in healthy individuals was discussed in section 5.8.6 with specific reference to the 5-HTTLPR. This polymorphic region has also been studied in the context of IBS, whereby it has been shown that the *S/S* genotype corresponded to decreased IBS symptoms, whilst the *LS/SS* genotype was associated both with increased pain ratings in one study (Camilleri et al., 2008), but also the severity of symptoms as a whole in another (Colucci et al., 2013).

5.9.3 **Inflammatory bowel disease**

IBD refers to both ulcerative colitis (UC) and Crohn's disease (CD) which are chronic GI disorders frequently accompanied by abdominal pain. The neurobiology of this pain has been investigated by some groups. Using positron emission tomography and painful mechanical rectal distension, it has been shown that UC patients, whilst showing brain region activity comparable to the aforementioned pain neuromatrix including the ACC, insula, and PAG, also show greater activity in the frontal cortex and PAG circuits (Mayer et al., 2005). Interestingly, when comparing IBD to IBS cohorts, IBD patients additionally show greater activity in the pons and PAG in comparison to IBS patients. Conversely, IBS patients display greater activity in the ACC, PFC, and amygdala in comparison to UC patients (Tillisch & Labus, 2011). These findings may suggest that in IBS there is greater involvement of emotional arousal circuits to visceral pain, whilst UC patients appear to show greater activity of regions involved in descending analgesia (such as the PAG).

5.10 **Conclusion**

The neurobiology of gut feelings is a complex and ever-evolving field of interoception. Ascending signalling pathways include neural, humoral, neuroimmune, and endocrine, and culminate with intricate brain networks specific to a specific visceral state, including those of visceral pain, hunger, and nausea. With the brain–gut axis, a bi-directional communication between gut and brain is permitted to ensure gastrointestinal homeostasis, and to that end, inter-individual factors including genetics, demographic, the psychophysiological, and the neurophysiological influence its regulation at an individual level. Furthermore, this neurobiology is perturbed in common GI disorders such as IBS and IBD. Future avenues of visceral interoception research should further interrogate these inter-individual factors thus far identified, including autonomic neurophysiology and gut microbiota, and indeed how these interact with one another.

References

Altschuler, S. M., Bao, X. M., Bieger, D., Hopkins, D. A., and **Miselis, R. R.** (1989). Viscerotopic representation of the upper alimentary tract in the rat: Sensory ganglia and nuclei of the solitary and spinal trigeminal tracts. *Journal of Comparative Neurology, 283*(2), 248–68.

Apkarian, A. V., Bushnell, M. C., Treede, R. D., and **Zubieta, J. K.** (2005). Human brain mechanisms of pain perception and regulation in health and disease. *European Journal of Pain, 9*(4), 463–84.

Aziz, Q., Andersson, J. L., Valind, S., Sundin, A., Hamdy, S., Jones, A. K., et al. (1997). Identification of human brain loci processing esophageal sensation using positron emission tomography. *Gastroenterology, 113*, 50–59.

Aziz, Q. and **Thompson, D. G.** (1998). Brain–gut axis in health and disease. *Gastroenterology, 114*(3), 559–78.

Aziz, Q., Thompson, D. G., Ng, V. W., Hamdy, S., Sarkar, S., Brammer, M. J., et al. (2000). Cortical processing of human somatic and visceral sensation. *Journal of Neuroscience, 20*(7), 2657–63.

Babaei, A., Siwiec, R. M., Kern, M., Douglas Ward, B., Li, S. J., and **Shaker, R.** (2013). Intrinsic functional connectivity of the brain swallowing network during subliminal esophageal acid stimulation. *Neurogastroenterology and Motility, 25*(12), 992–e779.

Bantick, S. J., Wise, R. G., Ploghaus, A., Clare, S., Smith, S. M., and **Tracey, I.** (2002). Imaging how attention modulates pain in humans using functional MRI. *Brain, 125*(Pt 2), 310–19.

Bercik, P., Denou, E., Collins, J., Jackson, W., Lu, J., Jury, J., et al. (2011). The intestinal microbiota affect central levels of brain-derived neurotropic factor and behavior in mice. *Gastroenterology, 141*(2), 599–609, 609 e1–3.

Berman, S. M., Naliboff, B. D., Suyenobu, B., Labus, J. S., Stains, J., Ohning, G., et al. (2008). Reduced brainstem inhibition during anticipated pelvic visceral pain correlates with enhanced brain response to the visceral stimulus in women with irritable bowel syndrome. *Journal of Neuroscience*, *28*(2), 349–59.

Bishop, S., Duncan, J., Brett, M., and **Lawrence, A. D.** (2004). Prefrontal cortical function and anxiety: Controlling attention to threat-related stimuli. *Nature Neuroscience*, *7*(2), 184–8.

Blankstein, U., Chen, J., Diamant, N. E., and **Davis, K. D.** (2010). Altered brain structure in irritable bowel syndrome: Potential contributions of pre-existing and disease-driven factors. *Gastroenterology*, *138*(5), 1783–9.

Bonaz, B., Picq, C., Sinniger, V., Mayol, J. F., and **Clarencon, D.** (2013). Vagus nerve stimulation: From epilepsy to the cholinergic anti-inflammatory pathway. *Neurogastroenterology and Motility*, *25*(3), 208–21.

Botha, C., Farmer, A. D., Nilsson, M., Brock, C., Gavrila, A. D., Drewes, A. M., et al. (2015). Preliminary report: Modulation of parasympathetic nervous system tone influences oesophageal pain hypersensitivity. *Gut*, *64*(4), 611–17.

Browning, K. N. and **Travagli, R. A.** (2011). Plasticity of vagal brainstem circuits in the control of gastrointestinal function. *Autonomic Neuroscience*, *161*(1–2), 6–13.

Camilleri, M., Busciglio, I., Carlson, P., McKinzie, S., Burton, D., Baxter, K., et al. (2008). Candidate genes and sensory functions in health and irritable bowel syndrome. *American Journal of Physiology-Gastrointestinal and Liver Physiology*, *295*(2), G219–25.

Carrive, P. and **Bandler, R.** (1991). Viscerotopic organization of neurons subserving hypotensive reactions within the midbrain periaqueductal grey: A correlative functional and anatomical study. *Brain Research*, *541*(2), 206–15.

Ceunen, E., Vlaeyen, J. W., and **Van Diest, I.** (2016). On the origin of interoception. *Froniers in Psychology*, *7*, 743.

Coen, S. J., Gregory, L. J., Yaguez, L., Amaro Jr., E., Brammer, M., Williams, S. C., et al. (2007). Reproducibility of human brain activity evoked by esophageal stimulation using functional magnetic resonance imaging. *American Journal of Physiology, Gastrointestinal and Liver Physiology*, **293**, G188–97.

Coen, S. J., Aziz, Q., Yaguez, L., Brammer, M., Williams, S. C., and **Gregory, L. J.** (2008). Effects of attention on visceral stimulus intensity encoding in the male human brain. *Gastroenterology*, *135*(6), 2065–74, 2074 e1.

Coen, S. J., Kano, M., Farmer, A. D., Kumari, V., Giampietro, V., Brammer, M., et al. (2011). Neuroticism influences brain activity during the experience of visceral pain. *Gastroenterology*, *141*(3), 909–17 e1.

Coen, S. J., Hobson, A. R. and **Aziz, Q.** (2012). Processing of Gastrointestinal Sensory Signals in the Brain. In: L. R. Johnson (ed.), *Physiology of the Gastronintestinal Tract*, 5th edn. Oxford: Academic Press, pp. 689–702.

Colucci, R., Gambaccini, D., Ghisu, N., Rossi, G., Costa, F., Tuccori, M., et al. (2013). Influence of the serotonin transporter 5HTTLPR polymorphism on symptom severity in irritable bowel syndrome. *PLoS One*, *8*(2), e54831.

Craig, A. D., Bushnell, M. C., Zhang, E. T., and **Blomqvist, A.** (1994). A thalamic nucleus specific for pain and temperature sensation. *Nature*, *372*(6508), 770–3.

Craig, A. D. (2002). How do you feel? Interoception: The sense of the physiological condition of the body. *Nature Reviews Neuroscience*, *3*(8), 655–66.

Craig, A. D. (2003). Pain mechanisms: Labeled lines versus convergence in central processing. *Annual Review of Neuroscience*, **26**, 1–30.

Cryan, J. F. and **O'Mahony, S. M.** (2011). The microbiome–gut–brain axis: From bowel to behavior. *Neurogastroenterology and Motility*, *23*(3), 187–92.

Cryan, J. F. and **Dinan, T. G.** (2012). Mind-altering microorganisms: The impact of the gut microbiota on brain and behaviour. *Nature Reviews Neuroscience*, *13*(10), 701–12.

Dagher, A. (2009). The neurobiology of appetite: Hunger as addiction. *International Journal of Obesity (London)*, **33** Suppl. 2, S30–3.

De Vadder, F., Kovatcheva-Datchary, P., Goncalves, D., Vinera, J., Zitoun, C., Duchampt, A., et al. (2014). Microbiota-generated metabolites promote metabolic benefits via gut-brain neural circuits. *Cell*, *156*(1–2), 84–96.

De Wandele, I., Rombaut, L., Leybaert, L., Van de Borne, P., De Backer, T., Malfait, F., et al. (2014). Dysautonomia and its underlying mechanisms in the hypermobility type of Ehlers–Danlos syndrome. *Seminars in Arthritis and Rheumatism*, *44*(1), 93–100.

Derbyshire, S. W. (2003). A systematic review of neuroimaging data during visceral stimulation. *American Journal of Gastroenterology*, *98*(1), 12–20.

Dominguez-Bello, M. G., Blaser, M. J., Ley, R. E., and **Knight, R.** (2011). Development of the human gastrointestinal microbiota and insights from high-throughput sequencing. *Gastroenterology*, *140*(6), 1713–19.

Drossman, D. A. and **Hasler, W. L.** (2016). Rome IV-functional GI disorders: Disorders of gut–brain interaction. *Gastroenterology*, *150*(6), 1257–61.

Dunckley, P., Wise, R. G., Fairhurst, M., Hobden, P., Aziz, Q., Chang, L., et al, . (2005). A comparison of visceral and somatic pain processing in the human brainstem using functional magnetic resonance imaging. *Journal of Neuroscience*, *25*(32), 7333–41.

Fairhurst, M., Wiech, K., Dunckley, P., and **Tracey, I.** (2007). Anticipatory brainstem activity predicts neural processing of pain in humans. *Pain*, *128*(1–2), 101–10.

Farmer, A. D., Coen, S. J., Kano, M., Paine, P. A., Shwahdi, M., Jafari, J., et al. (2013). Psychophysiological responses to pain identify reproducible human clusters. *Pain*, *154*(11), 2266–76.

Farmer, A. D. and **Aziz, Q.** (2014). Mechanisms of visceral pain in health and functional gastrointestinal disorders. *Scandinavian Journal of Pain*, *5*(2), 51–60.

Farmer, A. D., Coen, S. J., Kano, M., Naqvi, H., Paine, P. A., Scott, S. M., et al. (2014a). Psychophysiological responses to visceral and somatic pain in functional chest pain identify clinically relevant pain clusters. *Neurogastroenterology and Motility*, *26*(1), 139–48.

Farmer, A. D., Randall, H. A., and **Aziz, Q.** (2014b). It's a gut feeling: How the gut microbiota affects the state of mind. *Journal of Physiology*, *592*(14), 2981–8.

Farmer, A. D. and **Ruffle, J. K.** (2015). Irritable bowel syndrome. *Hamdan Medical Journal*, **8**(3).

Farmer, A. D., Ban, V. F., Coen, S. J., Sanger, G. J., Barker, G. J., Gresty, M. A., et al. (2015). Visually induced nausea causes characteristic changes in cerebral, autonomic and endocrine function in humans. *Journal of Physiology*, *593*(5), 1183–96.

Farmer, A. D., Albu-Soda, A., and **Aziz, Q.** (2016). Vagus nerve stimulation in clinical practice. *British Journal of Hospital Medicine (London)*, *77*(11), 645–51.

Frokjaer, J. B., Bergmann, S., Brock, C., Madzak, A., Farmer, A. D., Ellrich, J., et al. (2016). Modulation of vagal tone enhances gastroduodenal motility and reduces somatic pain sensitivity. *Neurogastroenterology and Motility*, **28**, 592–8.

Fukudo, S., Kanazawa, M., Mizuno, T., Hamaguchi, T., Kano, M., Watanabe, S., et al. (2009). Impact of serotonin transporter gene polymorphism on brain activation by colorectal distention. *Neuroimage*, *47*(3), 946–51.

Fukudo, S. and **Kanazawa, M.** (2011). Gene, environment, and brain–gut interactions in irritable bowel syndrome. *Journal of Gastroenterology and Hepatology*, **26** Suppl 3, 110–15.

Gregory, L. J., Yaguez, L., Williams, S. C., Altmann, C., Coen, S. J., Ng, V., et al. (2003). Cognitive modulation of the cerebral processing of human oesophageal sensation using functional magnetic resonance imaging. *Gut*, *52*(12), 1671–7.

Harkins, S. W., Price, D. D., and **Braith, J.** (1989). Effects of extraversion and neuroticism on experimental pain, clinical pain, and illness behavior. *Pain*, *36*(2), 209–18.

Hazlett-Stevens, H., Craske, M. G., Mayer, E. A., Chang, L., and **Naliboff, B. D.** (2003). Prevalence of irritable bowel syndrome among university students: The roles of worry, neuroticism, anxiety sensitivity and visceral anxiety. *Journal of Psychosomatic Research*, *55*(6), 501–5.

Hoff, D. A., Brock, C., Farmer, A. D., Dickman, R., Ruffle, J. K., Shaker, A., and **Drewes, A. M.** (2016). Pharmacological and other treatment modalities for esophageal pain. *Annals of the New York Academy of Sciences*, *1380*(1), 58–66.

Holland, P. C. and **Gallagher, M.** (2004). Amygdala-frontal interactions and reward expectancy. *Current Opinions in Neurobiology*, *14*(2), 148–55.

Kano, M., Farmer, A. D., Aziz, Q., Giampietro, V., Brammer, M. J., Williams, S. C., et al. (2013). Sex differences in brain activity to anticipated and experienced visceral pain in healthy subjects. *American Journal of Physiology–Gastrointestinal and Liver Physiology*, *304*(8), G687–99.

Kano, M., Coen, S. J., Farmer, A. D., Aziz, Q., Williams, S. C., Alsop, D. C., et al. (2014). Physiological and psychological individual differences influence resting brain function measured by ASL perfusion. *Brain Structure and Function*, *219*(5), 1673–84.

Kern, M. K. and **Shaker, R.** (2002). Cerebral cortical registration of subliminal visceral stimulation. *Gastroenterology*, *122*(2), 290–8.

Kern, M., Chai, K., Lawal, A., and **Shaker, R.** (2009). Effect of esophageal acid exposure on the cortical swallowing network in healthy human subjects. *American Journal of Physiology–Gastrointestinal and Liver Physiology*, *297*(1), G152–8.

Kilpatrick, L. A., Mayer, E. A., Labus, J. S., Gupta, A., Hamaguchi, T., Mizuno, T., et al. (2015). Serotonin transporter gene polymorphism modulates activity and connectivity within an emotional arousal network of healthy men during an aversive visceral stimulus. *PLoS One*, *10*(4), e0123183.

Kringelbach, M. L. (2005). The human orbitofrontal cortex: Linking reward to hedonic experience. *Nature Reviews Neuroscience*, *6*(9), 691–702.

Kulkarni, B., Bentley, D. E., Elliott, R., Youell, P., Watson, A., Derbyshire, S. W., et al. (2005). Attention to pain localization and unpleasantness discriminates the functions of the medial and lateral pain systems. *European Journal of Neuroscience*, *21*(11), 3133–42.

Kumari, V., ffytche, D. H., Das, M., Wilson, G. D., Goswami, S., and **Sharma, T.** (2007). Neuroticism and brain responses to anticipatory fear. *Behavioral Neurosciences*, *121*(4), 643–52.

Labus, J. S., Naliboff, B. N., Fallon, J., Berman, S. M., Suyenobu, B., Bueller, J. A., et al. (2008). Sex differences in brain activity during aversive visceral stimulation and its expectation in patients with chronic abdominal pain: A network analysis. *Neuroimage*, *41*(3), 1032–43.

Labus, J. S., Vianna, E., Jarcho, J. M., Tillisch, K., Bueller, J. A., and **Mayer, E. A.** (2010). 858 reduced structural connectivity between amygdala and prefrontal cortex in patients with irritable bowel syndrome: A diffuse tensor imaging study. *Gastroenterology*, *138*(5), S-118.

Lechan, R. M. and **Toni, R.** (2016). *Functional Anatomy of the Hypothalamus and Pituitary*. South Dartmouth, MA: MDText.com.

Ley, R. E., Peterson, D. A., and **Gordon, J. I.** (2006). Ecological and evolutionary forces shaping microbial diversity in the human intestine. *Cell*, *124*(4), 837–48.

Mayer, E. A., Berman, S., Suyenobu, B., Labus, J., Mandelkern, M. A., Naliboff, B. D., and **Chang, L.** (2005). Differences in brain responses to visceral pain between patients with irritable bowel syndrome and ulcerative colitis. *Pain*, *115*(3), 398–409.

Melzack, R. and **Wall, P. D.** (1965). Pain mechanisms: A new theory. *Science*, *150*(3699), 971–9.

Miller, A. D., Nonaka, S., and **Jakus, J.** (1994). Brain areas essential or non-essential for emesis. *Brain Research*, *647*(2), 255–64.

Moisset, X., Bouhassira, D., Denis, D., Dominique, G., Benoit, C., and **Sabate, J. M.** (2010). Anatomical connections between brain areas activated during rectal distension in healthy volunteers: A visceral pain network. *European Journal of Pain*, *14*(2), 142–8.

Omran, Y. A. and **Aziz, Q.** (2014). Functional brain imaging in gastroenterology: To new beginnings. *Nature Reviews Gastroenterology and Hepatology, 11*(9), 565–76.

Paine, P., Kishor, J., Worthen, S. F., Gregory, L. J., and **Aziz, Q.** (2009a). Exploring relationships for visceral and somatic pain with autonomic control and personality. *Pain, 144*(3), 236–44.

Paine, P., Worthen, S. F., Gregory, L. J., Thompson, D. G., and **Aziz, Q.** (2009b). Personality differences affect brainstem autonomic responses to visceral pain. *Neurogastroenterology and Motility, 21*(11), 1155–e98.

Pezawas, L., Meyer-Lindenberg, A., Drabant, E. M., Verchinski, B. A., Munoz, K. E., Kolachana, B. S., et al. R. (2005). 5-HTTLPR polymorphism impacts human cingulate-amygdala interactions: A genetic susceptibility mechanism for depression. *Nature Neurosciences, 8*(6), 828–34.

Ploghaus, A., Narain, C., Beckmann, C. F., Clare, S., Bantick, S., Wise, R., et al. (2001). Exacerbation of pain by anxiety is associated with activity in a hippocampal network. *Journal of Neuroscience, 21*(24), 9896–903.

Ploner, M., Lee, M. C., Wiech, K., Bingel, U., and **Tracey, I.** (2011). Flexible cerebral connectivity patterns subserve contextual modulations of pain. *Cerebral Cortex, 21*(3), 719–26.

Rhee, S. H., Pothoulakis, C., and **Mayer, E. A.** (2009). Principles and clinical implications of the brain-gut -enteric microbiota axis. *Nature Reviews Gastroenterology and Hepatology, 6*(5), 306–14.

Ruffle, J., Shah, M., Monro, J., and **Julu, P.** (2015a). Pattern of dysautonomia in patients with functional gastrointestinal disorders. *Autonomic Neuroscience: Basic and Clinical, 192*(Complete), 119.

Ruffle, J. K., Farmer, A. D., Kano, M., Giampietro, V., Aziz, Q., and **Coen, S. J.** (2015b). The influence of extraversion on brain activity at baseline and during the experience and expectation of visceral pain. *Personality and Individual Differences, 74*(0), 248–53.

Ruffle, J. K., Coen, S. J., Giampietro, V., Williams, S. C. R., Farmer, A. D., and **Aziz, Q.** (2017a). Higher baseline cardiac vagal tone implicates a subcortical functional brain network during acute oesophageal pain. *Neurogastroenterology and Motility, 29*((Suppl. 2)), 47–8.

Ruffle, J. K., Coen, S. J., Giampietro, V., Williams, S. C. R., Farmer, A. D., and **Aziz, Q.** (2017b). OC-054 Pain endophenotypes can be accurately predicted by whole brain connectivity during painful oesophageal stimulation. *Gut, 66*(Suppl. 2), A28.

Ruffle, J. K., Coen, S. J., Giampietro, V., Williams, S. C. R., Apkarian, A. V., Farmer, A. D., et al. (2018). Morphology of subcortical brain nuclei is associated with autonomic function in healthy humans. *Human Brain Mapping*, January *39*(1), 381–92.

Sanger, G. J. and **Andrews, P. L.** (2006). Treatment of nausea and vomiting: Gaps in our knowledge. *Autonomic Neuroscience, 129*(1–2), 3–16.

Schaub, N., Kano, M., Farmer, A. D., Aziz, Q., and **Coen, S. J.** (2013). Su2109 The Influence of the 5-HTTLPR Genotype on the cerebral processing of esophageal pain—A pilot study. *Gastroenterology, 144*(5), S-560.

Seminowicz, D. A., Labus, J. S., Bueller, J. A., Tillisch, K., Naliboff, B. D., Bushnell, M. C., et al. (2010). Regional gray matter density changes in brains of patients with irritable bowel syndrome. *Gastroenterology, 139*(1), 48–57 e2.

Sommer, F. and **Backhed, F.** (2013). The gut microbiota—Masters of host development and physiology. *Nature Reviews Microbiology, 11*(4), 227–38.

Spaziani, R., Bayati, A., Redmond, K., Bajaj, H., Mazzadi, S., Bienenstock, J., et al. (2008). Vagal dysfunction in irritable bowel syndrome assessed by rectal distension and baroreceptor sensitivity. *Neurogastroenterology and Motility, 20*(4), 336–42.

Spiller, R. and **Lam, C.** (2012). An update on post-infectious irritable bowel syndrome: Role of genetics, immune activation, serotonin and altered microbiome. *Journal of Neurogastroenterology and Motility, 18*(3), 258–68.

Stein, J. L., **Wiedholz, L. M.**, **Bassett, D. S.**, **Weinberger, D. R.**, **Zink, C. F.**, **Mattay, V. S.**, et al. (2007). A validated network of effective amygdala connectivity. *Neuroimage*, *36*(3), 736–45.

Tack, J., **Bisschops, R.**, and **Sarnelli, G.** (2004). Pathophysiology and treatment of functional dyspepsia. *Gastroenterology*, *127*(4), 1239–55.

Tack, J., **Broekaert, D.**, **Fischler, B.**, **Van Oudenhove, L.**, **Gevers, A. M.**, and **Janssens, J.** (2006). A controlled crossover study of the selective serotonin reuptake inhibitor citalopram in irritable bowel syndrome. *Gut*, *55*(8), 1095–103.

Tillisch, K. and **Labus, J. S.** (2011). Advances in imaging the brain–gut axis: Functional gastrointestinal disorders. *Gastroenterology*, *140*(2), 407–11 e1.

Tillisch, K., **Mayer, E. A.**, and **Labus, J. S.** (2011). Quantitative meta-analysis identifies brain regions activated during rectal distension in irritable bowel syndrome. *Gastroenterology*, *140*(1), 91–100.

Tracey, I., **Ploghaus, A.**, **Gati, J. S.**, **Clare, S.**, **Smith, S.**, **Menon, R. S.**, et al. (2002). Imaging attentional modulation of pain in the periaqueductal gray in humans. *Journal of Neuroscience*, *22*(7), 2748–52.

Tracey, I. and **Bushnell, M. C.** (2009). How neuroimaging studies have challenged us to rethink: Is chronic pain a disease? *Journal of Pain*, *10*(11), 1113–20.

Tracey, I. (2011). Can neuroimaging studies identify pain endophenotypes in humans? *Nature Reviews Neurology*, *7*(3), 173–81.

Van Oudenhove, L., **Coen, S. J.**, and **Aziz, Q.** (2007). Functional brain imaging of gastrointestinal sensation in health and disease. *World Journal of Gastroenterology*, *13*(25), 3438–45.

Winkelmann, T., **Thayer, J. F.**, **Pohlack, S.**, **Nees, F.**, **Grimm, O.**, and **Flor, H.** (2016). Structural brain correlates of heart rate variability in a healthy young adult population. *Brain Structure and Function*, *222*(2), 1061–8.

Chapter 6

The cutaneous borders of interoception: Active and social inference of pain and pleasure on the skin

Mariana von Mohr and Aikaterini Fotopoulou

6.1 Introduction

Humans are capable of conscious feelings that concern the state of the body, such as pain, itch, muscular and visceral sensations, hunger, thirst, sexual desire, and air need. The classification of such feelings, and particularly their relation to the more classical sensory systems for vision, audition, and touch, as well as to emotions such as anger and happiness, has been a matter of ongoing debate. Unlike sight, smell, and hearing that have dedicated sensory organs, there are no dedicated bodily organs for position and movement sense, pain, and many other modalities. Instead, developments in physics, anatomy, and physiology since the nineteenth century have given rise to a wide interest in mapping and classifying the senses with reference to criteria such as the nature of the stimulus, anatomy and location of receptors across body parts, the pathways to and the representation of the signal at the central nervous system (CNS), as well as the quality of the experience. This interest led to a number of classifications of the senses; for example, in exteroceptive (their receptive field "lies freely open to the numberless vicissitudes and agencies of the environment" Sherrington, 1910, p. 132), interoceptive (sensory receptors located within the body and primarily in the viscera), and proprioceptive sensations (receptors in muscles, tendons, and joints detecting position and movement of the body). Since this influential classification (see Ceunen, Vlaeyen, & Van Diest, 2016 for a review), exteroceptive and proprioceptive systems have received far more attention than interoceptive modalities. However, as this volume exemplifies, this has changed in the two last decades. On the one hand, theories and studies in affective neuroscience (e.g. Damasio, 2010) have brought to the foreground William James's older idea that interoceptive sensations may lie at the heart of our emotions and self-awareness. On the other hand, progress in anatomy and physiology has urged certain researchers (e.g. Craig, 2002) to propose alternative classifications of the senses that include a more encompassing definition of interoception as the sense of the physiological condition of the entire body, not just the viscera.

Bud Craig's proposal relies in synthesizing findings regarding the functional anatomy of a lamina I spinothalamocortical pathway that is portrayed as the long-missing afferent complement of the efferent autonomic nervous system, underlying distinct, conscious, affective bodily feelings such as cool, warm, itch, first (pricking) pain, second (burning) pain, pleasant or sensual touch, muscle burn, joint ache, visceral fullness, flush, nausea, cramps, hunger, thirst, and visceral taste (Craig, 2002). Specifically, he proposes that the primate brain has evolved a direct sensory pathway to the thalamus that provides a modality-specific representation of various individual aspects of the physiological condition of the body (interoception redefined; Craig 2002, 2003a). This pathway is thought to originate in lamina I of the spinal dorsal horn and in the nucleus of the solitary tract in the caudal medulla, and to represent the afferent inputs from sympathetic (somatic) and parasympathetic nerves, respectively, and to terminate with a posterior-to-anterior somatotopic organization in a specific thalamic structure (the posterior and basal parts of the ventral medial nucleus, Craig 2002). He has further proposed that the functional role of this pathway is to represent the sensory aspects of homeostatic emotions (Craig 2003a, 2008) and their accompanying motivations (represented in anterior cingulate cortex) that serve to maintain the body in relative stability despite ongoing internal and external changes (e.g. variabilities in metabolic energy levels and the availability of food). This proposal brings the concept of interoception into a tight relation to the notion of homeostasis (Cannon, 1929, see also Chapter 1 and Chapter 15 by Corcoran and Jakob Hohwy in the present volume), so that interoception is the sensory representation of the physiological condition of the whole body allowing homeostatic, and ultimately 'allostatic' control (i.e. self-initiated temporary change in homeostatic imperatives to prepare for a predicted external change). In other words, interoceptive signals provide information regarding current homeostatic levels (e.g. reduced glucose levels in the blood), which are used as motivations to steer action (e.g. ingest food to restore glucose levels). This definition of interoception, which subsumes cutaneous pain, itch, and pleasant touch, differs greatly from the classic association of these modalities with exteroception and particularly discriminatory touch. Moreover, in addition to this "spinal pathway," there are also other proposed interoceptive pathways (Critchley & Harrison, 2013), and more broad proposals regarding the role of higher order processing in interoception (Ceunen et al., 2016).

We will here focus on pleasant touch and cutaneous pain, which are two interoceptive (Craig, 2003a, 2003b) sub-modalities of touch that have contrasting affective qualities (pleasantness/unpleasantness) and social meanings (care/harm). Although the source of the skin stimulation lies outside the body and the resulting sensations can be used to gain information about how, where, and by what one is touched, we also assume that these modalities are of fundamental homeostatic importance, signalling physiological safety (i.e. the pleasantness of touch signifies a homeostatically safe environment in is contact with the body) or threat (i.e. pain signifies the reverse) to the organism and leading to certain behavioral and physiological reactions of homeostatic and allostatic significance. In the present chapter, we first briefly outline the current literature on the peripheral and central neurophysiology of unpleasant, cutaneous pain and affective, pleasant touch. Subsequently, we make use of recent neurocomputational theories of perception and action, as applied to both exteroceptive and interoceptive modalities, to put forward a unifying model of how bottom-up and top-down signals can be integrated to give rise to these modalities. We speculate that the understanding of these modalities within the Bayesian predictive coding framework of "active inference" (Friston, 2010) offers a unique opportunity to unify various insights into a common framework that emphasizes particularly: (a) the deep interdependence between bottom-up and top-down mechanisms in any modality; (b) the deep interdependence of perception and action in any modality; (c) the special role of these modalities in homeostatic and allostatic control; and (d) the particular relevance of social developmental factors in determining the salience of interoceptive modalities such as pain and pleasant touch.

6.2 The peripheral and central neurophysiology of cutaneous pain and pleasant touch

Surrogate animal models and human studies have revealed that nociceptors are distinctive afferent units rather than the extremes of a single class of receptors with a continuum of features (reviewed by Marks et al., 2006). While low-threshold, mechanoreceptive, or thermoreceptive afferent neurons cannot discriminate reliably between noxious and non-noxious (innocuous) stimulation, nociceptors can (Bessou et al., 1971). These two classes of fibers also differ in their termination patterns in the spinal cord (Sugiura, Lee, & Perl, 1986), their membrane constituents (Caterina et al., 1997), and properties, including their action potential shape (Ritter & Mendell, 1992). Broadly, nociceptors can be divided into two types: A- (most in the Aδ- range) and C-fibers, which are mediated by myelinated fast (5–30 m/s) and unmyelinated slow (0.4–1.4m/s) conductive axons (Dubin & Patapoutian, 2010), corresponding to initial fast-onset pain (sharp pain sensation) and slow second pain (pervasive burning pain sensation), respectively. Nociceptors, particularly in musculoskeletal tissue, have been mostly thought to be electrically 'silent', transmitting all or no action potentials only when excited, and thus give rise to pain (Marks et al., 2006).

Different pathways on how the nociceptor is conveyed to the CNS have been suggested, including different spinal neural features and their functional role. First, it is thought that an afferent volley is produced upon activation of the nociceptor. The nociceptive volley travels along the periphery and enters the dorsal horn of the spinal cord (Brooks & Tracey, 2005) and mostly terminates in laminae I where they synapse with relay neurons and local interneurons important for signal modification (see Dubin & Patapoutian, 2010 for the specific role of laminae I, IV, and V in relation to A- and C- fibers). Via spinal ascending pathways, the relay neurons project to the thalamus and brainstem, which in turn project to large distributed brain networks (Dubin & Patapoutian, 2010). However, a different type of multimodal spinal neurons located deeper in the dorsal horn, namely the wide dynamic (WDR) neurons, has also been implicated in nociceptive and pain-related mechanisms (Perl, 2007).

More generally, peripheral neurophysiological specificity does not seem to lead to a direct relation between nociception and conscious pain perception. While the activation of nociceptors and nociceptive pathways can lead to pain (Marks et al., 2006), it is also known that nociceptors can be active in the absence of pain perception and pain can occur without known nociceptive activity. Indeed, there have been observations of a lack of reported pain by soldiers during battle, despite severe injuries, as well as experimental evidence suggesting that pain perception varies with psychological state and context (Head & Holmes, 1911; Melzack, Wall, & Ty, 1982). In fact, since the proposal of the influential "gate control theory" (inhibition of nociceptive excitatory signalling at the level of the spinal cord), and more recent insights regarding the heightened sensitivity of afferent signals at the same level, known as "central sensitization," it is widely accepted that although much pain is a consequence of stimulation of peripheral nociceptors, the CNS plays a major role in the processing of noxious sensations (Melzack & Wall, 1965).

Furthermore, more potent neuroscientific methods in recent decades have provided corroborating evidence for the role of the brain in pain (Rainville et al., 1997; Ploghaus et al., 1999; Ploner, Freund, & Schnitzler, 1999). For example, novel cortical stimulation studies have qualified Penfield's inability to detect 'pain cortical areas' (Mazzola et al., 2011). Moreover, functional neuroimaging studies indicate that noxious stimulation involves large distributed brain networks (Brooks & Tracey, 2005; Talbot et al., 1991). The so-called pain matrix has been subdivided into a medial and lateral pain system, based on their respective projection sites from the thalamic structures to the cortex. The lateral pain system involves the S1 and secondary somatosensory cortex (S2) and is thought to play a role in the sensory-discriminative aspect of pain (i.e. where is the stimulus and how intense it is), whereas the medial pain system, including areas such as the AAC, the insula, and the amygdala, is thought to be involved in the affective-cognitive aspect of pain. However, the insular cortex may play a role in facilitating the integration of information between the lateral and medial pain systems (Brooks & Tracey, 2005) and some studies suggest that the functional role of these areas may not be pain-specific but rather relating to the processing of all sensory-salient events (see Legrain et al., 2011). Nevertheless, it is assumed that a top-down descending circuitry modulates ascending nociceptive information and consequently, influences pain perception. Hence, scientific and health organizations such as the International Association for the Study of Pain stress the difference between nociception and pain. However, debates regarding the bottom-up versus the top-down contributions to pain and their corresponding definitions remain. Similar debates surround the study of pleasant touch.

Recent research suggests that slow conducting unmyelinated (non-nociceptive) afferent CT fibers mediate the affective, pleasant component of touch. These C-fiber tactile afferents were first identified in a cat in 1939 by showing low spike heights using the skin-nerve preparation technique (Zotterman, 1939). More recently, low threshold mechanosensitive C-fibers (C-LTMs; detected by cutaneous sensory neurons, i.e. C-low threshold mechanoreceptors, C-LTMRs) have been found in the hairy skin of rodents and primates (Bessou et al., 1971). C-LTMs are now acknowledged also to exist in human skin, termed CT afferents (Vallbo, Olausson, & Wessberg, 1999). CTs have different characteristics than myelinated fast conducting Aβ-fibers associated with discriminative touch, including their conduction axon velocity (0.6–1.3 m/s) and skin location (i.e. found in hairy but not glabrous skin).

Microneurography studies have shown that CTs are highly sensitive mechanoreceptors responding to stimuli that are clearly innocuous, and their firing rate seems to be distinct from myelinated afferents, reflecting an inverted U-shaped relationship between the stroking velocity and mean firing rate with the most vigorous responses being at 1–10 cm/s (Löken et al., 2009). Moreover, subjective responses of perceived pleasantness in response to stroking also showed an inverted U-shape relationship, with the highest pleasantness responses found at 1–10 cm/s stroking velocities (Löken et al., 2009), indicating that CT afferents may carry a positive hedonic quality. Furthermore, CTs are also temperature sensitive (i.e. preferentially discharged ≈ 32°C, the typical skin temperature; Ackerley et al., 2014). However, one main difficulty in our understanding of selective CT stimulation is related to the fact that to date, we cannot stimulate CT fibers without stimulating Aβ-fibers in healthy subjects. Nevertheless, insights have been provided from patients with sensory neuropathy, as these patients are thought to lack Aβ afferents while their CTs afferents remain intact (Olausson et al., 2002, 2008). Research has shown that CT stimulation in these patients activates the insula (i.e. the preferential cortical target for CT afferents), but not somatosensory regions associated with the sensory discriminative processing of touch (Olausson et al., 2002). Moreover, these patients were able to detect, although poorly, slow brushing on the forearm (where CTs are abundant; Olausson et al., 2008). Given the sensory discriminative properties associated with Aβ-fibers and the lack thereof in these patients, it is possible to presume that CT afferents may follow a separate neurophysiological route than Aβ mediated discriminative touch (Olausson et al., 2008).

Unfortunately, our knowledge of how CTs peripheral information reaches spinal, brainstem, and cortical areas in humans remains scarce, yet meaningful insights regarding the spinal processing of CTs have been obtained from animal studies. Mice studies suggest that C-LTMS enter the laminae II of the dorsal horn, with axons arborizing in lamina I, where they would synapse with secondary afferent neurons (reviewed by McGlone, Wessberg, & Olausson, 2014). Secondary afferent neurons then project to higher centers such as the insula via spinal pathways (Andrew, 2010). Furthermore, as with pain, there could be different classes of spinal neurons responsive to gentle touch, including WDR neurons (Andrew, 2010). Finally, yet controversially, recent findings using mice genetic tools indicate the dorsal horn as the key initial focus for integration of Aβ and C-LTMRs (Abraira & Ginty, 2013). Together, these lines of inquiry suggest that there may be different pathways through which CT peripheral information is conveyed to higher centers, although these pathways may likely vary across species.

Similar to pain, neuroimaging research has shown that gentle stroking activates the posterior superior temporal sulcus, medial prefrontal cortex, orbitofrontal cortex (OFC), and ACC, which are typically implicated in the cognitive-affective aspects of pleasant touch (Gordon et al., 2013). Further, while investigating the cortical areas that represent pleasant touch, painful touch, and neutral touch, studies have also found increased activity in the OFC in response to pleasant and painful touch, highlighting the role of the OFC on the affective aspects of the touch. In contrast, the somatosensory cortex was less activated by pleasant and painful touch, relative to neutral touch (Rolls et al., 2003; see also Gordon et al., 2013; Olausson et al., 2002). These studies suggest that CT-based touch may not be involved in the discriminative aspects of touch. Importantly, slow gentle touch on CT skin has also been shown to preferentially activate the insula (Olausson et al., 2002; Gordon et al., 2013), although the insula also plays a critical role in integrating sensory-discriminative and affective-cognitive aspects of the touch (McCabe et al., 2008; Rolls, 2010).

6.3 An integration: The predictive, active, and social components of pain and pleasant touch

The history of the study of pain, and more recently of pleasant touch can be said to be steeped in the debates between bottom-up, neurophysiological specificity at the periphery versus top-down convergence and gating at the spinal and brain levels. In this section, we make use of a Bayesian, predictive coding framework, namely the Free Energy Principle, also referred to as "active inference" (Friston, 2010) to put forward a unifying model of how bottom-up and top-down signals can be integrated to give rise to affective, pleasant touch and unpleasant, cutaneous pain.

6.3.1 Action–perception loops and the control of physiological states

Recent neurocomputational theories of perception and action assume that the brain is an organ that learns and self-improves a generative model of the organism and its environment based on sensory signals and action (Friston, 2010). A basic tenet of such accounts is that perception is an active process, whereby top-down mechanisms are activated to make predictions about the upcoming bottom-up sensory signals. Thus, perception is an inferential process, whose aim is to minimize prediction errors or the difference between top-down hypotheses about the most likely causes of sensations (termed "empirical prior beliefs") and current sensations. Recurrent message passing among several levels of the sensorimotor hierarchy allows the suppression of (small or irrelevant) prediction errors by priors, or the adjustment of (empirical) prior expectations by (large or highly salient) prediction errors. Furthermore, the relative influence of predictions versus prediction errors across several layers in this hierarchical organization is determined by the weighting (precision) of predictions versus prediction errors at each level. Precision can be regarded as a measure of signal-to-noise ratio or confidence, or mathematically, as the inverse variance, uncertainty, or reliability of a signal (Feldman & Friston, 2010; Friston et al., 2012). Uncertainty is thought of as encoded mainly by neuromodulations of synaptic gain (such as dopamine and acetylcholine) that encode the precision of random fluctuations about predicted states — the context in which sensory data is encountered (Quattrocki &

Friston, 2014). For example, cholinergic or dopaminergic neuromodulatory mechanisms can optimize the attentional gain of populations encoding prediction errors, so that greater attention is allocated to certain salient events in the environment, influencing the relative weighting or importance of prediction errors.

Importantly, prediction errors can also be minimized through action. At the simplest control loop level, peripheral reflexes are engaged to suppress proprioceptive prediction errors (Feldman & Friston, 2010), generated by comparing primary afferents from receptors in muscles, tendons, and joints with proprioceptive predictions regarding body position that descend to alpha motor neurons in the spinal cord and cranial nerve nuclei. Thus, action is driven by such predictions rather than descending motor commands. Ultimately, action is seen as a prediction-driven tendency to re-sample the world to generate more sensory evidence for one's predictions (active inference). Critically, the organism could solve a discrepancy between prediction and error (e.g. unexpected noxious stimulation) by either changing its predictions (effectively convincing oneself that one is not in pain) or by generating protecting action (moving to avoid the noxious source of the prediction error). Both of these can be adaptive depending on the magnitude as well as the context of the noxious stimulation and hence, their relation needs to be optimized by weighting in each case. This framework emphasizes the tight interconnection of perception and action as well as the fundamental integration of bottom-up and top-down factors in all perceptual and active inference.

Recently several proposals have applied this framework to interoception (Paulus & Stein, 2006; Barrett & Simmons, 2015; Gu et al., 2013; Pezzulo, Rigoli, & Friston, 2015; Seth, 2013; Seth, Suzuki, & Critchley, 2011), and by extension to the concepts of "homeostatic" and "allostatic" control (see also Chapter 15 in the present volume). "Homeostasis" (Cannon, 1929) refers to the maintenance of a relative stability in one's physiological states despite ongoing internal and external changes. "Allostasis" refers to the idea that physiological changes need to be anticipated by adaptive changes and choices across different spatial and temporal scales, for example adjusting one's metabolic needs in certain environments where foraging is dangerous (Sterling & Eyer, 1988). In predictive coding frameworks, both homeostatic and allostatic control can be cast formally as active inference (e.g. Pezzulo et al., 2015; Stephan et al., 2016). Homeostatic control enslaves reflexes to produce corrective actions that fulfill beliefs about bodily states, and allostatic control entails changing homeostatic beliefs under guidance by higher predictive models about future perturbations of bodily states.

Moreover, as in the case of exteroceptive perception and action, the balance between homeostatic and allostatic regulation rests upon the precision (i.e. weighting) placed in deeper expectations about the organism and its environment. For example, during conditions of bodily threat or psychological stress, such as the anticipated pain from a sharp object approaching one's face, noxious signals on one's body may induce low-level proprioceptive predictions that mobilize withdrawal movements away from the source of the stimulation. However, high-precision predictions at a higher level of the neurocognitive hierarchy may indicate that the source of the noxious stimulation is actually our dentist, and then predictions of tooth pain can be fulfilled without engaging low-level motor reflexes and instead engage allostatic changes in the form of updated beliefs about the "safety" and tolerance (i.e. attenuated pain) of nociceptive signals in this context, in order to ensure future pain-free and healthy teeth.

6.3.2 Active, interoceptive inference, and feelings on the skin

Despite these proposals of interoceptive predictive coding, there is currently no direct evidence for the proposal that interoceptive predictions, prediction errors, and their relation rest on a common neurocomputational framework (for a first step, see Kleckner et al., 2017). There are, however, ample circumstantial findings in the pain and pleasant touch literature that can be cast in this light and importantly, the framework can allow some specific predictions regarding the nature of pain and pleasant touch, and their modulation by cognitive and social factors, that we will focus on here.

First, this framework suggests that peripheral signals, such as nociceptive and CT tactile channels, do not cause homeostatic perceptions or emotions (e.g. pain or the affectivity of touch), or vice versa. Instead, there is a circular and multi-layered causality, where on one end of the neural hierarchy, neuronally encoded predictions about bodily states, including in this case states of the skin, engage autonomic, somatic, and motor reflexes in a top-down fashion. On the other end of the hierarchy, specialized skin organs and their spinal cord circuitry carry interoceptive signals in a bottom-up way that informs and updates predictions at the levels above. These aspects can be linked to the cognitive and sensory aspects of pain, respectively. Moreover, the affective component of pain or touch can be seen as an attribute of the weighting (precision, see earlier) of any representation that generates predictions and prediction errors about the physiological state of the skin (see also Ainley et al., 2016; Fotopoulou, 2013). In other terms, the subjective feelings of pain or pleasant touch can be linked to the neuromodulatory weighting of the corresponding sensory prediction errors in relation to higher-order predictions regarding these sensory states. Typically, the optimization of precision is linked with the function of neuromodulators in the brain (see section 6.3.1) but similar processes of synaptic gain modulation have long been described in the spinal cord, particularly in the context of pain (see section 6.2.). We have previously proposed that in interoceptive modalities, optimizing the precision of internal body signals can be seen as optimizing *interoceptive sensitivity and related feelings* in perceptual inference (see also Ainley et al., 2016; Fotopoulou, 2013). We propose here that concepts such as "precision" and its reverse, uncertainty, relate to the affective, conscious components of pain and pleasant touch. The intensity of painful or pleasurable aspects of touch can be thus understood as our sensitivity to such tactile, interoceptive signals in a given context (e.g. a measurement of our subjective pain threshold in the lab) and our corresponding behavioral tendency to approach the world to gather more information (uncertainty) or to avoid resampling (the certainty of pain and pleasant touch). This view can offer a new integration of previous theories of pain and hence potentially also pleasant touch, as we specify in the following.

Specifically, classic theories may view cutaneous pain and the affectivity of touch as signals of danger or safety to the organism respectively, starting in the periphery and reaching consciousness if a "threshold" is surpassed at the spinal cord level, allowing the brain to "read" them as pain or pleasure. For example, this threshold may be equated to the "gate control theory" (Melzack & Wall, 1965) or more modern "central sensitization" theories, where the gain of the spinal cord nociceptive synapse is amplified and hence "travels up" the hierarchy to elicit conscious pain (Woolf & Salter, 2000). On the contrary, more "active," alternative theories of pain suggest that acute pain is not a warning signal but rather is the failure of the "aversion" machinery (nociceptor activity) designed to operate unconsciously in order to avoid harm and ultimately also conscious pain (Baliki & Apkarian, 2015). In such accounts, most nociceptive activity is designed to remain "subconscious" and protect the organism from harm without necessarily eliciting conscious pain. Conscious pain instead only emerges when subconscious pain is converted to conscious pain in subcortical areas in the brain. In such accounts, it is conscious pain that has the capacity to modulate spinal nociceptive sensitivity and thus actively determine "gate control" and/or "central sensitization" spinal nociceptive processes, mediated through descending pathways (Vera-Portocarrero et al., 2006).

From the point of view of active inference models, these are not competing but supplementary views. Allostatic control is an extension of homeostatic control and they both work to minimize prediction errors. Thus, these two perspectives can be integrated in the following way, illustrated here with specific reference to cutaneous pain and pleasant touch. For homeostatic control purposes, the organism entails (in an embodied manner) a set of inherited prior expectations of the state of the skin. Any stimulation of the skin that deviates from the range of such predicted states generates a prediction error. This prediction error is corrected in simple, unconscious loops, by reflexive motor or autonomic reactions that fulfil the initial beliefs about the state of the skin. If, however, these "homeostatic corrections" fail (i.e. the prediction error persists), then the prediction error travels up the hierarchy to generate posterior beliefs (updated predictions) at the above hierarchical level. These updated beliefs act as priors towards future positive or negative events, thus attempting to anticipate and avoid danger, or anticipate and approach pleasure, before these occur (allostasis). Specifically, more complex, generative, predictive models of the organism's needs are better able to predict stimuli at the levels below and at different time-scales and hence 'suppress' any future, anticipated prediction errors at the level below by guiding autonomic function and action more effectively and under the control of higher-order predictive models. Please note that these homeostatic and allostatic control operations are understood to be processes of unconscious inference for the most part, so conscious feelings of skin pain and pleasure are not necessary for such processes. This conclusion, however, raises the question of why should we have conscious feelings such as pain and pleasure, if we can predict and control our sensations unconsciously? We speculatively propose that it is important that the organism registers the core feelings that relate to the specificity of innate, homeostatic needs (in this case safe or dangerous contact on the skin), so that the cognitive resources available for scanning the world and the body for novelty and salience are always constrained by, and in competition with, the high precision of our innate expectations. In other terms, conscious pain and pleasant touch are there to ensure that we do not habitually update, or ignore our predictions about what is safe versus dangerous for the skin.

Interestingly, although these two modalities, pain and unpleasant touch, appear opposite in hedonic content and behavior tendencies towards their particular sensory stimulus (i.e. avoidance versus approach), from the point of view of the certainty–uncertainty axis described here, they are of similar characteristics. The greater the pain, or the felt pleasure of touch, the more one's attention and behavior is captured in the experience and the less one is likely to engage in active, exploration of new sensations. Instead, the organism's resources are focused on controlling or escaping pain, and enjoying or prolonging the feelings of pleasant touch. This view goes against the intuitive, long-standing view of core affective consciousness, pain and pleasure, as monitoring hedonic quality. Instead, the core quality of affective consciousness is a kind of certainty–uncertainty, or disambiguation principle (Fotopoulou, 2013). Pain and pleasant touch therefore are a measure of how important is for a given organism, in a given context, to be "certain" about what was predicted versus what occurred.

This view of the conscious feelings of pain and pleasant touch tallies with long-standing insights regarding the dissociation between sensory and affective aspects of pain and, more recently, pleasant touch, as well as with the fact that the physiology of nociception has a well-known specificity at the periphery which is not mirrored at the brain (see section 6.2). The unique feeling qualities of painful or pleasant touch may be associated with the CNS's capacity for synaptic gain modulation and large-scale integration of information arising from the body and the world in different time-scales. This is consistent with the fact that no single area or network in the brain has been reliably associated with the conscious perception of pain (Baliki & Apkarian, 2015). Instead, the various networks that have been associated with pain and its modulation, and with pleasant touch and its modulation, are not only common to these two modalities, but seem relevant to the processing of the salience of any sensory modality (Legrain et al., 2011). Indeed, several recent neuroimaging studies have included such areas and their observed functional connectivity in various hypothesized "salience networks" (Legrain et al., 2011; Medford & Critchley, 2010; Wiech et al., 2010). For instance, predictive signals from such a "salience network" process and integrate information about the significance of an impending noxious stimulus and determine whether or not such a stimulus will be consciously perceived as painful (Wiech et al., 2010).

More generally, a plethora of neuroimaging studies have shown that cognitive, affective, and social factors modulate our perception of cutaneous pain, with emerging evidence also making a case for these factors modulating the pleasantness of CT-optimal touch. For example, expectations may help an individual to adjust sensory, cognitive, and motor systems in order to process the noxious stimuli in terms of neural and behavioral responses optimally (Wiech, Ploner, & Tracey, 2008; see also Villemure & Brushnell, 2002 for review). Most consistently with the present proposal, expectations in which there is a high level of certainty regarding the stimulus may activate descending control systems to attenuate pain, whereas in contrast, uncertainty may increase pain (Ploghaus et al., 2003).

Although there is less evidence on the neural mechanisms underlying the cognitive and social factors that modulate pleasant CT-optimal touch, studies suggest that a person's beliefs about the stimulus (McCabe et al., 2008) or the person (Ellingsen et al., 2015) providing the pleasant touch influences the perceived pleasantness of the touch. We use the example of the social modulation of pain in the following to unpack and illustrate these ideas further.

6.3.3 The mentalization of nociception and CT stimulation: homeostatic and allostatic control by proxy

The long-observed fact that conscious pain is modulated by social context has received experimental support in recent years (see Krahé et al., 2013 for review). In the last decade, similar observations have also been made regarding the modulation of pleasant touch by social context. In this section, we will apply these insights from the active inference framework to propose some mechanisms by which this social modulation takes place. This application has the advantage that it can provide a mechanistic, unified account of the relation between bottom-up (e.g. neurophysiological) and top-down (e.g. psychosocial) influences on homeostasis and allostasis. Existing biopsychosocial models of pain offer similar insights but the current model has the advantage of offering direct links between these different bottom-up and top-down determinants of pain and pleasant touch instead of treating them as merely additive variables.

Specifically, we propose that the perception of the social environment of pain or pleasant touch can affect inferential processes about the perception of these modalities, as well as related active tendencies, by influencing the certainty or precision of an individual's predictions about an impending stimulus versus the certainty or precision of related prediction errors. As mentioned earlier, top-down predictions do not represent just the content of lower level representations but also predict their context, defined in mathematical terminology as the *precision* of a probability distribution (inverse variance or uncertainty). For example, the allocation of attention toward specific events can optimize their salience and ultimately influence the relative weighting or importance of prediction errors against predictions. This kind of top-down prediction in sensory cortices is thought to be mediated by cholinergic neuromodulatory mechanisms that optimize the attentional gain of populations encoding prediction errors (Feldman & Friston, 2010), as well as by dopamine in fronto-striatal circuits (Fiorillo, Tobler, & Schultz, 2003) and by neuropeptides such as oxytocin in social contexts (Quatrokki & Friston, 2014). In interoception, precision may relate to attention to signals from the body or interoceptive sensitivity (Ainley et al., 2016; Fotopoulou, 2013) and may be modulated by several contextual factors. Therefore, factors such as active social support or empathy may modulate pain or pleasant touch by changing the precision of top-down predictions about nociception or CT stimulation. In such social contexts, individuals have learned to anticipate social support and thus the optimization of the weight allocated to bottom-up signals versus top-down predictions maybe different than in conditions of experiencing similar stimuli alone, or in hostile environments. For example, in previous studies we have shown that the administration of intranasal oxytocin versus placebo, or the provision of high versus low empathy, or social support may modulate the subjective, behavioral and neural responses to noxious stimulation (Hurter et al., 2014; Krahé et al., 2015; Paloyelis et al., 2016). More generally, based on a systematic review of the experimental pain literature (Krahé et al., 2013), we have concluded that precision modulation by interpersonal interactions takes several forms, including two main categories: (a) social signals about the safety or threat and thus the salience of the impending stimulus itself, and (b) social signals about the threat or safety and thus the salience of the environment in which the stimulus occurs. In turn, the perception and interpretation of such interpersonal variables themselves may in turn depend on (a) their own salience, as well as (b) an individual's prior beliefs about interpersonal relating and associated behaviors (see following for further details).

This notion of social modulation as precision modulation is compatible with previous theories such as the social baseline theory, which proposes that the presence of other people helps individuals to conserve metabolically costly somatic and neural resources through the social regulation of emotion (Beckes & Coan, 2011; see also Decety & Fotopoulou, 2015). Integrating such notions within a predictive coding model has the advantage of placing them in a wider and neurobiologically plausible framework and hence integrating findings across many fields, as well as generating novel hypotheses, as we outline here.

6.3.3.1 Developmental considerations: The social origins of interoceptive inference

The active inference framework we propose allows us to observe that the social modulation of pain and pleasant touch is not a simple "add-on" in our understanding of such modalities. Rather, it appears that interpersonal interactions are necessary in shaping all interoceptive modalities from the onset. This claim is supported by several observations (presented in detail elsewhere, Fotopoulou & Tsakiris, 2017), the most important of which we outline here: namely, in early infancy, when the human motor system is not yet developed, interoceptive function and homeostasis are wholly dependent on embodied interactions with other bodies. Action and perception do not mature at the same time. As human infants are born without a fully matured motor system, and hence they cannot regulate their own homeostasis unaided, the actions of their caregivers necessarily determine how they come to update their beliefs by active inference and ultimately how they experience all their sensations and particularly those requiring purposeful actions. For example, young infants cannot position, balance, feed, thermoregulate, or protect themselves from accidentally cutting or burning their skin (beyond some reflexive avoidance movements). Thus, in the case of these interoceptive modalities, *no available movement on the part of the infant alone can change certain key neurophysiological states relating to homeostasis and allostasis*. As such, the young infant cannot use action to collect evidence about the causes of interoceptive experience to test its interoceptive predictions against the world.

Instead, infants use autonomic and motor reflexes in response to unpredicted physiological states (e.g. crying when hypothalamic function detect that glucose level are not within the predicted viable range) to elicit caregivers' actions that can change the infant's physiological state (e.g. by feeding it) until the homeostatic needs are met (i.e. glucose levels are within the predicted range). Thus, updating interoceptive predictions in infants (close the action–perception loop) includes multisensory signals regarding the reaction of caregivers to infants' initial autonomic and proprioceptive predictions; a process we have termed as the "mentalization" of physiological states elsewhere; Fotopoulou & Tsakiris, 2017). In other words, the origins of interoceptive active inference are always by necessity social, and thus core subjective feelings such as hunger and satiation, pain and relief, cold or warmth, have actually social origins.

6.3.3.2 Adult predictions about the role of others in pain and pleasant touch

These conclusions about the social origins of interoceptive feelings such as pain and pleasant touch are also consistent with the literature on the relation between these modalities and social attachment (see also Panksepp, 1998). As we mentioned earlier, pain and pleasant touch may be modulated by social factors. In turn, the perception and interpretation of social variables themselves may depend on individual prior beliefs, or generative models about interpersonal relating and associated behaviors. One influential way of conceptualizing prior beliefs about relating to others is attachment theory. Attachment theory posits that from early in life, attachment partners can serve as a "secure base" from which the infant explores the world (Bowlby, 1969). If a secure attachment bond is formed over repeated instances of responsive caregiving, the "secure base" signals safety to the infant, while insecure bonds lead to more ambivalent or even threatening signals from others. These bonds lead to the formation of attachment styles, which remain relatively stable into adulthood.

Individual differences in attachment style have been linked directly with the perception of pain and related reactions (e.g. Hurter et al., 2014; Meredith, Ownsworth, & Strong, 2008; Sambo et al., 2010). Moreover, in the clinical pain literature, insecure attachment has been proposed as a vulnerability factor for developing chronic pain (Meredith et al., 2008), supporting its importance as a pain-relevant prior. In a series of pain studies by our lab, we have shown that differences in attachment style influence the effects of interpersonal variables on subjective, behavioral, physiological and neural responses to pain. For example, social contextual factors and individual differences in attachment style determine the amount of subjective report, facial expressions, heart-rate, skin conductance and neural responses people show in response to experimental pain (Sambo et al., 2010; Hurter et al., 2014; Krahe et al., 2015, 2016).

Using laser-evoked potentials (LEPs) we further found that pleasant touch, as a form of active social support, can reduce both subjective and neural pain-related outcomes (Krahe et al., 2016; von Mohr et al., under review). However, contrary to other neuroimaging studies on passive forms of social support between couples (e.g. Coan, Schaefer,

& Davidson, 2006; Eisenberger et al., 2011), our neural effects indicate that the effects of active support by one's romantic partner may begin at earlier stages of cortical nociceptive processing, as reflected by changes in the N1 local peak amplitude (von Mohr et al., under review). The N1 component is thought to reflect pre-perceptual sensory response (outside of conscious awareness), with activation in the operculoinsular and primary somatosensory cortex (Garcia-Larrea, Frot, & Valeriani, 2003; Valentini et al., 2012). Given that LEPs have been recently proposed to detect environmental threat to the body in response to sensory salient events (Legrain et al., 2011), we speculate that pleasant touch by one's romantic partner seems to reduce the sensory salience of impending noxious stimulation.

Similar findings have been reported in relation to the perception of pleasantness and attachment style in response to CT-optimal touch (Krahé et al., under review). Nevertheless, the field of pleasant touch is still at its infancy and further neuroscientific studies are needed in both humans and other animals before firm conclusions can be drawn about the social nature of this modality.

6.4 Conclusion

Cutaneous pain and pleasant touch have been recently classified by some researchers as interoceptive modalities, even if their stimulation site lies outside the body. This reclassification is the basis of a more encompassing definition of interoception itself as the sense of the physiological condition of the entire body, not just the viscera. However, this reclassification lies at the heart of long-standing debates regarding the nature of such modalities and particularly the question of whether they should be defined as sensations on their basis of their bottom-up, neurophysiological specificity at the periphery or as homeostatic emotions on the basis of top-down convergence and modulation at the spinal and brain levels. In the present chapter, we speculatively recast this current state of knowledge within a recent Bayesian predictive coding framework of brain function, namely the active inference model. This framework suggests that peripheral signals, such as nociceptive and CT tactile channels, do not cause homeostatic perceptions or emotions (e.g. pain or pleasant touch), or vice versa. Instead, there is a circular and multilayered causality, where on one end of the neural hierarchy, neuronally encoded predictions about bodily states, including in this case states of the skin, engage autonomic, somatic, and motor reflexes in a top-down fashion. At the other end of the hierarchy, specialized skin organs and their spinal cord circuity carry interoceptive signals in a bottom-up way that informs and updates predictions at the levels above. These aspects can be linked to the cognitive and sensory aspects of pain, respectively. The affective component of pleasant or painful touch is a third component of this circular causality. Such affects are an attribute of the optimisation of the weighting (precision) of any representation that generates predictions and prediction errors about the physiological state of the skin (see also Ainley et al., 2016; Fotopoulou, 2013). This weighting is further not only determined by such specialized modalities and pathways but also necessarily contextualized by concurrent proprioceptive signals, as well as by concurrent exteroceptive cues about the body itself and about the physical, material, and social environment currently and across different time-scales (for allostatic control purposes). The painful or pleasurable aspects of touch can be thus understood as our sensitivity to bottom-up signals in given interoceptive, exteroceptive, cognitive, social, and time contexts and our corresponding behavioral and anticipatory tendencies.

These assumptions have received some empirical support in adult studies from our lab, as well as many other labs, that show that "on-line" social factors such as active social support or empathy, as well as "off-line" predictions about the availability of social help (e.g. individual differences in attachment style), may modulate pain or pleasant touch by changing the precision of top-down predictions versus prediction errors from nociception or CT stimulation. Finally, such claims are supported by the developmental observation that in early infancy, when the human motor system is not yet developed, interoceptive function and homeostasis are dependent on embodied interactions with other bodies. It is the adult's actions that will generate changes in interoceptive states and hence ultimately close the action–perception loop. Thus, the origins of interoceptive active inference are always, by necessity social, and core subjective feelings, such as hunger and satiation, pain and relief, cold or warmth, actually have social origins.

Acknowledgments

This work was supported by the European Research Council (ERC) Starting Grant ERC-2012-STG GA313755 (to AF) and the National Council on Science and Technology (CONACyT- 538843) scholarship (to MVM).

References

Abraira, V. E. and **Ginty, D. D.** (2013). The sensory neurons of touch. *Neuron*, *79*(4), 618–39.

Ackerley, R., Wasling, H. B., Liljencrantz, J., Olausson, H., Johnson, R. D., and **Wessberg, J.** (2014). Human C-tactile afferents are tuned to the temperature of a skin-stroking caress. *Journal of Neuroscience*, *34*(8), 2879–83.

Ainley, V., Apps, M. A., Fotopoulou, A., and **Tsakiris, M.** (2016). "Bodily precision": A predictive coding account of individual differences in interoceptive accuracy. *Philosophical Transactions of the Royal Society B*, *371*(1708), 20160003.

Andrew, D. (2010). Quantitative characterization of low-threshold mechanoreceptor inputs to lamina I spinoparabrachial neurons in the rat. *Journal of Physiology*, *588*(1), 117–24.

Baliki, M. N. and **Apkarian, A. V.** (2015). Nociception, pain, negative moods, and behavior selection. *Neuron*, *87*(3), 474–91.

Barrett, L. F. and **Simmons, W. K.** (2015). Interoceptive predictions in the brain. *Nature Reviews. Neuroscience*, *16*(7), 419.

Beckes, L. and **Coan, J. A.** (2011). Social baseline theory: The role of social proximity in emotion and economy of action. *Social and Personality Psychology Compass*, *5*(12), 976–88.

Bessou, P., Burgess, P. R., Perl, E. R., and **Taylor, C. B.** (1971). Dynamic properties of mechanoreceptors with unmyelinated (C) fibers. *Journal of Neurophysiology*, *34*(1), 116–31.

Bowlby, J. (1969). *Attachment and Loss: Vol. 1. Attachment*. New York, NY: Basic Books.

Brooks, J. and **Tracey, I.** (2005). From nociception to pain perception: Imaging the spinal and supraspinal pathways. *Journal of Anatomy*, *207*(1), 19–33.

Cannon, W. B. (1929). *Bodily Changes in Pain, Hunger, Fear and Rage*, 2nd edn. New York, NY: Appleton.

Caterina, M. J., Schumacher, M. A., Tominaga, M., and **Rosen, T. A.** (1997). The capsaicin receptor: A heat-activated ion channel in the pain pathway. *Nature, 389*(6653), 816.

Ceunen, E., Vlaeyen, J. W., and **Van Diest, I.** (2016). On the origin of interoception. *Frontiers in Psychology, 7*, 743.

Coan, J. A., Schaefer, H. S., and **Davidson, R. J.** (2006). Lending a hand: Social regulation of the neural response to threat. *Psychological Science, 17*(12), 1032–9.

Craig, A. D. (2002). Opinion: How do you feel? Interoception: The sense of the physiological condition of the body. *Nature Reviews Neuroscience, 3*(8), 655.

Craig, A. D. (2003a). Interoception: The sense of the physiological condition of the body. *Current Opinion in Neurobiology, 13*(4), 500–5.

Craig, A. D. (2003b). A new view of pain as a homeostatic emotion. *Trends in Neurosciences, 26*(6), 303–7.

Craig, A. D. (2008). Interoception and emotion: A neuroanatomical perspective. *Handbook of Emotions, 3*(602), 272–88.

Critchley, H. D. and **Harrison, N. A.** (2013). Visceral influences on brain and behavior. *Neuron, 77*(4), 624–38.

Damasio, A. (2010). *Self Comes to Mind: Constructing the Conscious Brain*. New York, NY: Vintage.

Decety, J. and **Fotopoulou, A.** (2015). Why empathy has a beneficial impact on others in medicine: Unifying theories. *Frontiers in Behavioral Neuroscience, 8, 457.*

Dubin, A. E. and **Patapoutian, A.** (2010). Nociceptors: The sensors of the pain pathway. *Journal of Clinical Investigation, 120*(11), 3760.

Eisenberger, N. I., Master, S. L., Inagaki, T. K., Taylor, S. E., Shirinyan, D., Lieberman, M. D., et al. (2011). Attachment figures activate a safety signal-related neural region and reduce pain experience. *Proceedings of the National Academy of Sciences, 108*(28), 11721–6.

Ellingsen, D. M., Leknes, S., Løseth, G., Wessberg, J., and **Olausson, H.** (2015). The neurobiology shaping affective touch: Expectation, motivation, and meaning in the multisensory context. *Frontiers in Psychology, 6*, 1986.

Feldman, H. and **Friston, K. J.** (2010). Attention, uncertainty, and free-energy. *Frontiers in Human Neuroscience, 4*, 215.

Fiorillo, C. D., Tobler, P. N., and **Schultz, W.** (2003). Discrete coding of reward probability and uncertainty by dopamine neurons. *Science, 299*(5614), 1898–1902.

Fotopoulou, A. (2013). Beyond the reward principle: Consciousness as precision seeking. *Neuropsychoanalysis, 15*(1), 33–38.

Fotopoulou, A. and **Tsakiris, M.** (2017). Mentalizing homeostasis: The social origins of interoceptive inference. *Neuropsychoanalysis, 19*(1), 3–28.

Friston, K. (2010). The free-energy principle: A unified brain theory? *Nature Reviews Neuroscience, 11*(2), 127–38.

Friston, K. J., Shiner, T., FitzGerald, T., Galea, J. M., Adams, R., Brown, H., et al. (2012). Dopamine, affordance and active inference. *PLoS Computational Biology, 8*(1), e1002327.

Garcia-Larrea, L., Frot, M., and **Valeriani, M.** (2003). Brain generators of laser-evoked potentials: From dipoles to functional significance. *Clinical Neurophysiology, 33*(6), 279–92.

Gordon, I., Voos, A. C., Bennett, R. H., Bolling, D. Z., Pelphrey, K. A., and **Kaiser, M. D.** (2013). Brain mechanisms for processing affective touch. *Human Brain Mapping, 34*(4), 914–22.

Gu, X., Hof, P. R., Friston, K. J., and **Fan, J.** (2013). Anterior insular cortex and emotional awareness. *Journal of Comparative Neurology, 521*(15), 3371–88.

Head, H. and **Holmes, G.** (1911). Sensory disturbances from cerebral lesions. *Brain*, **34**, 102–254.

Hurter, S., Paloyelis, Y., Williams, A. C. D. C., and **Fotopoulou, A.** (2014). Partners' empathy increases pain ratings: Effects of perceived empathy and attachment style on pain report and display. *Journal of Pain*, *15*(9), 934–44.

Kleckner, I., Zhang, J., Touroutoglou, A., Chanes, L., Xia, C., Simmons, W. K., et al. (2017). Evidence for a large-scale brain system supporting allostasis and interoception in humans. *Nature Human Behaviour*, *1*(5), 0069.

Krahé, C., Springer, A., Weinman, J. A., and **Fotopoulou, A.** (2013). The social modulation of pain: Others as predictive signals of salience—a systematic review. *Frontiers in Human Neuroscience*, *7*, 386.

Krahé, C., Paloyelis, Y., Condon, H., Jenkinson, P. M., Williams, S. C., and **Fotopoulou, A.** (2015). Attachment style moderates partner presence effects on pain: A laser-evoked potentials study. *Social Cognitive and Affective Neuroscience*, *10*(8), 1030–7.

Krahé, C., Drabek, M. M., Paloyelis, Y., and **Fotopoulou, A.** (2016). Affective touch and attachment style modulate pain: A laser-evoked potentials study. *Philosophical Transactions of the Royal Society B*, *371*(1708), 20160009.

Krahé, C., von Mohr, M., Gentsch, A., Vari, C., Fidler, L., Nolte, T., et al. (under review). Sensitivity to affective touch depends on adult attachment style.

Legrain, V., Iannetti, G. D., Plaghki, L., and **Mouraux, A.** (2011). The pain matrix reloaded: A salience detection system for the body. *Progress in Neurobiology*, *93*(1), 111–24.

Löken, L. S., Wessberg, J., McGlone, F., and **Olausson, H.** (2009). Coding of pleasant touch by unmyelinated afferents in humans. *Nature Neuroscience*, *12*(5), 547–8.

Marks, L. E., Ringkamp, M., Campbell, J. N., and **Raja, S. N.** (2006). *Peripheral Mechanisms of Cutaneous Nociception*. London: Elsevier.

Mazzola, L., Isnard, J., Peyron, R., and **Mauguière, F.** (2011). Stimulation of the human cortex and the experience of pain: Wilder Penfield's observations revisited. *Brain*, *135*(2), 631–40.

McCabe, C., Rolls, E. T., Bilderbeck, A., and **McGlone, F.** (2008). Cognitive influences on the affective representation of touch and the sight of touch in the human brain. *Social Cognitive and Affective Neuroscience*, *3*(2), 97–108.

McGlone, F., Wessberg, J., and **Olausson, H.** (2014). Discriminative and affective touch: Sensing and feeling. *Neuron*, *82*(4), 737–55.

Medford, N. and **Critchley, H. D.** (2010). Conjoint activity of anterior insular and anterior cingulate cortex: Awareness and response. *Brain Structure and Function*, *214*(5-6), 535–49.

Melzack, R. and **Wall, P. D.** (1965). Pain mechanisms: A new theory. *Science*, *150*(3699), 971–9.

Melzack, R., Wall, P. D., and **Ty, T. C.** (1982). Acute pain in an emergency clinic: Latency of onset and descriptor patterns related to different injuries. *Pain*, **14**(1), 33–4.

Meredith, P., Ownsworth, T., and **Strong, J.** (2008). A review of the evidence linking adult attachment theory and chronic pain: Presenting a conceptual model. *Clinical Psychology Reviews*, **28**, 407–29. doi:10.1016/j.cpr.2007.07.009

Olausson, H., Lamarre, Y., Backlund, H., Morin, B. G., Wallin, G., Starck, S., Ekholm, S., et al. (2002). Unmyelinated tactile afferents signal touch and project to insular cortex. *Nature Neuroscience*, *5*(9), 900.

Olausson, H., Cole, J., Rylander, K., McGlone, F., Lamarre, Y., Wallin, B. G., et al. (2008). Functional role of unmyelinated tactile afferents in human hairy skin: Sympathetic response and perceptual localization. *Experimental Brain Research*, *184*(1), 135–40.

Paloyelis, Y., Krahé, C., Maltezos, S., Williams, S. C., Howard, M. A., and **Fotopoulou, A.** (2016). The analgesic effect of oxytocin in humans: A double-blind, placebo-controlled cross-over study using laser-evoked potentials. *Journal of Neuroendocrinology*, *28*(4). <https://doi.org/10.1111/jne.12347>

Panksepp, J. (1998). *Affective Neuroscience: The Foundations of Human and Animal Emotions*. New York, NY: Oxford University Press

Paulus, M. P. and **Stein, M. B.** (2006). An insular view of anxiety. *Biological Psychiatry, 60*(4), 383–7.

Perl, E. R. (2007). Ideas about pain, a historical view. *Nature Reviews Neuroscience, 8*(1), 71–80.

Pezzulo, G., Rigoli, F., and **Friston, K.** (2015). Active inference, homeostatic regulation and adaptive behavioural control. *Progress in Neurobiology, 134*, 17–35.

Ploghaus, A., Tracey, I., Gati, J. S., Clare, S., Menon, R. S., Matthews, P. M., et al. (1999). Dissociating pain from its anticipation in the human brain. *Science, 284*(5422), 1979–81.

Ploghaus, A., Becerra, L., Borras, C., and **Borsook, D.** (2003). Neural circuitry underlying pain modulation: Expectation, hypnosis, placebo. *Trends in Cognitive Sciences, 7*(5), 197–200.

Ploner, M., Freund, H. J., and **Schnitzler, A.** (1999). Pain affect without pain sensation in a patient with a postcentral lesion. *Pain, 81*(1), 211–14.

Quattrocki, E. and **Friston, K.** (2014). Autism, oxytocin and interoception. *Neuroscience & Biobehavioral Reviews, 47*, 410–30.

Rainville, P., Duncan, G. H., Price, D. D., Carrier, B., and **Bushnell, M. C.** (1997). Pain affect encoded in human anterior cingulate but not somatosensory cortex. *Science, 277*(5328), 968–71.

Ritter, A. M. and **Mendell, L. M.** (1992). Somal membrane properties of physiologically identified sensory neurons in the rat: Effects of nerve growth factor. *Journal of Neurophysiology, 68*(6), 2033–41.

Rolls, E. T., O'Doherty, J., Kringelbach, M. L., Francis, S., Bowtell, R., and **McGlone, F.** (2003). Representations of pleasant and painful touch in the human orbitofrontal and cingulate cortices. *Cerebral Cortex, 13*(3), 308–17.

Rolls, E. T. (2010). The affective and cognitive processing of touch, oral texture, and temperature in the brain. *Neuroscience & Biobehavioral Reviews, 34*(2), 237–45.

Sambo, C. F., Howard, M., Kopelman, M., Williams, S., and **Fotopoulou, A.** (2010). Knowing you care: Effects of perceived empathy and attachment style on pain perception. *Pain, 151*(3), 687–93.

Seth, A. K., Suzuki, K., and **Critchley, H. D.** (2011). An interoceptive predictive coding model of conscious presence. *Frontiers in Psychology, 2*, 395.

Seth, A. K. (2013). Interoceptive inference, emotion, and the embodied self. *Trends in Cognitive Sciences, 17*(11), 565–73.

Sherrington, C. (1910). *The Integrative Action of the Nervous System*. Cambridge: Cambridge University Press.

Stephan, K. E., Manjaly, Z. M., Mathys, C. D., Weber, L. A., Paliwal, S., Gard, T., et al. (2016). Allostatic self-efficacy: A metacognitive theory of dyshomeostasis-induced fatigue and depression. *Frontiers in Human Neuroscience, 10*, 550.

Sterling, P. and **Eyer, J.** (1988). Allostasis: A new paradigm to explain arousal pathology. In: K. Fisher and J. Reason (eds), *Handbook of Life Stress, Cognition and Health*. Hoboken, NJ: John Wiley & Sons, pp. 629–49.

Sugiura, Y., Lee, C. L., and **Perl, E. R.** (1986). Projections of identified, unmyelinated (C) afferent fibers innervating mammalian skin. *Science, 234*, 358–62.

Talbot, J. D., Marrett, S., Evans, A. C., Meyer, E., Bushnell, M. C., and **Duncan, G. H.** (1991). Multiple representations of pain in human cerebral cortex. *Science, 251*(4999), 1355–9.

Valentini, E., Hu, L., Chakrabarti, B., Hu, Y., Aglioti, S. M., and **Iannetti, G. D.** (2012). The primary somatosensory cortex largely contributes to the early part of the cortical response elicited by nociceptive stimuli. *Neuroimage, 59*(2), 1571–81.

Vallbo, Å. B., Olausson, H., and **Wessberg, J.** (1999). Unmyelinated afferents constitute a second system coding tactile stimuli of the human hairy skin. *Journal of Neurophysiology, 81*(6), 2753–63.

Vera-Portocarrero, L. P., Zhang, E. T., Ossipov, M. H., Xie, J. Y., King, T., Lai, J., et al. (2006). Descending facilitation from the rostral ventromedial medulla maintains nerve injury-induced central sensitization. *Neuroscience*, *140*(4), 1311–20.

Villemure, C. and **Bushnell, C. M.** (2002). Cognitive modulation of pain: How do attention and emotion influence pain processing? *Pain*, *95*(3), 195–9.

von Mohr, M., Krahé, C., Beck, B., and **Fotopoulou, A.** (under review). The social buffering of pain by affective touch in romantic couples: A laser-evoked potentials study.

Wiech, K., Ploner, M., and **Tracey, I.** (2008). Neurocognitive aspects of pain perception. *Trends in Cognitive Sciences*, *12*(8), 306–13.

Wiech, K., Lin, C. S., Brodersen, K. H., Bingel, U., Ploner, M., and **Tracey, I.** (2010). Anterior insula integrates information about salience into perceptual decisions about pain. *Journal of Neuroscience*, *30*(48), 16324–16331.

Woolf, C. J. and **Salter, M. W.** (2000). Neuronal plasticity: Increasing the gain in pain. *science*, *288*(5472), 1765–1768.

Zotterman, Y. (1939). Touch, pain and tickling: An electro-physiological investigation on cutaneous sensory nerves. *Journal of Physiology*, *95*(1), 1–28.

PART III

From health to disease

Interoception in physical and mental health

Chapter 7

Interoception and emotion: Shared mechanisms and clinical implications

Lisa Quadt, Hugo D. Critchley, and Sarah N. Garfinkel

7.1 Introduction

Emotions are often accompanied by bodily changes. We experience this when we blush with embarrassment, feel our heart beat faster, and our breath go shallow when we are in fear. The view that emotion and body are intimately related was first formulated by William James (James, 1884) who claimed that peripheral autonomic changes *constitute* emotions. The sensing of autonomic changes is referred to as interoception, the afferent processing of signals that originate within the body. Involved in interoception are different classes and channels (e.g. cardiovascular, gastric) of information that are distinct with respect to their afferent pathway (neural, humoral) and the generation of the signal (mechanoreceptive organ stretching, chemoreception). These channels share neural substrates, that is, brain mechanisms, in which integrative processes take place. These allow for the generation of representations that predict internal states, which might steer adaptive behavior (e.g. when blood sugar levels drop below a specific threshold, find food). Changes in bodily states and their interoceptive signalling can be constitutive of emotional feelings, leading to the possibility that the affective style (e.g. the intensity of emotions) of a person reflects differences in conscious and unconscious processing of interoceptive information.

Individual interoceptive differences manifest themselves in different psychological dimensions of interoception that comprise objective, subjective, and metacognitive measures (Canales-Johnson et al., 2015; Garfinkel et al., 2015). Quantifications of interoceptive abilities include objective measures such as behavioral performance accuracy during heartbeat detection tasks (Schandry, 1981). Subjective (i.e. sensibility) measures include self-reports about interoceptive proficiency, such as evaluations of how well internal signals can be sensed using questionnaires (Porges, 1993). An enhanced mismatch between subjective and objective measures of interoception is associated with anxiety symptomatology (Garfinkel et al., 2016).

A way in which bodily and emotional processes merge can be found within the brain, where they share a similar neural architecture (Zaki, Davis, & Ochsner, 2012). Specific cortical regions, especially the anterior insular cortex (AIC), are activated when individuals focus their attention on changes in internal bodily states, highlighting the role of AIC in the perception of autonomic changes (Critchley, 2004; Peyron, Laurent, & Garcia-Larrea, 2000; Williams et al., 2000). The insular cortex is thus of special interest to both interoception and emotion. In the brain, fibers from lamina 1 project into the NTS (nucleus of the solitary tract), parabrachial nucleus, periaqueductal grey, and other brainstem autonomic output nuclei. However, the ventromedial posterior nucleus of the thalamus is the main relay of viscerosensory information within the spinothalamic tract projecting onto insular cortex (see Critchley & Harrison, 2013). The insular cortex is located in the brain bilaterally underneath frontal and temporal lobes and is part of the cerebral cortex. It is divided into posterior and anterior insular cortex, where each part has its own cellular and functional structure. Its cytoarchitecture changes from granular in the posterior region to agranular in the anterior insula. The insular cortex is bi-directionally connected to parietal, frontal, and limbic regions (Deen, Pitskel, & Pelphrey, 2011). While the posterior regions of the insula are reciprocally connected with the second somatosensory cortex (SII) and receive input from the thalamus, conveying information such as pain, temperature, and oxygen status, AIC is closely connected with the anterior cingulate cortex (ACC). AIC and ACC together engage subcortical regions such as the amygdala and orbitofrontal cortex (OFC). It has thus been suggested that the posterior parts of the insula support primary, objective representations of bodily signals, while AIC re-represents and integrates these signals with exteroceptive and motivational information (Seth, 2013). AIC is also engaged in emotion elicitation tasks (Kober et al., 2008; Wicker et al., 2003), and neuroscientific models posit that the processing of visceral information in AIC supports an overlap between interoceptive and emotional states (Lamm & Singer, 2010).

Appraisal theories of emotion (Schachter & Singer, 1962) add another component to the mix of interoception and emotion, namely that of cognitive appraisal. According to this view, emotional states are elicited by bodily changes and subsequent contextualization. Modern theories of the embodiment of emotion (Craig, 2002; Critchley et al., 2004) adopt a similar approach, by also integrating findings about the shared neural underpinnings of interoception and emotion with the idea of contextualization. Together they highlight the role of bodily signals in shaping emotional experience and the role of cognitive appraisal in shaping the type of emotion felt.

These theoretical and empirical advances on the interplay of emotional and interoceptive processes have recently been put together within the unifying perspective of predictive processing (Clark, 2016). Predictive processing (PP) views the brain as a hierarchical generator of predictions about its most likely next states. These predictions are then compared against actual sensory input (generating a *prediction error*), which either leads to a change of predictions in light of the new evidence (perception), or to action that changes brain-external circumstances (active inference). This principle not only applies to exteroceptive information processing but also to predicting and controlling bodily interoceptive states. This can be described as interoceptive inference (Seth, 2013), which has also been called "interoceptive predictive processing" (IPP). IPP claims that emotional states are brought forth in the process of minimizing interoceptive prediction error and the top-down (i.e. from higher to lower levels in the processing hierarchy) predictive inference of causes of interoceptive signals. The network of AIC and other cortical regions is thought to underlie this process of generating emotions via interoceptive inference (Seth, Suzuki, & Critchley, 2011).

In this chapter, we will elaborate on the IPP perspective to frame findings about the relationship between emotion and interoception. We will detail shared mechanisms of emotional and interoceptive processing, focusing on the role of the insular cortex as a central hub in addition to core regions such as ACC and amygdala. In a next step, we describe how differences in interoceptive processing can lead to individual differences in emotional expression, behavior, and experience. Finally, we show how impairments in interoception relate to affective psychopathology, with particular focus on autism spectrum conditions (ASCs), anxiety disorders, depression, and eating disorders (EDs).

7.2 **Shared mechanisms**

The relation between emotion and interoception is reflected in their neural counterparts. Previous findings support the description of a joint network of interoceptive and emotional processing that has AIC and ACC at its center. Imaging studies show that emotions are mediated by a matrix of subcortical and cortical structures whose activity is also correlated to alterations in internal bodily states (Phan et al., 2002). Specifically, ventral prefrontal, anterior cingulate, and insular cortices, amygdala, ventral striatum, and dorsal brainstem are identified as relevant structures for emotions, which also have been related to changes in heart rate (Critchley et al., 2005), temperature (Nummenmaa et al., 2014), and blood pressure (Critchley et al., 2000).

The insula and ACC play an especially important role for the joint processing of emotion and interoception. AIC is seen as mediating both interoceptive accuracy (i.e. how well individuals perceive inner states; Critchley et al. 2004) and deficits in emotion processing (Berthoz et al., 2002). This is in line with the claim that integration processes in the anterior insula allow the uncovering of internal bodily states which then informs emotional processing (Terasawa et al., 2013). Thus there appears to be a triadic relationship between activity in AIC, emotional and interoceptive processing. Specifically, heightened activity in the insula is associated with both interoceptive processing and the processing of emotional intensity (Zaki et al., 2012), supporting the view that judgments of emotional intensity are informed by the sensing of internal bodily sensations.

An instance of how interoceptive signalling influences emotion processing is how responses to emotional stimuli vary depending on when in the cardiac cycle they are presented (Critchley & Garfinkel, 2017). Fear stimuli, for example, are more easily detected and perceived as more intense when presented at systole when baroreceptors (interoceptors that encode blood vessel and cardiac chamber stretch due to pressure change) are active compared to presentation at diastole when baroreceptors are inactive (Critchley & Garfinkel, 2015; Garfinkel & Critchley, 2016; Garfinkel et al., 2014). Cardiovascular arousal thus can enhance the experience of fear and anxiety.

Another example of the interacting relationship between interoception and emotion can be found in the influence of inflammation on emotional states. Inflammatory processes can lead to "sickness behaviors" like fatigue, social withdrawal, and irritability (Harrison, 2017). Interoceptive pathways to insula are involved in conveying inflammation signals, thus suggesting an interoceptive mechanism in the shared relation between inflammatory and emotional states.

These findings show that emotional and interoceptive processing have a common underlying neural architecture, which comprises AIC, ACC, and other functionally connected regions. Bodily arousal and emotional intensity are tightly correlated, which points towards shared mechanisms beyond the brain.

7.3 Individual differences

People differ with respect to how intensely they experience emotions in general, and it is particularly interesting that this might be due to individual differences in interoceptive performance. It is typically assumed that a heightened ability to detect internal bodily changes is associated with more intensely felt emotions, a hypothesis that has been confirmed in several studies (Wiens, Mezzacappa, & Katkin, 2000).

Quantifying interoceptive performance involves a variety of methods, ranging from questionnaires to behavioral tests that look for fluctuations in physiological signals or experimentally alter organ physiology. Among the most widely used methods are heartbeat detection tasks, where individuals either count their heartbeats silently for a given amount of time (Schandry, 1981) or judge whether an external signal is in or out of synchrony with their heartbeat (Katkin et al., 1982). In order to grasp these different measures, novel conceptual tools have been introduced to describe different psychological dimensions of interoception; viz. objective performance accuracy, subjective sensibility, and metacognitive awareness (Garfinkel et al., 2016).

Interoceptive accuracy refers to the objective measure of how well people perform on interoceptive tasks, such as heartbeat discrimination or counting tasks. This dimension is dissociable from sensibility, which refers to the subjective impression of how well individuals think they are able to perceive internal signals. This can be measured by questionnaires such as the Body Perception Questionnaire (Porges, 1993). The third dimension describes the relationship between subjective and objective measures; that is, the metacognitive awareness of individuals regarding how well they performed on an interoceptive task (e.g. knowing they performed well when they actually performed well or knowing they performed poorly when they did perform poorly). Interoceptive awareness can be quantified through measures such as confidence-accuracy correspondence (Garfinkel et al., 2015). Thus metacognitive awareness can be conceptualized as an interoceptive insight measure. Deficits within these dimensions can predict emotional states and affective psychopathology. In line with this, individuals with higher alexithymia—a sub-clinical condition that is characterized by impairments in recognizing and describing one's emotions (Nemiah, 1976)—show impoverished interoceptive accuracy (Ernst et al., 2014).

The three-level model of interoceptive dimensions was recently extended (Critchley & Garfinkel, 2017) to include lower levels that exhibit afferent neural trafficking and the preconscious impact of interoceptive signals on sensory processing (Figure 7.1). Good heartbeat perceivers, for example, experience greater arousal for emotional pictures than poor heartbeat perceivers and also show greater heartbeat-evoked potentials (HEP) for emotional pictures (Herbert, Pollatos, & Schandry, 2007). Within brain, individual differences in insula activation correlate with levels of negative emotional states expressed as anxiety and neuroticism (Terasawa et al., 2013). This again points into the direction of a link between interoceptive and emotional performance. Additionally, higher levels beyond

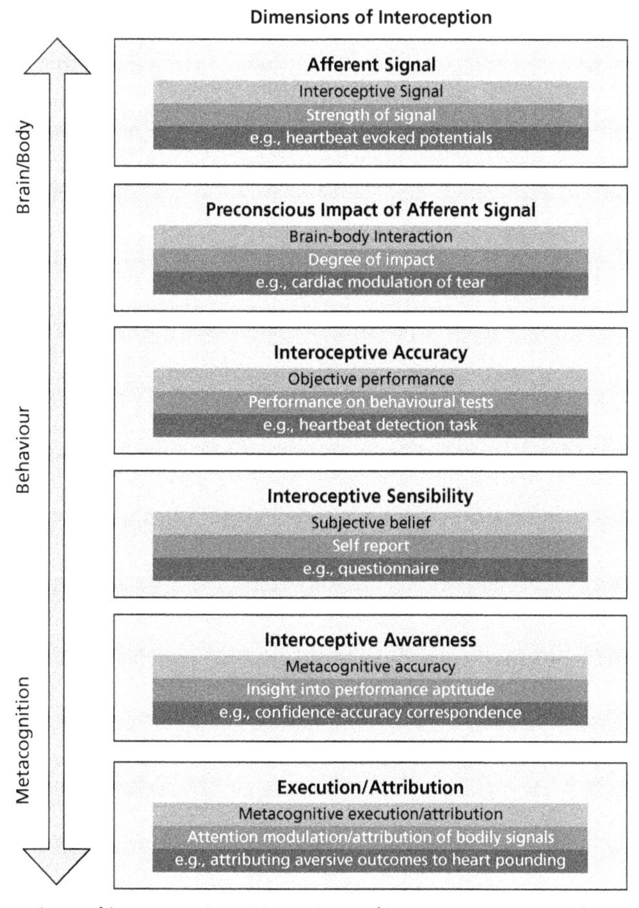

Figure 7.1 Dimensions of interoception: Dimensions of interoception range from the level of brain and body, to behavior, and metacognition. At each dimension, individual differences manifest themselves and can have an impact on emotional processes and states. These dimensions are though to interact with each other, for example in the alignment of interoceptive accuracy and sensibility.

metacognition are added to the model, which include executive processes like the modulation of attention (Critchley & Garfinkel, 2017). Individual differences could manifest in the ability to attend flexibly to either interoceptive or exteroceptive signals or switching between interoceptive tasks. This in turn may be related to focusing on and consciously detecting one's own emotional state.

The ability to detect emotion and its relationship to interoceptive performance may also extend into the social domain and influence how accurately emotions of others are perceived. Empirical results on this topic are, however, conflicting, possibly due to different measurement methods. On the one hand, it was found that the higher the interoceptive accuracy, the more sensitive one is to the emotions of another person (Terasawa et al., 2014). In line with this finding is a study showing that people who score high on alexithymia questionnaires show reduced activation in insular cortex both when they try to access their own emotions and when empathizing with another person's pain (Bird et al., 2010; Silani et al., 2008). Another indication for a close relationship between interoception and empathy is a finding that shows enhanced neural activity during empathy in brain regions related to both interoception and empathy after participants completed an interoceptive performance task (Ernst et al., 2013). The insula cortex underlies both current and predictive representations, which are crucial for learning processes of uncertainty and emotional states (Singer, Critchley, & Preuschoff, 2009). In this learning process, predictions about feeling states in self and others are compared to actual incoming signals and then updated depending on the discrepancy between prediction and signal. Integrative processes within the insula cortex support this error-based learning process in which empathic and subjective feeling states are generated.

On the other hand, Ainley, Maister, and Tsakiris (Ainley et al., 2015) did not find any correlations between interoceptive accuracy and empathy scores on questionnaires that focus on cognitive, rather than affective, aspects of empathy. The relationship between empathy and interoceptive performance thus is still open to debate, however there seems to be a consensus that levels of interoceptive accuracy may positively correlate with higher levels of affective empathy (see Bird, Shah, & Catmur, 2017; Tsakiris, 2017).

In summary, these findings strongly suggest that the degree to which one is able to detect and attend to internal states determines how well emotions are recognized in self and others. These individual differences can be found along different dimensions of interoception, which interact with and influence emotional experience.

7.4 Interoceptive predictive processing (IPP) and emotion

Predictive processing (PP; Clark, 2013, 2016) is ultimately a theory about how the brain makes sense of the world and body in which it is embedded. While it has historically been exclusively applied to perception and action, it has recently been extended to include interoception and emotion (Seth et al., 2011).

7.4.1 Predictive processing

The rationale of PP is that there are hidden causes in the world—hidden from the brain in the skull—that need to be inferred. All the brain can access are its own states: it can neither directly access the external world, nor the body it is embedded in, nor other agents. It thus has to solve an *inverse problem*, viz. how do the effects on the brain relate to causes in the external world (Hohwy, 2013). The solution to this problem presents itself in the form of inference; in order to find out about what lies behind the effects the brain receives, the causes must be inferred. It is proposed that this happens within a hierarchy where predictions about the most likely state of the level below are generated and then compared to actual sensory input.[1] While low levels predict basic sensory properties of incoming signals at fast timescales, higher levels predict more complex regularities at slower timescales (Hohwy, 2010). The crucial information, that is, the mismatch (i.e. error) between prediction and signal, is then conveyed via feedforward connections in order to improve the model. This process of updating the model is called *perceptual inference* and is contrasted against *active inference* (Friston, 2010). In active inference, instead of changing models, biological agents act so to change sensory input to make it accommodate predictions better. Both perceptual and active inference serve the brain's main task: minimizing prediction error.

One question that arises, though, is the following: How does the brain "decide" which of these strategies to choose? This is determined by how precise the expectations and error signals are deemed to be. The "job" of prediction errors, as we have seen, is to improve the generative model. However, it is important that errors are not simply taken to be "trustworthy" (i.e. reliably informing the system about external states) and change the model or motivate to act. Error signals are taken into account depending on an estimation of how reliable they will be. If prediction errors are, for example, estimated as highly precise, they are likely to change the hypothesis; that is, the impact of an error signal depends on how precise it is estimated to be. At the same time, the reliability of predictive models needs to factored in too. Thus, "we are, in effect, estimating the uncertainty of our own representations of the world." (Clark, 2015, p. 12)

7.4.2 Interoceptive predictive processing (IPP)

This PP scheme was recently applied to interoception (Barrett & Simmons, 2015; Seth, 2013b; Seth et al., 2011). In general, IPP follows the same principle as inference of exteroceptive states as described earlier. Predictive models of the next most probable interoceptive signals are generated and compared to actual input. This mechanism serves to

[1] There might be confusion in the PP scheme about what is considered a "signal" and what counts as a "representation" (thanks to our reviewer for bringing up this important issue). A helpful distinction could be that representations exist even at very low levels, if representations are defined as abstractions from the actual signal. As soon as there is a prediction about what the signal (e.g. mechanoreceptive organ stretching) might be, there is an abstraction from the signal itself, thus making it a representation (for a more detailed discussion, see Quadt, 2017, Chapter 6, and Quadt, 2018).

keep bodily states in their expected range and to adapt flexibly to external and internal changes. Instead of simply comparing inputs to homeostatic setpoints and changing the internal environment accordingly, the idea is that the system anticipates demands that deviate from the average and thus efficiently regulates needs and resources. The terms "allostasis" and "predictive regulation" were introduced to conceptualize this process of optimizing regulation in a predictive manner (Sterling, 2012). According to the size and estimated reliability of the prediction error, prediction errors can be minimized in several ways; namely by updating generative models of interoceptive states; by engaging hormonal, visceral, immunological, and autonomic mechanisms to change interoceptive signals via active inference; or by actions that change external conditions which have an impact on the body (see Figure 7.2; Seth, 2015).

The engagement of autonomic, hormonal, visceral, and immunological mechanisms serves to maintain homeostasis or to enable allostasis (see also Chapter 15 in the present volume).[2] Throughout the process of monitoring its own states, the system keeps updating and changing its states in order to keep them in an expected range. Active interoceptive inference describes the process of how internal systems use autonomic, immunological, and metabolic resources depending on the difference (prediction error) between predicted (demanded) and actual signal (Barrett & Simmons, 2015).

Throughout the process of adjusting interoceptive predictions and bodily states, emotional contents may arise (Barrett, 2017; Seth, 2013a). Visceromotor cortices engender autonomic, hormonal, and immunological predictions which underlie the system's allostatic responses. These predictions are not only forwarded to the body where they cause internal changes, they are also sent to the insula, termed the "primary interoceptive cortex" (Barrett & Simmons, 2015). Here, these predictions are compared to afferent signals resulting from visceral, muscular, and skin changes. The ensuing error signal is propagated back up to visceromotor regions where the prediction originated. Once interoceptive input is accounted for, that is, once it is sufficiently explained by predictive models, emotional content arises (Barrett, 2017).

This model of emotions draws on the James–Lange theory, which assumes that emotional experiences are first and foremost constituted by the monitoring of interoceptive states. However, one shortcoming of this theory, which has been adopted and refined widely (e.g. the somatic marker hypothesis, Damasio, 1996), is that it (at least implicitly) asserts a one-to-one mapping of emotional effect and interoceptive cause (Clark, 2016). This means that it is assumed that there is one change in interoception (that can probably be marked, hence "somatic *marker* hypothesis") that leads to the perceived emotion.

[2] The difference between homeostasis and allostasis is that the former refers to the maintenance of specific and rather rigid setpoints, while the latter describes a highly flexible demand-regulated change of states. Rather than committing to homeostatic setpoints (e.g. keeping blood pressure around a specific value), allostasis anticipates the changing needs of the system and adjusts bodily states accordingly (e.g. adjusting blood pressure relative to moment-by-moment demands). For a much more detailed discussion, see Sterling, 2012).

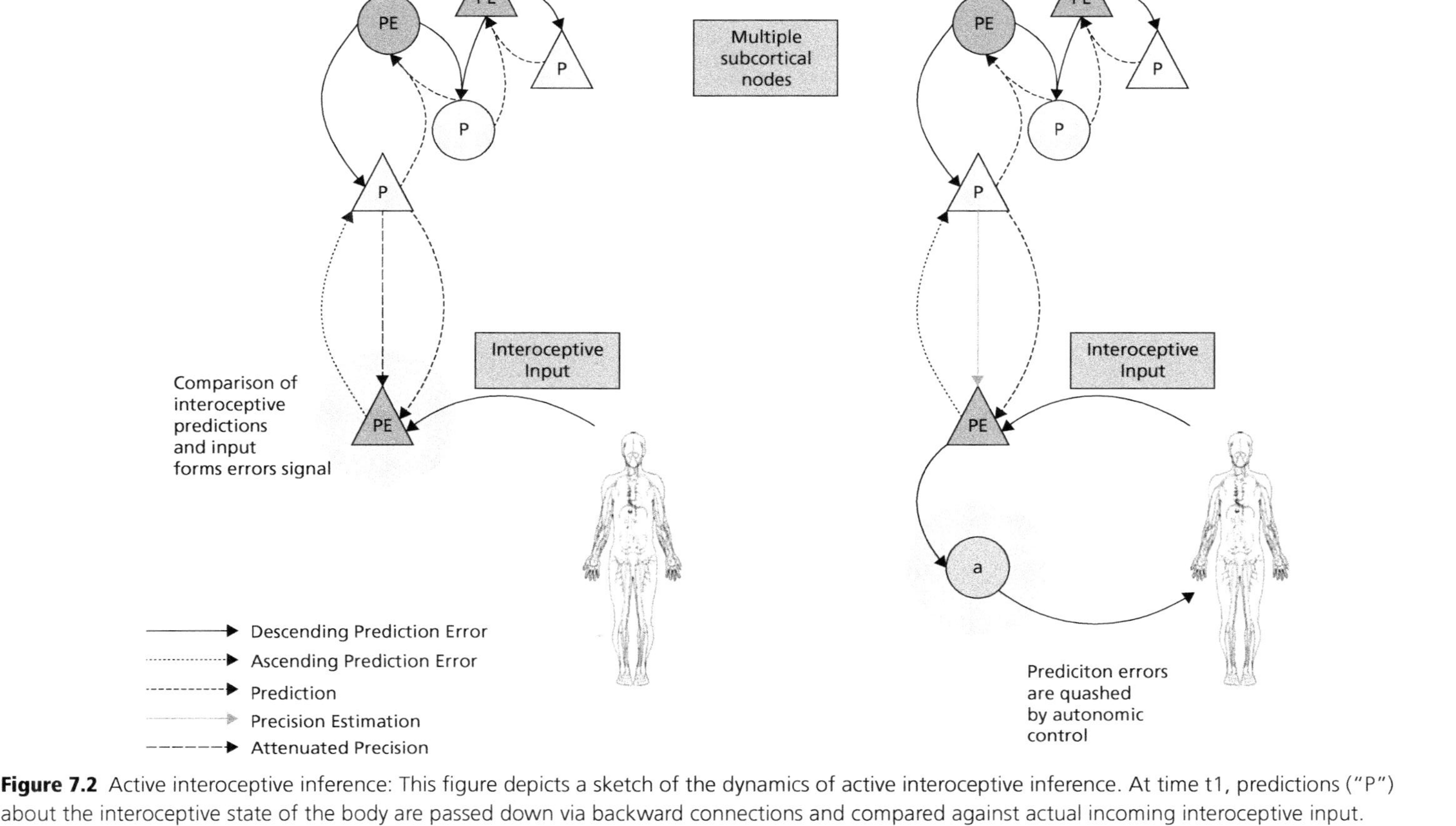

Figure 7.2 Active interoceptive inference: This figure depicts a sketch of the dynamics of active interoceptive inference. At time t1, predictions ("P") about the interoceptive state of the body are passed down via backward connections and compared against actual incoming interoceptive input. When there is a mismatch between predicted and actual body state, a prediction error ("PE") is generated. Note that precision of this ascending error signal must be attenuated, so not to change predictions and thus to inhibit autonomic control. At time t2, prediction errors are quashed by autonomic control. The changed interoceptive input is again fed forward to now inform predictions.

However, it is more likely that there are several possible causes that bring forth an emotion. Viewing this basic idea within an IPP perspective, though, promises to alleviate this problem of former theories in the sense that the *most probable* of a *variety of likely reasons* is actively inferred.

IPP furthermore describes a strong relation between exteroceptive, proprioceptive, and interoceptive processes in that it assumes that information from all three channels is integrated at hierarchically higher levels. It is this "context-reflecting amalgam" (Clark, 2016) that then presents itself as an experienced emotion. Emotions, in this view, integrate low-level uni-modal information (i.e. interoceptive, exteroceptive, or proprioceptive information) with higher-level predictions of probable causes. In other words, emotions occur in the process of integrating information from several sources in order to form interoceptive predictions. These predictions, which then contain contextual information from exteroception, interoception, and proprioception, are compared to actual incoming signals. Emotional states arise throughout this process. Note that this implies an intimate and most likely interacting relation between interoceptive and exteroceptive processing. For one, both external and internal events shape emotional response. Additionally, when external events trigger a cascade of interoceptive processing, these events will be "affectively colored" (Clark, 2016).

One important consequence of adopting such a view is that it updates appraisal or two-factor theories of emotional experience (Schachter & Singer, 1962). These theories suggest that emotions have two components: a bodily and a cognitive one. The latter is needed to appraise the former and thus leaves the emotion subjectively colored. However, IPP now claims that subjective emotional states simply occur in virtue of the single mechanism just described. Multimodal higher-level top-down predictions entail contextual information, which frames how interoceptive signals are interpreted and transformed into emotions. This means that in the process of interoceptive predictive processing, cognitive appraisal is already "built in", and shapes emotional experience.

The role of the insular cortex, especially the AIC, undoubtedly plays a key role in this coordinating process. Seth (2013) claims that emotional responses crucially rely on predictions of causes of interoceptive input that are continually updated. These predictions are generated, compared to actual input, and then updated within a salience network that consists of insular cortex, ACC, and several other functional connections to the brainstem.

IPP is a promising theory to frame the relationship between emotion and interoception because it proposes a single principle—prediction error minimization—to underlie the generation of emotional and bodily states. It also provides novel ways to look at psychopathology, which we will detail in section 7.5.

7.5 **Clinical implications**

Many psychiatric conditions come with emotional impairments—ranging from prevalent negative affect in depression to feelings of high alert and arousal in anxiety. A clear example of how emotion and interoception are related in psychopathology is the connection between interoceptive performance and occurrence of alexithymia. It has been proposed that where there is alexithymia, there is poor interoceptive accuracy (Murphy et al., 2016). Indeed, many clinical conditions come with both alexithymia and impairments in interoceptive processing. Here, we will focus on autism spectrum conditions (ASCs), anxiety disorders, depression, and eating disorders (EDs; see also Chapter 9 in the present volume), all of which show an interesting relation between emotional and interoceptive processing.

7.5.1 Autism spectrum conditions

Autism spectrum conditions are characterized as neurodevelopmental lifelong conditions that come with alterations in social cognition and emotion processing, as well as restrictions in interest and activities, and stereotyped patterns of behavior (Frith, 2014). ASCs express high rates of alexithymia (Bird et al., 2010), which indicate difficulties in processing and detecting own emotional states. This extends into the social realm where the detection of emotions in others can be exacerbated.

A predictive processing perspective has been used to explain several aspects of the symptomology of ASCs, including unusual perception and sensation (Pellicano & Burr, 2012), and impairments in social cognition (Palmer, Seth, & Hohwy, 2015). Aiming at an overarching predictive processing account of autism, it was claimed that sensory processing in individuals with ASCs is characterized by an unusually high weighting of sensory prediction errors (Palmer, Lawson, & Hohwy, 2017).

An aberrant oxytocin system in early infancy may play a role in the development of autistic traits (Quattrocki & Friston, 2014). The neuromodulatory effects of oxytocin perform a major part in the processing of interoceptive information and their association with exteroceptive stimuli, and may also be involved in the neuromodulations that are necessary to elicit emotions. The functional anatomy of oxytocin is situated in the brain in such a way that it is involved in interoceptive paths that also mediate emotions. Oxytocin is thought to play an important role in the modulation of associative learning between interoceptive and exteroceptive cues. To learn emotional affordances (e.g. caregiver means warmth and comfort) during infancy, associations between exteroceptive cues (touch) and interoceptive signals (warmth) need to be established. Neuromodulatory mechanisms are involved in making these associations. For example, the interoceptive change of body temperature is associated with the bodily presence of a caregiver due to neuromodulatory mechanisms that underlie the establishment of this association. This is thought to be done via selective augmentation and attenuation of interoceptive prediction errors, most likely mediated by oxytocin. If these mechanisms go awry, however, the context-sensitive adjustment of prediction errors is disrupted, resulting in a disturbance of the necessary mechanisms to acquire generative models for interoceptive inference, which target the emotional states of self and other. In other words, the failure to associate the interoceptive consequence (warmth and comfort) with the exteroceptive cause (caregiver) may lead to an incorrect attribution of agency in prosocial actions. Impaired interoceptive inference, following this logic, could thus lead to difficulty in recognizing emotions in self and others. The faulty modulation of precision of interoceptive prediction error may thus result in hypersensitivity to interoceptive cues ("autonomic hypersensitivity"). This is because when interoceptive signals are always weighted as precise, they will have an increased propensity to be propagated back up the hierarchy, and consequently they have the power to change predictions. This, in turn, could lead to difficulties in both emotional and interoceptive processing.

Viewing autism as a consequence of an abnormal neuromodulatory system (including oxytocin) provides an interesting perspective on well-known symptoms like emotional echopraxia (which can be interpreted as interoceptive hypersensitivity) and the tendency not to engage with exteroceptive cues in social settings. This explanation points to aberrant precision control in brain systems that mediate interoceptive inference, such as anterior insular and cingulate cortex (Seth & Friston, 2016).

On a neural level, autism studies report altered activity in regions that underlie emotion processing, as well as impoverished functional connectivity in regions important to both interoception and emotion. Ebisch, Gallese, Willems, and colleagues (Ebisch et al., 2011) quantified aberrant functional connectivity between posterior insula and somatosensory cortices, as well as between anterior insula and amygdala. These regions are hubs for interoception and emotion (Critchley, Mathias, & Dolan, 2002), suggesting not only a link between the two in healthy individuals but also in individuals with ASCs. Based on this evidence, it was shown that impairments in interoceptive processing are related to aberrant emotional processing in ASCs (Garfinkel et al., 2016). This appears to confirm theories of emotion which state that the detection of internal signals informs emotional experience, since it shows that when detection is disrupted, emotional impairments follow. Another indication of a relationship between aberrant interoception, emotion and ASCs is that these conditions often co-occur with heightened alexithymia. Interestingly, it was shown, however, that levels of alexithymia and not ASC severity are predictive of low interoceptive accuracy (Shah et al., 2016). Thus poor interoceptive accuracy may serve as a general feature of alexithymia as well as underscore alexithymic traits in individuals with ASCs.

A discrepancy between levels of interoception, that is, enhanced interoceptive sensibility and low interoceptive accuracy, is predictive of anxiety symptomology. This discrepancy was termed "interoceptive trait prediction error" (ITPE) and was found to be enhanced in individuals with ASCs (Garfinkel et al., 2016). This finding is in line with the proposal that the development of anxiety is due to both noisy interoceptive input and noisily amplified self-referential interoceptive belief states (Paulus & Stein, 2010). Viewing the relation between anxiety and autism in terms of ITPE is based on the fine-grained distinction of psychological dimensions of interoception. Where previous findings suggest that there is heightened sensitivity to bodily signals in autism, the differentiation between interoceptive sensibility and accuracy helps identify how interoceptive processing is altered autism.

The accounts of autism described here assign an important role of prediction error processing to symptoms of ASC. However, there are crucial differences between the types of prediction errors mentioned. While in general IPP, prediction errors refer to error signals occurring on a moment-to-moment basis in interoceptive processing, ITPE describes a relationship between subjective and objective traits. They thus characterize relevant error signals on different time scales, both of which could contribute to the occurrence of autistic characteristics.

Taken together, these results suggest that alignment and misalignment of interoceptive dimensions are fundamental to affective symptoms in autism, and—as will be detailed in following sections—other clinical conditions.

7.5.2 Anxiety disorders

The misalignment of interoceptive dimensions may be especially important for the development of anxiety disorders (ADs; see also Chapter 8 in the present volume). The misattribution of bodily sensations is a factor underlying the development of panic and related anxiety symptoms (Clark et al., 1997). The basis for misinterpreted bodily signals forms a heightened tendency to detect internal physiological changes. Indeed, several studies show that higher interoceptive accuracy is related to higher anxiety traits (Domschke et al., 2010).

In a model of anxiety that focuses on the role of insula in the processing of bodily signals, the ability to detect sub-threshold interoceptive signals is identified as one major mechanism in the expression of anxiety (Paulus & Stein, 2006, 2010). These signals are then amplified and associated with potential aversive outcomes, thus forming the basis for anxious thought. Individuals with high anxiety traits are thought to be particularly sensitive to changes in interoceptive state when they anticipate ensuing aversive events. Belief-based thought with the tendency to focus on potential negative outcomes then strongly modifies the emotional valence of amplified bodily signals and leads to anxiety symptoms.

From an IPP perspective, it is likely that anxiety symptoms stem from abnormal precision weighting processes. In line with previous theories, aberrantly large interoceptive prediction errors lead to heightened anxiety. Whereas in healthy individuals these errors get attenuated, this mechanism might fail in anxious individuals, causing an abnormally high sensitivity to afferent interoceptive signals. In other words, bodily signals are weighted high much more often in anxious than healthy individuals. This means that these signals are more likely to be propagated back up the hierarchy and update predictions at higher levels. Where interoceptive input is usually attenuated and does not reach awareness, this mechanism might be impaired in anxiety, leading to a hypersensitivity to interoceptive signals. This is then also reflected in higher interoceptive accuracy, where bodily signals are more readily detected and available to conscious perception.

7.5.3 Depression

Major depressive disorder (MDD) is marked by a range of somatic and affective symptoms, including loss of appetite, sleep disorders, aches and pains, changes in libido, loss of energy, pervasive negative affect, and intense feelings of loneliness and hopelessness (Tylee &

Gandhi, 2005). Somatic symptoms are universal cross-culturally (Kirmayer, 2001) and associated with disruptions in physiological regulatory processes, including hypoactivity of the autonomic nervous system (Dawson, Schell, & Catania, 1977). Over the past decade, there has been growing recognition that somatic changes may drive alterations in emotion and cognition (Dunn et al., 2007; Pollatos, Traut-Mattausch, & Schandry, 2009). The role of interoception in low mood and clinical depression has been investigated in a number of studies; interoceptive accuracy is reduced in low to moderate, but not severe depression (Dunn et al., 2007). A negative correlation between heartbeat perception and depressive symptoms has been reported (Pollatos et al., 2009), where individuals with reduced interoceptive accuracy may experience emotions less intensely. These emotional impairments will impact social processes, as is often observed in MDD.

There is frequent comorbidity of depression and anxiety, possibly confounding interpretations. One subsequent study chose depressed subjects with no comorbid anxiety disorder (Furman et al., 2013). An association between interoceptive accuracy and positive affect intensity was observed. Moreover, worse performance was related to less affect intensity ratings in individuals with MDD, but not controls. The reduced autonomic reactivity to positive stimuli in depression (Bylsma, Morris, & Rottenberg, 2008), and the association between depressive symptoms and decreased responses to positive stimuli (Sloan & Sandt, 2010), indicate an aberrant interoceptive mechanism for positive reinforcement. In other words, physiological disruption in depression limits the intensity of interoceptive input. This in turn results in attenuated affective reactions to positive information.

Depression was recently framed in the PP framework and described as a disorder of predictive mechanisms that steer allostasis, that is, the ability to adapt flexibly to changing internal and external environments (Barrett, Quigley, & Hamilton, 2016). Affective feelings can inform the system about the state of bodily energy conditions, whereby the inefficient regulation of energy is coupled to affective, motor, autonomic, and metabolic dysregulations. In depression, the brain's internal model is negatively affected by this dysregulation. The brain is described as "locked in" in the sense that there is an insensitivity to interoceptive prediction errors which—coupled with energy dysregulation that is related to negative affect—leads to depression. In more detail, this means that when interoceptive prediction errors (i.e. bodily signals) are not used to update predictions, these predictions may result in inefficient energy regulation. This inefficiency could be related to negative affect, and the tendency to disengage in physical and mental activity. Pervasive negative affect, in turn, could lead to the generation of more and more negative internal models, resulting in both predictions and prediction errors to show a bias towards the negative and unpleasant.

Furthermore, peripheral endocrine immunological changes that accompany the onset of a depressive episode can perturb precision of interoceptive afferents (Seth & Friston, 2016). The attenuation of precision of ascending interoceptive signals, and greater reliance on interoceptive predictions, lead to dyshomeostasis. This process could engender a positive feedback loop in which higher reliance on predictions leads to larger and nosier prediction errors, which in turn increases the reliance on the now dysfunctional predictions. Since interoceptive predictions include "homeostatic setpoints," dysfunctional prediction will result in dysregulated homeostasis, which may trigger sickness behavior and fatigue, marking the onset of depression.

Taken together, these findings suggest that dysfunctions in interoception and autonomic regulation are strongly related to both somatic and emotional symptoms of depression. PP models of depression exhibit a strong connection between allostasis/homeostasis and the resulting dysbalance of affective processing.

7.5.4 Eating disorders

Both interoceptive and emotional processing appear impaired in eating disorders. Alexithymia often co-occurs with EDs, indicating a generally impaired recognition of own emotions. This extends into the social realm where it was found that emotion recognition in others is diminished in patients with eating disorders (Harrison et al., 2009). Emotion recognition performance, however, was predicted by alexithymia scores rather than eating disorder symptomology (Brewer et al., 2015). What still stands out, though, is the high co-occurrence of alexithymia and EDs, suggesting that emotional processing is indeed impaired in eating disorders.

When investigated directly, there appears to be a three-way relation between interoceptive performance, emotional intensity, and symptomology of eating disorders. So far, interoceptive abilities in EDs were tested by the Eating Disorder Inventory (EDI; Garner, Olmstead, & Polivy, 1983), in which the ability to discriminate sensations of hunger and satiety and to respond to emotional states ("interoceptive awareness")[3] was in focus. Interoceptive awareness, as measured by the EDI, was impaired in patients with eating disorders, where this is characterized as a low certainty in emotion recognition related to hunger and satiety (Fassino et al., 2004).

When using the heartbeat counting task (Schandry, 1981) to quantify interoceptive accuracy, decreased measures were found in patients with eating disorders compared to healthy controls (Pollatos et al., 2008). This shows that interoceptive ability is impaired in general and not just with respect to hunger and satiety, as measured by the EDI.

Together with findings that show altered autonomic functioning in eating disorders (Murialdo et al., 2007), which could lead to altered bodily feedback, this suggests that individuals with EDs experience emotions less intensely. Evidence in favor of this claim comes again from studies linking alexithymia to eating disorders (Berthoz et al., 2007) and showing diminished affect in patients (de Zwaan et al., 1996).

Eating disorders could be a result of aberrant precision weighting when viewed from an IPP perspective (Seth, 2015). In PP, only prediction errors that are deemed "reliable" will be propagated back up the hierarchy and update predictions. This means that in

[3] Note how the term "interoceptive awareness" here relates to the specific measure of discrimination of sensations and response to emotional states and is different from how we use the term in section 7.3 as a measure of the relationship between objective and subjective scores.

healthy individuals, interoceptive prediction errors related to blood sugar levels are generally weighted high in order to update predictions and lead to the sensation of hunger when the levels drop below a specific threshold. The desired, predicted bodily state thus is different from the actual state, which leads to the generation of interoceptive prediction errors. These in turn are forwarded to higher-level, multimodal models. Such models generate predictions of temporal sequences of exteroceptive and interoceptive inputs, which are propagated down the hierarchy. The ensuing prediction errors can then be resolved by either autonomic control, where fat stores are metabolized, or by engaging active movements to seek food resources. It is hypothesized that dysfunctions in precision weighting, which steers this process, may help understanding EDs. If, for example, it is constantly assumed that blood sugar will be low (i.e. high-level predictions of low blood sugar become aberrantly strong), behavior to find food may not be pursued.

Taken together, these findings suggest that problems in the discrimination of sensations like hunger and satiety, which are deemed at the core of the onset and maintenance of eating disorders, are mediated by a more general inability to regulate and describe emotions. This in turn can be traced back to impairments in interoceptive ability, showing a link between interoception and emotion in eating disorders.

7.6 **Conclusion**

Links between interoception and emotion can be found in the relationship between interoceptive performance and experience of emotional intensity, the ability to recognize one's own emotions (as measured in alexithymia scores) and interoceptive accuracy, and emotion and interoception in psychopathology.

The framework of IPP provides a means to put these findings together in terms of interoceptive inference and integration of multimodal information to generate interoceptive predictions. Aberrant precision weighting may be involved in psychopathology, as was hypothesized for depression and eating disorders.

Together, experimental and clinical findings support the proposal that interoception, including individual differences in interoceptive processing, guides the experience and expression of emotions. Altered interoceptive pathways may account for aberrant emotional processing in psychopathological disorders. These observations provide insights into potential body-centered therapies and pharmacological targets for novel interventions for clinical disorders of emotion. Where interoceptive dimensions diverge, leading to psychopathological symptoms like anxiety, training interoceptive accuracy could lead to a reduction in these symptoms. Thus insight into specific interoceptive deficits may offer a targeted therapeutic approach for clinical conditions with altered emotional and affective processing.

References

Ainley, V., Maister, L., and **Tsakiris, M.** (2015). Heartfelt empathy? No association between interoceptive awareness, questionnaire measures of empathy, reading the mind in the eyes task or the director task. *Frontiers in Psychology*, 6, 554. doi:10.3389/fpsyg.2015.00554.

Barrett, L. F. and **Simmons, W. K.** (2015). Interoceptive predictions in the brain. *Nature Reviews Neuroscience, 16*(7), 419.

Barrett, L. F., Quigley, K. S., and **Hamilton, P.** (2016). An active inference theory of allostasis and interoception in depression. *Philosophical Transaction of the Royal Society B, 371*(1708), 20160011.

Barrett, L. F. (2017). The theory of constructed emotion: An active inference account of interoception and categorization. *Social Cognitive and Affective Neuroscience, 12*(1), 1–13. doi:10.1093/scan/nsw154.

Berthoz, S., Artiges, E., Van De Moortele, P. F., Poline, J. B., Rouquette, S., Consoli, S. M., et al. (2002). Effect of impaired recognition and expression of emotions on frontocingulate cortices: An fMRI study of men with alexithymia. *American Journal of Psychiatry, 159*(6), 961–7. doi:10.1176/appi.ajp.159.6.961.

Berthoz, S., Perdereau, F., Godart, N., Corcos, M., and **Haviland, M. G.** (2007). Observer-and self-rated alexithymia in eating disorder patients: Levels and correspondence among three measures. *Journal of Psychosomatic Research, 62*(3), 341–7.

Bird, G., Silani, G., Brindley, R., White, S., Frith, U., and **Singer, T.** (2010). Empathic brain responses in insula are modulated by levels of alexithymia but not autism. *Brain, 133*(Pt 5), 1515–25. doi:10.1093/brain/awq060.

Bird, G., Shah, P., and **Catmur, C.** (2017). From heart to mind: Linking interoception, emotion, and theory of mind. *Cortex, 93*, 220–3. doi:10.1016/j.cortex.2017.02.010.

Brewer, R., Cook, R., Cardi, V., Treasure, J., and **Bird, G.** (2015). Emotion recognition deficits in eating disorders are explained by co-occurring alexithymia. *Royal Society Open Science, 2*(1), 140382.

Bylsma, L. M., Morris, B. H., and **Rottenberg, J.** (2008). A meta-analysis of emotional reactivity in major depressive disorder. *Clinical Psychology Review, 28*(4), 676–91.

Canales-Johnson, A., Silva, C., Huepe, D., Rivera-Rei, Á., Noreika, V., del Carmen Garcia, M., et al. (2015). Auditory feedback differentially modulates behavioral and neural markers of objective and subjective performance when tapping to your heartbeat. *Cerebral Cortex*, **25**, 4490–503. doi:10.1093/cercor/bhv076.

Clark, A. (2013). Whatever next? Predictive brains, situated agents, and the future of cognitive science. *Behavioral and Brain Sciences, 36*, 181–253. doi:10.1017/S0140525X12000477.

Clark, A. (2015). Embodied prediction. In: T. K. Metzinger and J. M. Windt (eds), *Open MIND*. Frankfurt am Main: MIND Group, pp. 1–21. doi:10.15502/9783958570115.

Clark, A. (2016). *Surfing Uncertainty: Prediction, Action and the Embodied Mind*. Oxford: Oxford University Press.

Clark, D. M., Salkovskis, P. M., Öst, L.-G., Breitholtz, E., Koehler, K. A., Westling, B. E., et al. (1997). Misinterpretation of body sensations in panic disorder. *Journal of Consulting and Clinical Psychology, 65*(2), 203.

Craig, A. D. (2002). How do you feel? Interoception: The sense of the physiological condition of the body. *Nature Reviews Neuroscience, 3*(8), 655–66. doi:10.1038/nrn894.

Critchley, H. D., Corfield, D., Chandler, M., Mathias, C., and **Dolan, R. J.** (2000). Cerebral correlates of autonomic cardiovascular arousal: A functional neuroimaging investigation in humans. *Journal of Physiology, 523*(1), 259–70.

Critchley, H. D., Mathias, C. J., and **Dolan, R. J.** (2002). Fear conditioning in humans: The influence of awareness and autonomic arousal on functional neuroanatomy. *Neuron, 33*(4), 653–63.

Critchley, H. D. (2004). The human cortex responds to an interoceptive challenge. *Proceedings of the National Academy of Sciences USA, 101*(17), 6333–4. doi:10.1073/pnas.0401510101.

Critchley, H. D., Wiens, S., Rotshtein, P., Ohman, A., and **Dolan, R.** (2004). Neural systems supporting interoceptive awareness. *Nature Neuroscience, 7*(2), 189–95. doi:10.1038/nn1176.

Critchley, H. D., Rotshtein, P., Nagai, Y., O'Doherty, J., Mathias, C. J., and **Dolan, R. J.** (2005). Activity in the human brain predicting differential heart rate responses to emotional facial expressions. *Neuroimage, 24*(3), 751–62. doi:10.1016/j.neuroimage.2004.10.013.

Critchley, H. D. and **Garfinkel, S. N.** (2015). Interactions between visceral afferent signaling and stimulus processing. *Frontiers in Neuroscience, 9*, 286. doi:10.3389/fnins.2015.00286.

Critchley, H. D. and **Garfinkel, S. N.** (2017). Interoception and emotion. *Current Opinion in Psychology, 17*, 7–14. <https://doi.org/10.1016/j.copsyc.2017.04.020>

Damasio, A. R. (1996). The somatic marker hypothesis and the possible functions of the prefrontal cortex. *Philosophical Transactions Royal Society London B, 351*(1346), 1413–20. doi:10.1098/rstb.1996.0125.

Dawson, M. E., Schell, A. M., and **Catania, J. J.** (1977). Autonomic correlates of depression and clinical improvement following electroconvulsive shock therapy. *Psychophysiology, 14*(6), 569–78.

de Zwaan, M., Biener, D., Bach, M., Wiesnagrotzki, S., and **Stacher, G.** (1996). Pain sensitivity, alexithymia, and depression in patients with eating disorders: Are they related? *Journal of Psychosomatic Research, 41*(1), 65–70.

Deen, B., Pitskel, N. B., and **Pelphrey, K. A.** (2011). Three Systems of Insular Functional Connectivity Identified with Cluster Analysis. *Cerebral Cortex, 21*(7), 1498–506. doi:10.1093/cercor/bhq186.

Domschke, K., Stevens, S., Pfleiderer, B., and **Gerlach, A. L.** (2010). Interoceptive sensitivity in anxiety and anxiety disorders: An overview and integration of neurobiological findings. *Clinical Psychology Review, 30*(1), 1–11. doi:10.1016/j.cpr.2009.08.008.

Dunn, B. D., Dalgleish, T., Ogilvie, A. D., and **Lawrence, A. D.** (2007). Heartbeat perception in depression. *Behavior Research and Therapy, 45*(8), 1921–30.

Ebisch, S. J., Gallese, V., Willems, R. M., Mantini, D., Groen, W. B., Romani, G. L., et al. (2011). Altered intrinsic functional connectivity of anterior and posterior insula regions in high-functioning participants with autism spectrum disorder. *Human Brain Mapping, 32*(7), 1013–28. doi:10.1002/hbm.21085.

Ernst, J., Northoff, G., Böker, H., Seifritz, E., and **Grimm, S.** (2013). Interoceptive awareness enhances neural activity during empathy. *Human Brain Mapping, 34*(7), 1615–24.

Ernst, J., Böker, H., Hättenschwiler, J., Schüpbach, D., Northoff, G., Seifritz, E., et al. (2014). The association of interoceptive awareness and alexithymia with neurotransmitter concentrations in insula and anterior cingulate. *Social Cognitive and Affective Neuroscience, 9*(6), 857–63. doi:10.1093/scan/nst058.

Fassino, S., Pierò, A., Gramaglia, C., and **Abbate-Daga, G.** (2004). Clinical, psychopathological and personality correlates of interoceptive awareness in anorexia nervosa, bulimia nervosa and obesity. *Psychopathology, 37*(4), 168–74.

Friston, K. (2010). The free-energy principle: A unified brain theory? *Nature Review Neuroscience, 11*(2), 127–38. <http://www.nature.com/nrn/journal/v11/n2/suppinfo/nrn2787_S1.html>

Frith, U. (2014). Autism—are we any closer to explaining the enigma? *Psychologist, 27*(10), 744–5.

Furman, D. J., Waugh, C. E., Bhattacharjee, K., Thompson, R. J., and **Gotlib, I. H.** (2013). Interoceptive awareness, positive affect, and decision making in major depressive disorder. *Journal of Affective Disorders, 151*(2), 780–5.

Garfinkel, S. N., Minati, L., Gray, M. A., Seth, A. K., Dolan, R. J., and **Critchley, H. D.** (2014). Fear from the heart: Sensitivity to fear stimuli depends on individual heartbeats. *Journal of Neuroscience, 34*(19), 6573–82. doi:10.1523/JNEUROSCI.3507-13.2014.

Garfinkel, S. N., Seth, A. K., Barrett, A. B., Suzuki, K., and **Critchley, H. D.** (2015). Knowing your own heart: Distinguishing interoceptive accuracy from interoceptive awareness. *Biological Psychology, 104*, 65–74. doi:10.1016/j.biopsycho.2014.11.004.

Garfinkel, S. N. and **Critchley, H. D.** (2016). Threat and the body: How the heart supports fear processing. *Trends in Cognitive Sciences, 20*(1), 34–46. doi:10.1016/j.tics.2015.10.005.

Garfinkel, S. N., **Tiley, C.**, **O'Keeffe, S.**, **Harrison, N. A.**, **Seth, A. K.**, and **Critchley, H. D.** (2016). Discrepancies between dimensions of interoception in autism: Implications for emotion and anxiety. *Biological Psychology*, *114*, 117–26. doi:10.1016/j.biopsycho.2015.12.003.

Garner, D. M., **Olmstead, M. P.**, and **Polivy, J.** (1983). Development and validation of a multidimensional eating disorder inventory for anorexia nervosa and bulimia. *International Journal of Eating Disorders*, *2*(2), 15–34.

Harrison, A., **Sullivan, S.**, **Tchanturia, K.**, and **Treasure, J.** (2009). Emotion recognition and regulation in anorexia nervosa. *Clinical Psychology & Psychotherapy*, *16*(4), 348–56.

Harrison, N. A. (2017). Brain structures implicated in inflammation-associated depression. In: R. Dantzer and L. Capuron (eds), *Inflammation-Associated Depression: Evidence, Mechanisms and Implications*. Cham: Springer International Publishing, pp. 221–48.

Herbert, B. M., **Pollatos, O.**, and **Schandry, R.** (2007). Interoceptive sensitivity and emotion processing: An EEG study. *International Journal of Psychophysiology*, *65*(3), 214–27.

Hohwy, J. (2010). The hypothesis testing brain: some philosophical applications. In: J. Sutton (ed.), *9th Conference of the Australasian Society for Cognitive Science*. Sydney, Sep 30–Oct 02, 2009. Sydney: Macquarie Centre for Cognitive Science, pp. 135–44.

Hohwy, J. (2013). *The Predictive Mind*. Oxford: Oxford University Press.

James, W. (1884). What is an emotion? *Mind*, *9*, 188–205.

Katkin, E. S., **Morell, M. A.**, **Goldband, S.**, **Bernstein, G. L.**, and **Wise, J. A.** (1982). Individual differences in heartbeat discrimination. *Psychophysiology*, *19*(2), 160–6.

Kirmayer, L. J. (2001). Cultural variations in the clinical presentation of depression and anxiety: Implications for diagnosis and treatment. *Journal of Clinical Psychiatry*, *62*, 22–30.

Kober, H., **Barrett, L. F.**, **Joseph, J.**, **Bliss-Moreau, E.**, **Lindquist, K.**, and **Wager, T. D.** (2008). Functional grouping and cortical-subcortical interactions in emotion: A meta-analysis of neuroimaging studies. *Neuroimage*, *42*(2), 998–1031. doi:10.1016/j.neuroimage.2008.03.059.

Lamm, C. and **Singer, T.** (2010). The role of anterior insular cortex in social emotions. *Brain Structure and Function*, *214*(5–6), 579–91. doi:10.1007/s00429-010-0251-3.

Murialdo, G., **Casu, M.**, **Falchero, M.**, **Brugnolo, A.**, **Patrone, V.**, **Cerro, P.**, et al. (2007). Alterations in the autonomic control of heart rate variability in patients with anorexia or bulimia nervosa: Correlations between sympathovagal activity, clinical features, and leptin levels. *Journal of Endocrinological Investigation*, *30*(5), 356–62.

Murphy, J., **Brewer, R.**, **Catmur, C.**, and **Bird, G.** (2016). Interoception and psychopathology: A developmental neuroscience perspective. *Developmental Cognitive Neuroscience*, **23**, 45–56. doi:10.1016/j.dcb2016.12.006.

Nemiah, J. C. (1976). Alexithymia: A view of the psychosomatic process. *Modern Trends in Psychosoamtic Medicine*, *3*, 430–9.

Nummenmaa, L., **Glerean, E.**, **Hari, R.**, and **Hietanen, J. K.** (2014). Bodily maps of emotions. *Proceedings of the National Academy of Sciences USA*, *111*(2), 646–51. doi:10.1073/pnas.1321664111.

Palmer, C. J., **Seth, A. K.**, and **Hohwy, J.** (2015). The felt presence of other minds: Predictive processing, counterfactual predictions, and mentalising in autism. *Consciousness and Cognition*, *36*, 376–89. doi:10.1016/j.concog.2015.04.007.

Palmer, C. J., **Lawson, R. P.**, and **Hohwy, J.** (2017). Bayesian approaches to autism: Towards volatility, action, and behavior. *Psychology Bulletin*, *143*(5), 521–42. doi:10.1037/bul0000097.

Paulus, M. P., and **Stein, M. B.** (2006). An insular view of anxiety. *Biological Psychiatry*, *60*(4), 383–7. doi:10.1016/j.biopsych.2006.03.042.

Paulus, M. P. and **Stein, M. B.** (2010). Interoception in anxiety and depression. *Brain Structure and Function*, *214*(5–6), 451–63. doi:10.1007/s00429-010-0258-9.

Pellicano, E. and **Burr, D.** (2012). When the world becomes "too real": A Bayesian explanation of autistic perception. *Trends in Cognitive Sciences, 16*(10), 504–10.

Peyron, R., Laurent, B., and **Garcia-Larrea, L.** (2000). Functional imaging of brain responses to pain. A review and meta-analysis (2000). *Clinical Neurophysiology, 30*(5), 263–88.

Phan, K. L., Wager, T., Taylor, S. F., and **Liberzon, I.** (2002). Functional neuroanatomy of emotion: A meta-analysis of emotion activation studies in PET and fMRI. *Neuroimage, 16*(2), 331–48.

Pollatos, O., Kurz, A.-L., Albrecht, J., Schreder, T., Kleemann, A. M., Schöpf, V., et al. (2008). Reduced perception of bodily signals in anorexia nervosa. *Eating Behaviors, 9*(4), 381–8.

Pollatos, O., Traut-Mattausch, E., and **Schandry, R.** (2009). Differential effects of anxiety and depression on interoceptive accuracy. *Depression and Anxiety, 26*(2), 167–73.

Porges, S. (1993). Body perception questionnaire. Laboratory of Developmental Assessment, University of Maryland, Baltimore, MD.

Quadt, L. (2017). Levels of social embodiment—towards a unifying perspective on social cognition. Mainz. Doctoral dissertation, Gutenberg Qualify. <http://d-nb.info/113138878X/34>.

Quadt, L. (2018). Commentary: First-order embodiment, second-order embodiment, third-order embodiment. *Frontiers of Psychology, 9*(445), 1–3. doi:10.3389/fpsyg.2018.0045.

Quattrocki, E. and **Friston, K.** (2014). Autism, oxytocin and interoception. *Neuroscience and Biobehavioral Reviews, 47*, 410–30. doi:10.1016/j.neubiorev.2014.09.012.

Schachter, S. and **Singer, J. E.** (1962). Cognitive, social, and physiological determinants of emotional state. *Psychological Review, 69*, 379–99.

Schandry, R. (1981). Heart beat perception and emotional experience. *Psychophysiology, 18*(4), 483–8.

Seth, A. K., Suzuki, K., and **Critchley, H. D.** (2011). An interoceptive predictive coding model of conscious presence. *Frontiers in Psychology, 2*, 395. doi:10.3389/fpsyg.2011.00395.

Seth, A. K. (2013). Interoceptive inference, emotion, and the embodied self. *Trends in Cognitive Sciences, 17*(11), 565–73. doi:10.1016/j.tics.2013.09.007.

Seth, A. K. (2015). The cybernetic bayesian brain. In: T. K. Metzinger and J. M. Windt (eds), *Open MIND*. Frankfurt am Main: MIND Group, pp. 1–24. doi: 10.15502/9783958570108.

Seth, A. K. and **Friston, K. J.** (2016). Active interoceptive inference and the emotional brain. *Philosophical Transaction of the Royal Society B, 371*(1708). doi:10.1098/rstb.2016.0007.

Shah, P., Hall, R., Catmur, C., and **Bird, G.** (2016). Alexithymia, not autism, is associated with impaired interoception. *Cortex, 81*, 215–20.

Silani, G., Bird, G., Brindley, R., Singer, T., Frith, C., and **Frith, U.** (2008). Levels of emotional awareness and autism: An fMRI study. *Social Neuroscience, 3*(2), 97–112. doi:10.1080/17470910701577020.

Singer, T., Critchley, H. D., and **Preuschoff, K.** (2009). A common role of insula in feelings, empathy and uncertainty. *Trends in Cognitive Sciences, 13*(8), 334–340. doi:10.1016/j.tics.2009.05.001.

Sloan, D. M. and **Sandt, A. R.** (2010). Depressed mood and emotional responding. *Biological Psychology, 84*(2), 368–74.

Sterling, P. (2012). Allostasis: A model of predictive regulation. *Physiology Behavior, 106*(1), 5–15.

Terasawa, Y., Shibata, M., Moriguchi, Y., and **Umeda, S.** (2013). Anterior insular cortex mediates bodily sensibility and social anxiety. *Social Cognitive and Affective Neuroscience, 8*(3), 259–266. doi:10.1093/scan/nss108.

Terasawa, Y., Moriguchi, Y., Tochizawa, S., and **Umeda, S.** (2014). Interoceptive sensitivity predicts sensitivity to the emotions of others. *Cognition and Emotion, 28*(8), 1435–1448. doi:10.1080/02699931.2014.888988.

Tsakiris, M. (2017). The multisensory basis of the self: From body to identity to others. *Quarterly Journal of Experimental Psychology, 70*(4), 597–609.

Tylee, A. and **Gandhi, P.** (2005). The importance of somatic symptoms in depression in primary care. *Primary Care Companion Journal of Clinical Psychiatry*, *7*(4), 167–76.

Wicker, B., Keysers, C., Plailly, J., Royet, J. P., Gallese, V., and **Rizzolatti, G.** (2003). Both of us disgusted in My insula: The common neural basis of seeing and feeling disgust. *Neuron*, *40*(3), 655–64.

Wiens, S., Mezzacappa, E. S., and **Katkin, E. S.** (2000). Heartbeat detection and the experience of emotions. *Cognition and Emotion*, *14*(3), 417–27. doi:10.1080/026999300378905.

Williams, L. M., Brammer, M. J., Skerrett, D., Lagopolous, J., Rennie, C., Kozek, K., et al. (2000). The neural correlates of orienting: An integration of fMRI and skin conductance orienting. *Neuroreport*, *11*(13), 3011–15.

Zaki, J., Davis, J. I., and **Ochsner, K. N.** (2012). Overlapping activity in anterior insula during interoception and emotional experience. *Neuroimage*, *62*(1), 493–99. doi:10.1016/j.neuroimage.2012.05.012.

Chapter 8

The somatic error hypothesis of anxiety

Sahib S. Khalsa and Justin S. Feinstein

8.1 Introduction

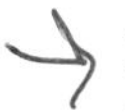

Interoceptive experiences are characterized by heightened physiological and psychological states, particularly when homeostatic deviations occur in response to threats—or potential threats—to the body. This chapter argues that anxiety disorders are fundamentally driven by somatic errors that fail to be adaptively regulated, leaving the organism in a state of dissonance where the predicted body state is perpetually out of line with the current body state as mapped within the interoceptive circuitry of the brain.

Classification models have clearly identified interoceptive symptoms as prominent features in the diagnosis of psychiatric disorders including anxiety, mood, eating, and somatic symptom disorders (APA, 2013), though they are likely to be present in many others. Despite the contribution of interoceptive disturbances in the clinical manifestations of these disorders, there are presently no interoceptive biomarkers that have been demonstrated to improve diagnosis, prognosis, or treatment reliably (Khalsa et al., 2018). Furthermore, interoception has not yet gained a foothold in alternative frameworks for biologically phenotyping mental illness, such as the Research Domain Criteria (RDoC) initiative (Kozak & Cuthbert, 2016). This stagnated progress is perhaps complicated by the fact that it remains unclear whether such patients process interoceptive sensations differently or whether they have a systematic bias toward reporting such feelings. Recent developments in computational neuroscience are spurring progress in interoception research by re-examining the traditional view that visceral sensations arise solely from perception of the body's internal milieu via ascending afferent pathways. Based on the notion of "active inference" (Friston, Daunizeau, & Kiebel, 2009), these models suggest that interoceptive perceptions are dynamically constructed by the brain, meaning that interoception occurs through an iterative process of comparing the brain's anticipation of sensation with concurrently incoming sensation (Paulus & Stein, 2006; Singer, Critchley, & Preuschoff, 2009; Seth et al., 2011; Barrett & Simmons, 2015; Pezzulo, Rigoli, & Friston, 2015; Stephan et al., 2016; Petzschner et al., 2017).

A consequence of active inference models may be that certain psychiatric disorders, especially those characterized by chronic and unrelenting anxiety, are exemplified by mismatches between the brain's ongoing comparison of anticipated and incoming signals. These mismatches have been previously referred to as altered prediction states or "interoceptive prediction errors" (Paulus & Stein, 2006; Seth et al., 2011). In particular, it has been proposed that sustained and exaggerated interoceptive prediction errors dysregulate the ability to accurately sense what is happening in the body, resulting in a turbulent reference state (i.e. a "noisy baseline") (Paulus & Stein, 2010), attentional bias toward threat (Hakamata et al., 2010), increased worry and self-related cognitions, dysfunctional learning about bodily states over time (Van den Bergh et al., 2017), and increased allostatic load (Sterling, 2012) leading to increased stress and mental illness (Sterling, 2014; Peters, McEwen, & Friston, 2017). Building upon this framework, a number of recent models have further elaborated how the brain computes interoceptive prediction errors, including which regions and cellular lamina are involved, and how these may be modeled using hierarchical Bayesian models (Seth, Suzuki, & Friston, 2011; Barrett & Simmons, 2015; Pezzulo, Rigoli, & Friston, 2015; Stephan et al., 2016; Petzschner et al., 2017). The purpose of this chapter is not to review these proposals in detail, and for further guidance the reader is encouraged to examine the cited references and other chapters in this edited volume. Instead, our aim is to juxtapose these perspectives against some clinical observations of how interoceptive dysfunction generates anxious psychopathology via a global mechanism of somatic errors.

8.2 What are somatic errors?

One way that anxiety disorders can be broadly characterized is by a dysfunction in the way the mind computes and integrates representations of the inner and outer worlds of the body across time. According to this view, anxiety results from the brain's distorted translation of what it anticipates will happen in these worlds versus what is actually happening in these worlds, producing discrepancy or error signals. These somatic errors are not simply the passive result of a dysfunctional transfer of afferent body-to-brain mapping. They are highly constructive. They reflect dynamic breakdowns in the brain's tightrope act of simultaneously mapping objects in the world external to the body, mapping objects in the world internal to the body, integrating these maps with neural representations of the predicted state of the world, and subsequently modifying these maps over time to maintain an updated representation of the self (Figure 8.1).

Thus, there are two very different worlds inside our brain: the internal world of our body and the external world in which that body lives. Each waking moment, the brain is in constant flux, attempting to pair what is happening on the outside with what is happening on the inside. A somatic error is produced whenever the body state predicted by the brain differs from the actual body signals being continuously delivered and mapped in viscerosensory regions of the brainstem, diencephalon, insular, and somatosensory cortices. Collectively, the brain's processing of these afferent body signals is critical for the computation of a neural map of the self. While there is an initial moment of sensory mapping of the self with no prior experience (i.e. the

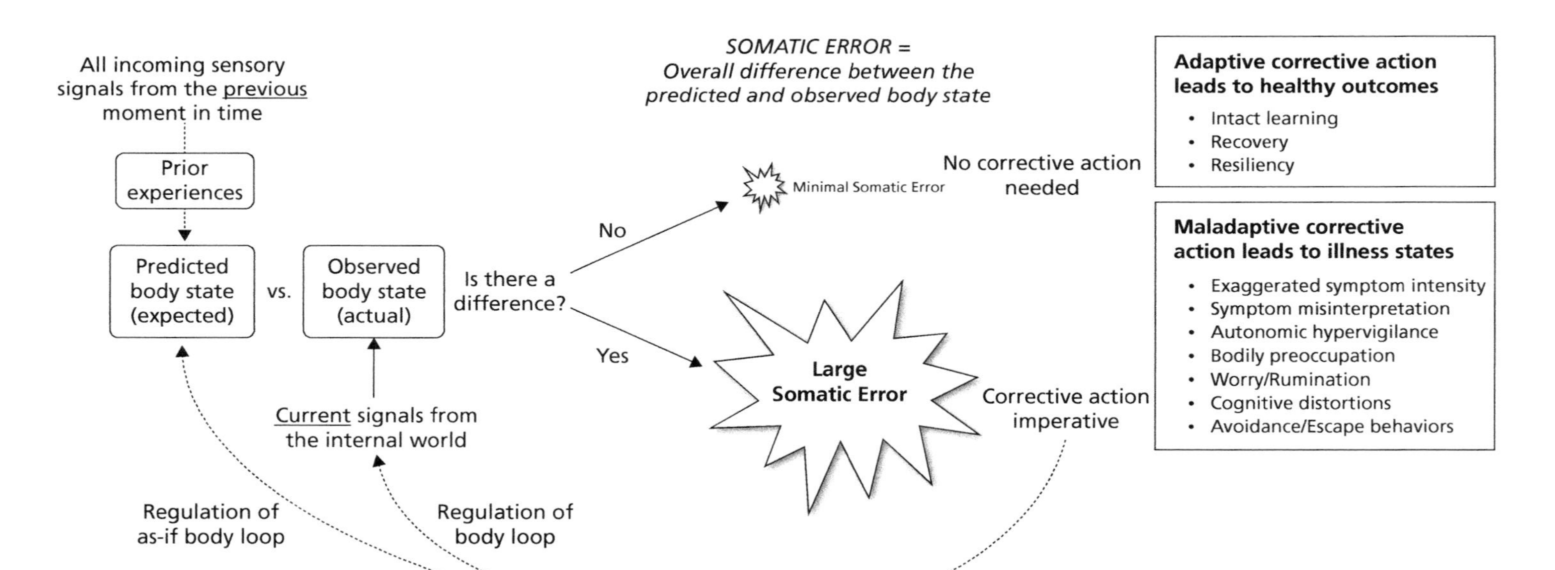

Figure 8.1 The somatic error hypothesis of anxiety. A regulatory battle for control ensues in the central nervous system following a mismatch between the current physiological state of an organism as mapped in viscerosensory brain regions, and the predicted body state as computed in visceromotor control regions. The discrepancy between the predicted and current body state (i.e., the 'somatic error') signals a need for corrective action, motivating changes in both cognition and behavior. The predicted body state is continuously constructed based on a moving snapshot of all the sensory signals encountered during the previous moment in time, filtered through the lens of past experience via conditioning. Notably, these conditioned sensory signals can emerge from both the internal world of the body, and the external world in which that body currently lives. The observed body state is a moment-to-moment mapping of all the incoming signals from the internal world of the body. The degree of discrepancy between the predicted and observed body state signals the need for corrective action, which can be achieved by either adjusting the predictions to better match the current physiological state (via regulation of the as-if body loop), or by modifying the current physiological state to more closely conform to the predictions (via regulation of the body loop). When somatic errors are small, corrective action is discretionary, whereas when somatic errors are large, corrective action is imperative. Adaptive corrective action leads to healthy outcomes whereas maladaptive corrective actions lead to anxiety, as described further in the text.

"inaugural moment" per Damasio, 1999), this initial neural map is quickly modified by life experience. The result is the gradual development over time of a set of prior experiences which inform expectations about the potential physiological impact of encountering specific sensory stimuli whether they be internal or external to the body. At the interface between these two worlds lies the brain's machinery for generating predicted body states, namely in anterior insula and visceromotor control regions such as the amygdala, anterior cingulate, and ventromedial prefrontal cortices (vmPFC), critical gatekeepers responsible for helping to merge the internal and external worlds so that the next time they collide, the body will be better prepared to cope with the challenges posed by the environment (we elaborate in further detail on the neural circuitry of somatic errors in section 8.5).

The predicted body state is continuously modified and constructed based on the sensory signals and cognitions from the previous moment in time. This ongoing modification inevitably results in discrepancies between the predicted and observed state of the body, that is, somatic errors. The occurrence of somatic errors are entirely normal biological events, and their successful detection and regulation is often critical for the maintenance of homeostatic conditions within the body. When somatic errors are minimal, no corrective action is needed and the preceding neural map of the self is maintained. When somatic errors are large, corrective action becomes imperative. Under normal circumstances successful corrective action flexibly modifies the neural model of the self. However, under abnormal circumstances somatic errors can persist for many years, reinforced by maladaptive behaviors (often in the form of avoidance and withdrawal behavior) and cognitions (often in the form of worry, rumination, and hypervigilance), resulting in distorted and rigid models of the self in the world.

8.3 Corrective action failure and its consequences

Corrective action in the presence of somatic error can be achieved by adjusting the predictions to match the current physiological state better, or by modifying the current physiological state to conform more closely to the predictions. A key proposition of this model is that successful corrective action reduces somatic error, promoting homeostatic balance within the nervous system, and reductions in feelings of anxiety. However, in cases of anxiety disorder, these reductions are often short-lived. The discrepancy between the predicted and observed body state is easily reinstated by a myriad of triggers, leading to long-term impairment in life functioning. Prolongation of somatic error for an unsustainable period of time will eventually force the system into making long-term allostatic adjustments, further promoting states of chronic and disordered anxiety, and leading to feelings of helplessness due to repeated failures to quell the somatic error, and often comorbid depression. In its most severe form, the somatic error becomes so pervasive that the only corrective action that seems to quell the error is avoidance of all perceived triggers (a condition known as *agoraphobia*).

This interoceptively focused model of anxiety is predicated on the assumption that a primary function of the nervous system is to develop accurate models of the world in an effort to establish conditions ideal for optimizing bodily functioning. These internal models rely upon sensory mapping of current signals (akin to the "body loop" described by Damasio)[1] and anticipated signals (akin to the "as-if body loop" also described by Damasio),[2] leading to the generation and experience of emotion. Corrective actions in response to somatic errors can be achieved via regulation of these body loops, and may be reflected by the adaptation of different patterns of thoughts, beliefs, or behaviors by an individual. Adaptive corrective action via regulation of body loop and as-if body loop signals results in adaptation, learning, and resilience. On the other hand, corrective action failure results in dysregulation of body loop and as-if body loop signaling. This can manifest via reports of sudden changes in symptom intensity, mislabeling of symptoms, a predominant focus on bodily signals in daily life, extreme hypervigilance towards disturbed body states, aberrant self-related thinking patterns, and attempts to reduce these aversive experiences via avoidance or escape behaviors. We propose that in the case of certain psychiatric disorders, a systematic failure to correct somatic errors leads individuals to make choices which fail to establish ideal conditions for optimizing internal bodily functioning and survival; that is, repeated attempts to reduce somatic error conflict lead to suboptimal functioning that is energetically costly to regulate, resulting in maladapative behaviors and cognitions, often leading to further discrepancies between predicted and observed body states. These discrepancies propagate and/or amplify the presence of somatic errors, leading to a positive feedback loop which often manifests as anxious psychopathology.

Most of the processing and regulation of somatic errors occurs beneath the surface of conscious awareness. However, if the somatic error magnitude becomes large enough, and the repeated failure to correct the error overwhelms the system, it can directly lead to subjective feeling states marked by prominent (often aversive) interoceptive symptoms, as well as an obligatory motivation to act to reduce the associated discomfort and distress. In the setting of psychopathology, this compensatory response generates a cascade of persisting predictions that, in future moments, are often disconnected from ongoing afferent body signals. Such "predictions gone astray" reflect an overregulation by the brain of repeatedly modifying the observed body state. In essence, the predicted body state hijacks the present moment, culminating in an observed body state that never quite matches the contingencies of the present moment.

When it comes to subjective feeling states, particularly in the setting of psychopathology, it may be very difficult for individuals to differentiate the past, present, and future, all of which are melded into a current feeling state. One way to consider these

[1] Damasio defined the body loop as a set of neural and humoral pathways by which "the body landscape is changed and is subsequently represented in somatosensory structures of the central nervous system, from the brainstem on up" (1999, p. 80).

[2] Damasio characterized the as-if body loop as a separate pathway for the brain to simulate the body, in which "the representation of body-related changes is created directly in sensory maps, under the control of other neural sites." In other words, "it is 'as if' the body had really been changed, but it has not." The primary benefit of operating directly at the as-if body loop was that "bypassing the body saves both time and energy, something that may be helpful in certain circumstances" (1999, p. 281).

temporal influences is to view the predicted body state as a merging of both the past (memories and conditioned associations between exteroceptive stimuli and their interoceptive consequences) and the future (Bayesian predictions based on a moving snapshot of all the sensory information from the previous moment in time, filtered through the lens of past experience). The subjective feeling state of each moment in time is then a balancing between an observed body state in the present and a predicted body state of the future that is grounded by past experience. Such a balancing act requires seamless integration and realistic weighting of all streams of information from the past, present, and future in order to maintain balance and homeostatic stability within the nervous system. Unfortunately, in the case of chronic anxiety, the weight given to the predicted body state of some future moment often dominates the present moment. In turn, this can lead to persistent and exaggerated somatic errors that fail to be sufficiently regulated and controlled. In the desperate search for a more stable state, a nervous system in constant disequilibrium and struggling to cope with the contingencies of life will initiate corrective actions, namely avoidance/withdrawal from all sensory cues that predict the onset of future disequilibrium. This behavior is a by-product of a sensitization process which we discuss in greater detail later in this chapter. Nevertheless, a nervous system alarmed about its own demise will strive to find ways to adapt, and anxiety is a natural outcome when it fails to make accurate predictions about its own future.

8.4 **Somatic errors in the brain**

Body sensing brain regions include those which play primary roles in directly mapping the autonomic, chemosensory, endocrine, and immune systems, which relay information via interoceptive sensory channels to the brainstem (e.g. nucleus tractus solitarius, NTS), hypothalamus, thalamus (e.g. ventromedial posterior thalamic nucleus), insula (mainly dorsal mid and posterior sectors), and somatosensory cortices (SI and SII) (Damasio, 1999; Craig, 2002; Critchley et al., 2004; Khalsa et al., 2009; Feinstein et al., 2013; Hassanpour et al., 2018). The processing of information across these channels occurs in a hierarchical fashion, with multiple feedback loops starting in early levels of the brainstem. Body prediction generators include agranular visceromotor brain regions such as the anterior cingulate, vmPFC, amygdala, and anterior insula (Barrett & Simmons, 2015), as well as granular neocortical regions implicated in other forms of motor and autonomic control including supplementary motor areas and premotor cortex.

A somatic error is fundamentally a summative reflection of the discrepancies in predicted and observed body states as information flows from lower to higher levels within the nervous system, and back (see Smith et al., 2017 for a detailed example of this pertaining to the autonomic nervous system and vagal control). Ultimately, the calculation of somatic errors occurs in brainstem nuclei such as NTS, and in cortical structures such as the dorsal mid-insula, both of which are uniquely situated, anatomically, to (a) compare incoming interoceptive information directly with the predictions of this sensory information submitted by nearby structures such as the parabrachial nucleus and anterior insula, and (b) transmit error signals to other closely connected structures, such as the periaqueductal gray and dorsal anterior cingulate, so that corrective action can be initiated and the error signal can be regulated. We propose that discrete cortical and subcortical networks underlie the prediction, detection, and regulation of somatic errors. Namely, the vmPFC (Barrett & Simmons, 2015), anterior insula (Simmons et al., 2011), amygdala/extended amygdala (Davis et al., 2010), and parabrachial nucleus (Herbert, Moga, & Saper, 1990) are important hubs for the generation of prediction signals, particularly faulty prediction signals in the context of anxious anticipation and subjective uncertainty and ambiguity. In contrast, important hubs for the detection of somatic errors include NTS, one of the primary recipients of interoceptive signals from the cranial nerves and spinal cord, and the dorsal mid/posterior insula, the first cortical recipient of afferent signals from the vagus nerve and lamina 1 spinothalamic neurons (Craig, 2002) and a region highly responsive to bottom-up physiological changes in the viscera (Gianaros et al., 2017; Hassanpour et al., 2018). Finally, the periaqueductal grey (Roy et al., 2014), amygdala (Feinstein, Adolphs, & Tranel , 2016), and dorsal anterior cingulate cortex (ACC) (Shackman et al., 2011; Gianaros et al., 2017) are important hubs for the regulation of somatic errors and inhibition of pain and panic. Differences in the laminar organization may explain how signal transmission flows between hubs, and more specifically why granular regions of the insula detect somatic errors (Barrett & Simmons, 2015), and agranular regions such as the anterior insula and ACC have outsized roles in the prediction and regulation of somatic errors. Based on this reasoning, it is plausible that sustained somatic error dysregulation may result in long-term brain alterations localized to the regions involved in the prediction, detection, and regulation of somatic errors. Supportive evidence comes from functional abnormalities seen in amygdala, insula, and ACC during emotion processing across multiple types of anxiety disorders (Etkin & Wager, 2007), as well as recent meta-analytic work observing volumetric reductions localized to the insula and ACC across multiple forms of mental illness, including anxiety (Goodkind et al., 2015). The presence of functional and structural brain alterations in the amygdala, insula, and ACC following sustained somatic error dysregulation in patients with anxiety suggests that somatic errors may be a core feature of anxious psychopathology.

8.5 How is a somatic error different from a somatic marker?

The somatic marker hypothesis (Damasio, 1994, 1996) proposed the idea that marker signals pertaining to the state of the body were integral to the process of decision-making. Much like interoceptive processes, these marker signals operate at both overt (conscious) and covert (unconscious) levels to rapidly guide decision-making, particularly under conditions of uncertainty (Bechara et al., 1997). The circuitry underlying somatic markers is postulated to overlap with brain circuits involved in the generation and experience of emotion, with initial evidence for the hypothesis based on observed deficits in autonomic responses to emotionally charged stimuli and abnormal decision-making behaviors in neurological lesion patients with damage to sectors of the vmPFC. However, somatic markers were theorized also to require the operation of other body-sensing and emotion-related brain structures such as the amygdala, insula, and somatosensory cortices, which collaborated with the ventromedial prefrontal cortex to establish an optimal decision signal via the body loop or the as-if body loop circuit. In this regard, there is considerable overlap between the somatic marker and somatic error hypotheses, with the latter critically building off the former. However, there are several key differences. First, the somatic marker hypothesis focuses specifically on predicting future body states in service of guiding advantageous decision-making, whereas the somatic error hypothesis concentrates on the comparison between predicted body states in relation to the observed body state in service of guiding corrective regulatory actions. In essence, somatic markers guide optimal decision-making, whereas sustained somatic errors obscure optimal decision-making. Thus, somatic errors may help to explain the process by which somatic marker signals become distorted or lost in translation during the decision-making process. Second, the somatic marker hypothesis provides no explication of psychiatric disturbances such as anxiety disorders, whereas the somatic error hypothesis is entirely aimed at addressing how anxiety is fundamentally driven by failures to adaptively regulate the error signal via the body loop or as-if body loop.

8.6 Somatic errors are prominent drivers of anxiety

The heightened experience of fear and anxiety, the pervasive avoidance of stimuli capable of inducing such an experience, and the compulsive worrying and rumination about future encounters with anxiety-inducing stimuli represent the emotional, behavioral, and cognitive sequelae of an anxious state. Within the framework of the somatic error hypothesis these sequelae are a consequence, or by-product, of the corrective actions aimed at attenuating somatic error. Thus, many instances of chronic anxiety are being fundamentally driven by somatic errors that fail to be adaptively regulated, leaving the individual in a state of dissonance where the predicted body state is perpetually out of line with the current body state.

Here we begin to outline the process by which chronic anxiety develops over time. The classic example is panic disorder, where an individual suddenly experiences an unprovoked panic attack marked by interoceptive sensations of sympathetic nervous system overdrive: they feel palpitations, dyspnea, dizziness, a feeling of separation from their self or surroundings, and a sense of impending doom or death. These feelings are typically accompanied by signs of sympathetic activation, although they can arise in the absence of bodily changes via dysregulated as-if body loop signaling. In the absence of any indicators of a source of threat, a search process ensues, and corrective action is taken, often in the form of escape and safety-seeking followed by future avoidance. Each panic-associated interoceptive sensation begins to take on further negative meaning and generates new abnormal beliefs about the self and the world, leading to abnormal behaviors.

To provide a more concrete example of this phenomenon in relation to the somatic error hypothesis, we discuss the case of "Freddy," a patient with severe panic disorder, so severe in fact that at its peak he was going to the emergency room over six times a month. Each visit was precipitated by a panic attack that Freddy misinterpreted as a heart attack. Upon arriving at the emergency room, the doctors would run him through the same battery of tests, including 12-lead electrocardiogram and myocardial enzyme assessments to detect damage to the heart. The outcome was always the same: Freddy's heart was healthy and there was absolutely no evidence for any cardiac abnormalities. Let us assume, for the moment, that at the onset of a panic attack, Freddy's observed body state was characterized by a heightened heart rate, pounding palpitations, and difficulty breathing. In the absence of any obvious sensory cues that could predict such sensations, a large somatic error is produced that compels corrective action. For Freddy, the corrective action often entailed a rapid adjustment of his predicted body state so that it more closely matched his observed body state. Consequently, the predicted body state became one of a heart attack, leading him, quite rationally, to rush to the emergency room. The fascinating aspect of Freddy's case is that despite repeated medical tests showing that nothing was wrong with his heart, the visceral feeling at the onset of a panic attack was so powerful that all rational thought processes and memories for these past visits to the emergency room became overshadowed by the somatic error. The only explanation that made sense to him at that moment in time was that he must be having a heart attack. Thus, being unable to dampen the error signal by downregulating his observed body state during the onset of a panic attack, Freddy often turned to upregulating his predicted body state such that he now had the feeling "as-if" he was having a heart attack. Freddy's repeated failures to regulate the somatic error adaptively after dozens of emergency room visits led him to even more aberrant corrective action. He began misattributing his panic attacks to other related aspects of the context that just so happened to be occurring at the same time, a process known as fear generalization (Dymond et al., 2015). For example, one day Freddy had a panic attack while driving to his mother's house, and he became convinced that his mother was somehow responsible for generating the panic attack. This aberrant belief caused him to avoid visiting his mother for an entire year. Another panic attack that occurred while he was at work made him to avoid going to his job, eventually leading him to be fired. These failed attempts to control the discomfort and distress associated with each panic attack interfered with his daily life, and were only temporarily successful at reducing the underlying error signal. Freddy continued to experience triggers of somatic error routinely (e.g. perturbations in interoceptive sensations and/or aberrant predictions), continued to have panic attacks, and continued to avoid an ever-growing list of perceived triggers, ultimately leading to the development of panic disorder with agoraphobia, a condition marked by substantially greater functional disability. This illustrates that corrective actions are not always adaptive. They do not always eradicate somatic error and can, in fact, perpetuate it.

8.7 The slippery slope of anxiety sensitivity

Anxiety sensitivity refers to an individual's fear of experiencing anxiety-related sensations, especially those arising from within the body (e.g. heart palpitations or dyspnea), and is a core construct underlying the initiation and maintenance of pathological anxiety (Taylor,

2014). Individuals with high levels of anxiety sensitivity often believe that these sensations can lead to adverse consequences such as death, insanity, or social rejection. Such catastrophic misinterpretations make anxiety sensitivity an anxiety amplifier; people with high levels of anxiety sensitivity are quickly alarmed by anxiety-related sensations, which further intensifies their anxiety and reinforces their avoidance. Consequently, most patients with pathological anxiety also have heightened anxiety sensitivity, including patients with panic disorder, agoraphobia, post-traumatic stress disorder (PTSD), generalized anxiety disorder, and social anxiety disorder (Olatunji & Wolitzky-Taylor, 2009; Naragon-Gainey, 2010).

In the context of the somatic error hypothesis, anxiety sensitivity can be conceptualized as the persistent triggering of an abnormally large predicted body state by sensory signals that have become associated with anxiety. Even small degrees of exposure to these sensory cues can generate an exaggerated body prediction, which will lead to a somatic error followed by corrective action that upregulates the observed body state to be more in line with the predicted body state. However, by upregulating the very signals which one is sensitized to, there is further amplification of the predicted body state, followed by additional amplification of the observed body state. The process can quickly escalate into a vicious cycle which often leads patients to avoid all sensory cues that have been associated with the experience of anxiety. Avoidance of perceived triggers quickly reduces the somatic error but this relief is only temporary as the vicious cycle returns whenever the trigger is again encountered, as was seen in the case of Freddy.

8.8 Somatic errors and altered thought

Distorted beliefs are not somatic errors but can lead to somatic errors by triggering alterations in the predicted body state. Distorted beliefs are thus a consequence of dysfunctional modeling of the bodily world by the brain, and do not necessarily require conscious appraisal. However, because an initial somatic error can reverberate alarmingly throughout networks in the brain critical for making inferences about the world, distorted beliefs can quickly reinforce or magnify somatic errors. This distinction was made by Paulus and Stein (2006) such that altered interoceptive prediction signals were viewed as the primary process underlying states of anxiety, with both cognitive features (e.g. worrying) and behavioral features (e.g. avoidance) being the resulting consequence of this dysfunction. Later, they argued for a stronger role of cognition and self-based beliefs such that negative schemas might drive a tendency to anticipate aversive body states through a process of alliesthesia (Paulus & Stein, 2010). Both views differ substantially from the cognitive-behavioral perspective because they emphasize that cognitions are typically a consequence rather than a cause of anxiety, and they arise out of interoceptive prediction error signaling. This is compatible with the general notion that maladaptive corrective actions can perpetuate somatic errors and lead to sensitized states of anxiety. We are not arguing at this juncture that somatic error is the sole generator of anxiety (e.g. for several models with a broader emphasis on deficits in cognitive, behavioral, and social processes; see Mineka & Zinbarg, 2006; Bystritsky et al., 2013; Beck & Haigh, 2014)). Nor do we claim that somatic error processing is necessarily unique to anxiety (e.g. for several models featuring allostatic dysregulation of interoceptive signals in depression; see Harshaw, 2015; Barrett, Quigley, & Hamilton, 2016; Stephan et al., 2016). However, we do assert that sustained somatic errors which lead to maladaptive corrective actions are the cause (rather than consequence) of the cognitive, behavioral, and emotional manifestations of anxiety.

8.9 **Somatic errors and visceral illusions**

While changes in observed body state can be routinely felt, it is also possible to feel changes in the predicted body state, so long as the prediction triggers a somatic error. To highlight this point, we previously examined interoceptive processing in anorexia nervosa (AN) by administering double-blinded infusions of either saline or isoproterenol, a peripherally acting beta-adrenergic agonist akin to adrenaline (Khalsa et al., 2015). The general notion was to perturb the observed body state systematically under different contexts, either shortly before or after a calorically dense meal. In general, AN patients reported feeling the isoproterenol sensations at the same rate as healthy comparison participants, suggesting preserved interoception for changes in their observed body state (Figure 8.2). However, there was one important exception. During saline infusions, which did not alter the observed body state, the patients reported feeling significantly more sensations of palpitations and dyspnea, but only during the pre-meal period (Figure 8.2). The fact that

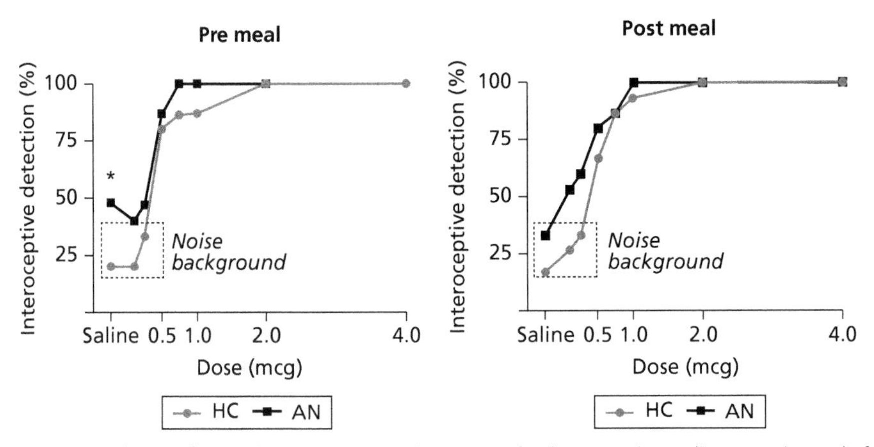

Figure 8.2 Evidence of somatic error in anorexia nervosa (AN). AN patients disproportionately felt sensations of heart palpitations and dyspnea during saline infusions, when no bodily modulation had occurred, but only during a pre-meal state when anticipating the consumption of a large meal (*$p < 0.05$). The shaded rectangles illustrate a hypothetical noise background as postulated by (Paulus & Stein, 2010). HC = healthy comparisons.

Adapted from *International Journal of Eating Disorders*, 48 (7), Sahib S. Khalsa, Michelle G. Craske, Wei Li, Sitaram Vangala, Michael Strober, Jamie D. Feusner, Altered interoceptive awareness in anorexia nervosa: Effects of meal anticipation, consumption and bodily arousal, pp. 889–97, doi:10.1002/eat.22387, © 2015 Wiley Periodicals, Inc.

no bodily modulation had actually occurred during the saline infusions suggests that AN patients were actually feeling cardiorespiratory "visceral illusions." Moreover, these visceral illusions were only present during the pre-meal state, a time period which is known to trigger strong feelings of fear and anxiety in patients with AN. This noisy baseline observed in AN is indicative of a somatic error being driven by their anxious predictions of the approaching meal. It seems possible that such visceral illusions permeate many aspects of these patients' lives, leading to maladaptive corrective actions that often include a profound avoidance of food.

Another instance of visceral illusion can occur when medical conditions cause potentially life-threatening changes to the observed body state. One such condition is known as atrial fibrillation, which is a cardiac arrhythmia affecting the upper chambers of the heart. Patients with atrial fibrillation frequently report interoceptive disturbances in the form of palpitations, shortness of breath, dizziness, fatigue, and chest pain, yet these symptoms only corroborate an observable heart rhythm disturbance in approximately one-third of active cases (Camm, Corbucci, & Padeletti, 2012). A fascinating study evaluated the accuracy of heart rhythm perception in such patients by fitting them with continuous electrical monitors for an entire week and recording self-perceived reports of irregular rhythms via button presses (Garimella et al., 2015). They found that the subset of patients with comorbid anxiety had a tendency to overestimate the presence of the irregular rhythm incorrectly (i.e. endorsing arrhythmia perception despite its absence). Once again, predicted body states were consciously felt as anxiety-inducing visceral illusions.

8.10 Iatrogenic somatic errors

Traumatic alterations to the observed body state are often a harbinger for corrective action that leads the predicted body into a highly anxious state. A prime example from cardiovascular medicine concerns the insertion of an implantable cardioverter defibrillator (ICD) within the body. ICD placement occurs when patients with cardiac pathology affecting the lower chambers of the heart are judged to be at increased risk of developing a fatal arrhythmia (Tracy et al., 2012). Although this intervention has well demonstrated survival benefits (Maron et al., 2000), the mechanism of treatment involves delivering a single or series of electrical discharges (i.e. "shocks") directly to neurons in the heart in order to resynchronize its rhythm. These shocks may be delivered appropriately (i.e. the discharge occurs in the presence of a detected arrhythmia) or inappropriately (i.e. the discharge occurs when there is no arrhythmia) (Sears & Conti, 2003). Even in the setting of positive treatment response, patients frequently develop clinically significant anxiety due to the large number of painful shocks to the heart, including approximately 10% that are due to false alarms (Magyar-Russell et al., 2011). Moreover, the amount of ICD shocks predicts the development of anxiety one year after implantation (Schulz et al., 2013).

We have treated numerous patients affected by these serious cardiac conditions (Khalsa et al., 2014) and found that the sensations elicited by ICD discharges in these individuals are indeed interoceptive in nature (Table 8.1). The somatic error generated by the ICD shock and subsequent corrective actions taken by patients are consistently reflective of

Table 8.1 Interoceptive symptoms and corrective actions following receipt of implantable cardioverter defibrillator (ICD) shocks in six patients referred for psychiatric treatment evaluation

Patient	Chief concern	Initial shock episode	Subsequent shock episodes	Feared sequelae	Corrective actions taken prior to consultation
ICD #l	*"I'm looking for some way to decrease my concerns about this thing firing off again."*	Pain intensity: 5 out of 10 Location: *"whole body": "like somebody hitting me in the stomach, only you can't prepare for it."* Radiation: throughout body Reported precipitating factors: dehydration, exertion	Total no. shocks: 4, single episode Pain intensity: 5 out of 10 Location: *"central core of the body"* Quality: *"like a jolt";* *"like getting punched in the chest."* Radiation: throughout the body Precipitating factors: walking *"a long distance"* *"I probably had some stress about getting on the plane"*	Hospitalization Cardiac surgery	Excessively checking radial pulse to determine whether heart is skipping Eating smaller meals due to concerns fullness caused shocks, then avoiding all restaurants Avoiding physical exertion such as swimming or playing with grandchildren
ICD #2	*"I've been fighting this for a long time now."*	Pain intensity: 8 out of 10 Location: chest Quality: *"like a horse kicked me in the chest."* Radiation: to shoulder Reported precipitating factors: hot day	Total no. shocks: > 30, multiple episodes Pain intensity: 8 out of 10 Location: chest Precipitating factors: unknown	Recurring dreams of being shocked. Feeling persisted upon waking. Lack of control over body symptoms	Avoiding physical positions believed to induce palpitations and arrhythmia sensation Extremely avoidant of any salt intake Will not walk any distance > l mile

ICD #3	Anxiety	Pain intensity : 10 out of 10 Location: chest Quality: *"like a kick to the chest"* Radiation: none Reported precipitating factors: none, was watching TV	Total no. shocks: *"too many to count"* (> 40), multiple episodes	Nightmares of getting shocked	Scanning body repeatedly for signals predicting shock Avoiding jogging for > 10 years Avoiding being alone for fear help won't arrive Avoiding being in public due to fear of embarrassment
ICD #4	*"Fear, I guess that I will die."*	Pain intensity: 8 out of 10 Location: chest Quality: *"It felt like I was in a head-on car collision . . . it felt like my brain was being scrambled."* Radiation: neck Reported precipitating factors: none	No further shocks; single episode	Nightmares about being shocked again. Fear of life-threatening condition	Avoiding approaching site of shock due to severe anxiety Avoiding sexual activity
ICD #5	*"I'm just living in a world where I can't walk 10 miles."*	Pain intensity: unable to report Quality: *"like every cell in your body is given a jolt from head to foot. It feels like your whole body has expanded by an inch."* Precipitating factors: none	Total no. shocks: 27, multiple episodes	*"It's kind of a consciousness. Every moment I'm worrying: 'is there going to be a trigger?'"*	Avoiding all exercise Avoiding stress
ICD #6	Anxiety	Pain intensity: none, but *"very unpleasant"*; *"kapow, kabang!"* Location: chest Precipitating factors: none	Total no. shocks: 12, multiple episodes	*"There's a sense of helplessness with it. I understand intellectually it's [ICD] keeping me alive, but physically it isn't pleasant"*	Frequently checking blood pressure and auscultating heart with stethoscope Repeated Emergency Department presentations

inflated body-state predictions and excessive avoidance behavior. One potent example of such maladaptive corrective action concerned "Sam," a cardiomyopathy patient who began spending all of his time in his local hospital after receiving recurrent ICD shocks. Sam would remain in the public visitation areas of the hospital throughout all hours for several months, and experienced significant fear upon leaving, under the rationale that this was the safest place to be to avoid further harm should another shock occur. Due to continued worry about being shocked, Sam even purchased a stethoscope in order to better listen to his own heartbeat. Upon perceiving the sensation of a racing heart, he would immediately auscultate it with the stethoscope for verification. Sam claimed he could distinguish between normal tachycardia and tachycardia associated with his arrhythmia, and predict the onset of a shock approximately three seconds later, although this did nothing to ameliorate his anxiety. Sam's corrective action here was maladaptive to the extreme, necessitating the neglect of all major functional domains (familial, occupational, and social), and against the reassurance and recommendations of his cardiologists. Even worse, it did not actually address the root cause of the anxiety, that the source of his somatic error was a prediction gone astray (i.e. "If I leave the hospital I will receive an ICD shock"). In this specific situation there was no actual bodily threat to respond to, just an aberrant prediction. Sam's case further illustrates how somatic errors triggered by aberrant body-state predictions can generate palpably real feelings. We speculate that they feel real because they are the result of aberrant activity in body-sensing brain regions (specifically, as-if body loops), resulting in a *de novo* or "simulated" perception indistinguishable from the real thing. Such cases, although uncommon, are not unique. Another corrective action failure involved a patient who refused to shower alone for three months out of fear that he would be shocked by his ICD and no one would find him. This same patient remained within a three-mile radius of his home for an entire year because it was located near a hospital, out of fear that he would be shocked and would not be evaluated and resuscitated in time.

8.11 Clinical implications of the somatic error hypothesis

By this point it should be clear that a somatic error can inspire both adaptive and maladaptive corrective actions. The ultimate goal of the corrective action is to minimize somatic error as quickly and efficiently as possible by temporarily returning the organism to a more stable homeostatic state, and thus, whether the action is adaptive or maladaptive is not actually taken into account during the regulatory process. For this reason, avoidance/withdrawal behavior is often the corrective action that initially wins the regulatory battle, as it is a highly effective technique for rapidly reducing somatic error. Unfortunately, avoidance/withdrawal behaviors fail to prevent the recurrence of somatic errors, nor do they confer enhanced regulatory control strategies over them. In this context it is not surprising that avoidance/withdrawal is the primary behavioral manifestation of most anxiety disorders, and the symptom that elicits the most impairment in life functioning.

It follows that the active ingredient of most psychotherapies for anxiety often involves learning to inhibit immediate maladaptive corrective actions triggered by somatic errors and experiencing the discrepancy long enough to develop a new adaptive model. A prime example is exposure-based therapies, which principally target avoidance behaviors by teaching individuals how to systematically approach the very things in life they have been avoiding including distressing experiences, thoughts, and memories. This requires placing the person in situations likely to exacerbate somatic errors, at least temporarily, but the main difference is that maintaining exposure to the aversive experience long enough requires the brain to adjust its regulatory strategy and develop a new setpoint (e.g. by changing the expectation of harm from an avoided situation). This happens primarily via inhibitory fear learning, which includes standard mechanisms such as habituation and desensitization, but importantly, seems to rely on the successful learning of new information via expectancy violations (Craske et al., 2008). Exposure therapy can be very effective, but is unfortunately highly underutilized in clinical practice (Deacon et al., 2013; Boettcher, Brake, & Barlow, 2015).

Interoceptive interventions that directly modify the observed state of the body can also help to acutely correct somatic errors. These interventions view the body as the entry point for modifying erroneous sensory experiences relevant to anxiety and can help reduce somatic errors being driven at the body loop level. Elicitation of the physiological relaxation response (Benson, 1993) is one way to attenuate the observed body state. Examples include progressive muscle relaxation, deep breathing, and autogenic guided imagery. These are often incorporated within cognitive-behavioral therapies due to small but reliable clinical effects, although they are only temporarily effective because they do not inherently induce new learning or address aberrant body predictions. Short-acting anxiolytic medications such as benzodiazepines also provide a temporary relief of somatic errors, but they do not change the brain's tendency to issue erroneous prediction signals about the inner and outer worlds of the body. Moreover, they do not introduce new learning, and in fact such medications are well known to hamper learning (Lister et al., 1988).

Given our emphasis on the role of interoceptive disturbances generating somatic errors, it is worth noting that there are several strategies on the horizon, some of which take the notion of interoceptive exposure therapy to a whole new level. These strategies, some newer and some older, may be effective at modulating interoceptive processing and attenuating somatic errors. The first strategy is referred to as Floatation-REST (Reduced Environmental Stimulation Therapy), an intervention which attenuates exteroceptive sensory input to the nervous system through the act of floating supine in a pool of water saturated with Epsom salt. The float experience is calibrated so that sensory signals from visual, auditory, olfactory, gustatory, thermal, tactile, vestibular, gravitational, and proprioceptive channels are minimized, as is most movement and speech. Subjectively, the effect appears to be one of both heightened interoceptive awareness and relaxation (Feinstein et al., 2018a), leading to lower levels of chronic anxiety in generalized anxiety disorder (Jonsson & Kjellgren, 2016) as well as lower levels of acute anxiety in patients with heightened anxiety sensitivity (Feinstein et al., 2018b). The floatation environment, which systematically reduces the nervous system's exposure to most external triggers of stress and anxiety, may provide a chronically anxious and hypervigilant nervous system with a rare respite from the daily barrage of external triggers, reducing the occurrence of exteroceptively triggered body predictions. Likewise, the heightened interoceptive awareness induced during Floatation-REST amplifies the observed body state and, in the context of physiological relaxation, the aversive association between visceral sensations and anxiety may be weakened. Subsequently, a competing association may be formed, one that links the experience of visceral sensations with a state of relaxation instead of anxiety. Another novel interoceptive approach is whole body hyperthermia (WBH), which involves the selective stimulation of heat-sensitive thermosensory pathways projecting from the skin to subcortical and cortical brain regions to achieve an elevated core body temperature of 38.5 degrees Celsius. A recent randomized sham-controlled trial found that a single session of WBH produced a significant antidepressant effect lasting up to six weeks in depressed patients (Janssen et al., 2016). While the underlying mechanism is uncertain, the study's effective sham-control suggests that the active antidepressant component was related to the heightened modulation of observed thermosensory and inflammatory signals from the body. From the perspective of somatic error, this intervention also relies heavily on modulation of current body state via the body loop, potentially forcing a recalibration of the prior setpoint. Other potential anxiety interventions involving interoceptive modulations of the observed body state include: modulation of muscle tension via Swedish massage (Rapaport et al., 2016), yoga (Jeter et al., 2015), exercise (Pedersen & Saltin, 2015) and cyclic activation of the sympathetic nervous system (Kox et al., 2014). In each case, these practices provide the brain with an intense inflow of salient and unambiguous bodily information, albeit across different sensory channels. The systematic application of these bodily inputs forces a shift in the mapping of the observed body state. These strategies may help to re-establish a new set point closer to a healthy physiological baseline, triggering a "reset" which ultimately reduces allostatic load. Other ways to reduce somatic errors at the as-if body loop level include psychotherapies, especially insight-oriented therapies such as cognitive therapy or psychodynamic therapy, that provide a means of belief-based attenuation of erroneous predictions. Finally, mindful meditation practices may help minimize somatic errors by refocusing attention on observed body-state processes and reducing attention to predicted body-state processes (Farb, Segal, & Anderson, 2013).

8.12 Conclusion

The somatic error hypothesis provides a point of understanding for both the genesis of anxiety, and the basis from which to explore novel interoceptive interventions that modulate body–brain communication. We anticipate that the concept of somatic error may be relevant to other forms of psychopathology characterized by aberrant body–brain signaling, and we hope this chapter has highlighted some of the ways in which corrective actions aimed at regulating somatic error can be the catalyst for anxiety in all its different varieties.

References

American Psychiatric Association (2013). *Diagnostic and Statistical Manual of Mental Disorders: DSM-5*. Washington, DC: American Psychiatric Association.

Barrett, L. F. and **Simmons, W. K.** (2015). Interoceptive predictions in the brain. *Nature Reviews Neuroscience, 16*, 419–29.

Barrett, L. F., Quigley, K. S., and **Hamilton, P.** (2016). An active inference theory of allostasis and interoception in depression. *Philosophical Transactions of the Royal Society of London B: Biological Sciences, 371*(1708), pii: 20160011. doi:10.1098/rstb.2016.0011.

Bechara, A., Damasio, H., Tranel, D., and **Damasio, A. R.** (1997). Deciding advantageously before knowing the advantageous strategy. *Science, 275*, 1293–5.

Beck, A. T. and **Haigh, E. A.** (2014). Advances in cognitive theory and therapy: The generic cognitive model. *Annual Review of Clinical Psychology, 10*, 1–24.

Benson, H. (1993). *The Relaxation Response*. New York, NY: Consumer Reports.

Boettcher, H., Brake, C. A., and **Barlow, D. H.** (2015). Origins and outlook of interoceptive exposure. *Journal of Behavior Therapy and Experimental Psychiatry, 53*, 41–51.

Bystritsky, A., Khalsa, S. S., Cameron, M. E., and **Schiffman, J. S.** (2013). Current diagnosis and treatment of anxiety disorders. *Pharmacy and Therapeutics, 38*, 30–57.

Camm, A. J., Corbucci, G., and **Padeletti, L.** (2012). Usefulness of continuous electrocardiographic monitoring for atrial fibrillation. *American Journal of Cardiology, 110*, 270–6.

Craig, A. D. (2002). How do you feel? Interoception: The sense of the physiological condition of the body. *Nature Reviews Neuroscience, 3*, 655–66.

Craske, M. G., Kircanski, K., Zelikowsky, M., Mystkowski, J., Chowdhury, N., and **Baker, A.** (2008). Optimizing inhibitory learning during exposure therapy. *Behavior Research Therapy*, **46**, 5–27.

Critchley, H. D., Wiens, S., Rotshtein, P., Ohman, A., and **Dolan, R. J.** (2004). Neural systems supporting interoceptive awareness. *Nature Neuroscience, 7*, 189–95.

Damasio, A. R. (1994). *Descartes's Error: Emotion, Reason, and the Human Brain*. New York, NY: Avon.

Damasio, A. R. (1996). The somatic marker hypothesis and the possible functions of the prefrontal cortex. *Philosophical Transactions of the Royal Society of London B, 351*, 1413–20.

Damasio, A. R. (1999). *The Feeling of What Happens: Body and Emotion in the Making of Consciousness*. New York, NY: Harcourt Brace.

Davis, M., Walker, D. L., Miles, L., and **Grillon, C.** (2010). Phasic vs sustained fear in rats and humans: Role of the extended amygdala in fear vs anxiety. *Neuropsychopharmacology, 35*, 105–35.

Deacon, B. J., Lickel, J. J., Farrell, N. R., Kemp, J. J., and **Hipol, L. J.** (2013). Therapist perceptions and delivery of interoceptive exposure for panic disorder. *Journal of Anxiety Disorders, 27*, 259–64.

Dymond, S., Dunsmoor, J. E., Vervliet, B., Roche, B., and **Hermans, D.** (2015). Fear generalization in humans: Systematic review and implications for anxiety disorder research. *Behavior Therapy, 46*, 561–82.

Etkin, A. and **Wager, T. D.** (2007). Functional neuroimaging of anxiety: A meta-analysis of emotional processing in PTSD, social anxiety disorder, and specific phobia. *American Journal of Psychiatry, 164*, 1476–88.

Farb, N. A., Segal, Z. V., and **Anderson, A. K.** (2013). Mindfulness meditation training alters cortical representations of interoceptive attention. *Social Cognitive and Affective Neuroscience, 8*, 15–26.

Feinstein, J. S., Buzza, C., Hurlemann, R., Follmer, R. L., Dahdaleh, N. S., Coryell, W. H., et al. (2013). Fear and panic in humans with bilateral amygdala damage. *Nature Neuroscience, 16*, 270–2.

Feinstein, J. S., Adolphs, R., and **Tranel, D.** (2016). *A Tale of Survival from the World of Patient SM*. New York, NY: Guilford Press.

Feinstein, J. S., Khalsa, S. S., Yeh, H., Al Zoubi, O., Arevian, A. C., Wohlrab, C., et al. (2018a). The elicitation of relaxation and interoceptive awareness using floatation therapy in individuals with high anxiety sensitivity. *Biological Psychiatry Cognitive Neuroscience and Neuroimaging, 3*, 555–62.

Feinstein, J. S., Khalsa, S. S., Yeh, H., Wohlrab, C., Simmons, W. K., Stein, M. B., et al. (2018b). Examining the short-term anxiolytic and antidepressant effect of Floatation-REST. *PLoS One, 13*, e0190292.

Friston, K. J., Daunizeau, J., and **Kiebel, S. J.** (2009). Reinforcement learning or active inference? *PLoS One, 4*, e6421.

Garimella, R. S., Chung, E. H., Gehi, A. K., Mounsey, J. P., Schwartz, J. D., Pursell, I., et al. (2015). Accuracy of patient perception of their prevailing rhythm: A comparative analysis of monitor data and questionnaire responses in patients with atrial fibrillation. *Heart Rhythm, 12*, 658–65.

Gianaros, P. J., Sheu, L. K., Uyar, F., Koushik, J., Jennings, J. R., Wager, T. D., et al. (2017). A brain phenotype for stressor-evoked blood pressure reactivity. *Journal of the American Heart Association, 6*.

Goodkind, M., Eickhoff, S. B., Oathes, D. J., Jiang, Y., Chang, A., Fox, P. T., et al. (2015). Identification of a common neurobiological substrate for mental illness. *JAMA Psychiatry, 72*, 305–15.

Hakamata, Y., Lissek, S., Bar-Heim, Y., Britton, J.C., Fox, N. A., Leibenluft, E., et al. (2010). Attention bias modification treatment: A meta-analysis toward the establishment of novel treatment for anxiety. *Biological Psychiatry, 68*, 982–90.

Harshaw, C. (2015). Interoceptive dysfunction: Toward an integrated framework for understanding somatic and affective disturbance in depression. *Psychological Bulletin, 141*, 311–63.

Hassanpour, M. S., Simmons, W. K., Feinstein, J. S., Luo, Q., Lapidus, R., Bodurka, J., et al. (2018). The insular cortex dynamically maps changes in cardiorespiratory interoception. *Neuropsychopharmacology, 43*, 426–34.

Herbert, H., Moga, M. M., and **Saper, C. B.** (1990). Connections of the parabrachial nucleus with the nucleus of the solitary tract and the medullary reticular formation in the rat. *Journal of Comparative Neurology, 293*, 540–80.

Janssen, C. W., Lowry, C. A., Mehl, M. R., Allen, J. J., Kelly, K. L., Gartner, D. E., et al. (2016). Whole-body hyperthermia for the treatment of major depressive disorder: A randomized clinical trial. *JAMA Psychiatry, 73*, 789–95.

Jeter, P. E., Slutsky, J., Singh, N., and **Khalsa, S. B.** (2015). Yoga as a therapeutic intervention: A bibliometric analysis of published research studies from 1967 to 2013. *Journal of Alternative and Complementary Medicine, 21*, 586–92.

Jonsson, K, and **Kjellgren, A.** (2016). Promising effects of treatment with flotation-REST (restricted environmental stimulation technique) as an intervention for generalized anxiety disorder (GAD): A randomized controlled pilot trial. *BMC Complementary and Alternative Medicine, 16*, 108.

Khalsa, S. S., Rudrauf, D., Feinstein, J. S., and **Tranel, D.** (2009). The pathways of interoceptive awareness. *Nature Neuroscience, 12*, 1494–6.

Khalsa, S. S., Shahabi, L., Ajijola, O. A., Bystritsky, A., Naliboff, B. D., and **Shivkumar, K.** (2014). Synergistic application of cardiac sympathetic decentralization and comprehensive psychiatric treatment in the management of anxiety and electrical storm. *Frontiers in Integrative Neuroscience, 7*, 98.

Khalsa, S. S., Craske, M. G., Li, W., Vangala, S., Strober, M., and **Feusner, J. D.** (2015). Altered interoceptive awareness in anorexia nervosa: Effects of meal anticipation, consumption and bodily arousal. *International Journal of Eating Disorders, 48*, 889–97.

Khalsa, S. S., Adolphs, R., Cameron, O. G., Critchley, H. D., Davenport, P. W., Feinstein, J. S., et al. (2018). Interoception and mental health: A roadmap. *Biological Psychiatry Cognitive Neuroscience and Neuroimaging, 3*, 501–13.

Kox, M., van Eijk, L.T., Zwaag, J., van den Wildenberg, J., Sweep, F. C., van der Hoeven, J. G., et al. (2014). Voluntary activation of the sympathetic nervous system and attenuation of the innate immune response in humans. *Proceedings of the National Academy of Sciences USA, 111*, 7379–84.

Kozak, M. J. and **Cuthbert, B. N.** (2016). The NIMH research domain criteria initiative: Background, issues, and pragmatics. *Psychophysiology, 53*, 286–97.

Lister, R. G., Weingartner, H., Eckardt, M. J., and **Linnoila, M.** (1988). Clinical relevance of effects of benzodiazepines on learning and memory. *Psychopharmacology Series, 6*, 117–27.

Magyar-Russell, G., Thombs, B. D., Cai, J., Baveja, T., Kuhl, E. A., Singh, P. P., et al. (2011). The prevalence of anxiety and depression in adults with implantable cardioverter defibrillators: A systematic review. *Journal of Psychosomatic Research, 71*, 223–31.

Maron, B. J., Shen, W. K., Link, M. S., Epstein, A. E., Almquist, A. K., Daubert, J. P., et al. (2000). Efficacy of implantable cardioverter-defibrillators for the prevention of sudden death in patients with hypertrophic cardiomyopathy. *New England Journal of Medicine, 342*, 365–73.

Mineka, S. and **Zinbarg, R.** (2006). A contemporary learning theory perspective on the etiology of anxiety disorders: It's not what you thought it was. *American Psychology, 61*, 10–26.

Naragon-Gainey, K. (2010). Meta-analysis of the relations of anxiety sensitivity to the depressive and anxiety disorders. *Psychology Bulletin, 136*, 128–50.

Olatunji, B. O. and **Wolitzky-Taylor, K. B.** (2009). Anxiety sensitivity and the anxiety disorders: A meta-analytic review and synthesis. *Psychology Bulletin, 135*, 974–99.

Paulus, M. P. and **Stein, M. B.** (2006). An insular view of anxiety. *Biological Psychiatry, 60*, 383–7.

Paulus, M. P. and **Stein, M. B.** (2010). Interoception in anxiety and depression. *Brain Structure and Function, 214*, 451–63.

Pedersen, B. K. and **Saltin, B.** (2015). Exercise as medicine—evidence for prescribing exercise as therapy in 26 different chronic diseases. *Scandinavian Journal of Medicine and Science in Sports*, J Med Sci Sports *25* Suppl. 3, 1–72.

Peters, A., McEwen, B. S., and **Friston, K.** (2017). Uncertainty and stress: Why it causes diseases and how it is mastered by the brain. *Progress in Neurobiology, 156*, 164–88.

Petzschner, F. H., Weber, L. A. E., Gard, T., and **Stephan, K. E.** (2017). Computational psychosomatics and computational psychiatry: *Toward* a joint framework for differential diagnosis. *Biological Psychiatry*, **82**, 421–30.

Pezzulo, G., Rigoli, F., and **Friston, K.** (2015). Active Inference, homeostatic regulation and adaptive behavioural control. *Progress in Neurobiology, 134*, 17–35.

Rapaport, M. H., Schettler, P., Larson, E. R., Edwards, S. A., Dunlop, B. W., Rakofsky, J. J., et al. (2016). Acute swedish massage monotherapy successfully remediates symptoms of generalized anxiety disorder: A proof-of-concept, randomized controlled study. *Journal of Clinical Psychiatry, 77*, e883–91.

Roy, M., Shohamy, D., Daw, N., Jepma, M., Wimmer, G. E., and **Wager, T. D.** (2014). Representation of aversive prediction errors in the human periaqueductal gray. *Nature Neuroscience, 17*, 1607–12.

Schulz, S.M., Massa, C. Grzbiela, A., Dengler, W., Wiedemann, G., and **Pauli, P.** (2013). Implantable cardioverter defibrillator shocks are prospective predictors of anxiety. *Heart and Lung, 42*(2), 105–11.

Sears, S. E., Jr. and **Conti, J. B.** (2003). Understanding implantable cardioverter defibrillator shocks and storms: Medical and psychosocial considerations for research and clinical care. *Clinical Cardiology, 26*, 107–11.

Seth, A. K., Suzuki, K., and **Critchley, H. D.** (2011). An interoceptive predictive coding model of conscious presence. *Frontiers in Psychology, 2*, 395.

Shackman, A. J., Salomons, T. V., Slagter, H. A., Fox, A. S., Winter, J. J., Davidson, R. J. (2011). The integration of negative affect, pain and cognitive control in the cingulate cortex. *Nature Reviews Neuroscience, 12*, 154–67.

Simmons, A. N., Stein, M. B., Strigo, I. A., Arce, E., Hitchcock, C., and **Paulus, M. P.** (2011). Anxiety positive subjects show altered processing in the anterior insula during anticipation of negative stimuli. *Human Brain Mapping, 32*, 1836–46.

Singer, T., Critchley, H. D., and **Preuschoff, K.** (2009). A common role of insula in feelings, empathy and uncertainty. *Trends in Cognitive Sciences, 13*, 334–40.

Smith, R., Thayer, J. F., Khalsa, S. S., and **Lane, R. D.** (2017). The hierarchical basis of neurovisceral integration. *Neuroscience and Biobehavioral Reviews, 75*, 274–96.

Stephan, K. E., Manjaly, Z. M., Mathys, C. D., Weber, L. A., Paliwal, S., Gard, T., et al. (2016). Allostatic self-efficacy: A metacognitive theory of dyshomeostasis-induced fatigue and depression. *Frontiers in Human Neuroscience, 10*, 550.

Sterling, P. (2012). Allostasis: A model of predictive regulation. *Physiology Behavior, 106*, 5–15.

Sterling, P. (2014). Homeostasis vs allostasis: Implications for brain function and mental disorders. *JAMA Psychiatry, 71*, 1192–3.

Taylor, S. (2014). *Anxiety Sensitivity: Theory, Research, and Treatment of the Fear of Anxiety*. London: Routledge.

Tracy, C. M., Epstein, A. E., Darbar, D., DiMarco, J. P., Dunbar, S. B., and **Mark Estes, N. A.**, et al. (2012). 2012 ACCF/AHA/HRS focused update of the 2008 guidelines for device-based therapy of cardiac rhythm abnormalities. *Circulation, 126*, 1784–800.

Van den Bergh, O., Witthoft, M., Petersen, S., and **Brown, R. J.** (2017). Symptoms and the body: Taking the inferential leap. *Neuroscience and Biobehavioral Reviews, 74*, 185–203.

Chapter 9

The relevance of interoception for eating behavior and eating disorders

Beate M. Herbert and Olga Pollatos

9.1 Introduction

The importance of interoception for adaptive and maladaptive behavior, as well as for psychopathology, has gained growing interest, and dysfunctional interoception has been increasingly recognized as representing a core impairment across psychosomatic and psychiatric disorders (e.g. Khalsa & Lapidus, 2016; Murphy et al., 2017). Recently its role in psychopathology has been related to a potential "p-factor" (Murphy et al., 2017) that may represent lesser-to-greater severity of psychopathology with associated dysfunction in interoceptive neural circuitry.

Eating is a fundamental behavior that reveals how we are intrinsically guided by interoceptive signals and that is most directly associated with homeostatic psychophysiological needs, survival, and well-being. Eating comprises perceiving and discriminating interoceptive sensations of hunger and satiety, and steering behavior according to these sensations. These processes are critically disturbed in obesity and eating disorders (ED), such as anorexia nervosa (AN) and bulimia nervosa (BN).

Disordered interoception and distorted body image (see section 9.3) have been recognized as core symptoms of ED from the beginnings of modern clinical research and are defining characteristics of these devastating disorders (Bruch, 1962, 1973). In the field of maladaptive eating and ED, dysfunction of interoception represents more than a potential p-factor; it is the pivot of these disorders.

Interoception is of multifaceted nature and comprises distinguishable dimensions (Garfinkel et al., 2016a), as well as different modalities, that is, different organ/visceral systems (Herbert et al., 2012a). We adopt the nomenclature of Garfinkel, Manassei, Hamilton-Fletcher, and colleagues (Garfinkel et al., 2016a) that differentiates among three major dimensions: "Interoceptive Accuracy" (IAcc) as reflected in objective performance on behavioral tests, such as heartbeat perception tests; "Interoceptive Sensibility" (IS), that is, the individuals' experience and subjective beliefs and perceptions as is assessed by self-report; and "Interoceptive Awareness" (IA), that is, the metacognitive insights into performance aptitude, as characterized by the degree to which interoceptive accuracy is predicted by subjective confidence in an individual's judgment about her task performance. These dimensions represent different levels of being aware of one's interoceptive body.

Additionally, we introduce the further dimension of "Interoceptive Emotional Evaluation" (IE) into a model of distinguishable facets of interoception that has been demonstrated to be of importance in shaping behavior and that is interacting with IAcc, especially in the eating domain (Herbert et al., 2012b; Herbert et al., 2013) (see Figure 9.1). Interoceptive emotional evaluation (IE) represents subjective appraisal related to sensations and perceptions of interoceptive signals. We usually assess IE as subjective ratings of affective evaluations of perceived interoceptive signals (e.g. arousal, valence, anxiety, as well as other affects) in situ, that is during specific behavioral paradigms measuring IAcc (Herbert et al. 2012a, 2012b, 2013; van Dyck et al., 2016). By using specific protocols, we demonstrated that IE can be modulated during short-term fasting (Herbert et al., 2012b), or after manipulation of insular cortex activity (Pollatos et al., 2016). IE has been linked to autonomic-nervous activity changes (heart rate variability measures) that reflect processes of top-down inhibition (Herbert et al., 2012a, 2012b, 2013). Additionally, IAcc and IE represent independent dimensions (Herbert et al., 2012a, 2012b, 2013; Pollatos et al., 2016). We suggest that IE is of relevance in understanding ED because profound negative evaluation of bodily signals—as show up in aversive and/or ambivalent

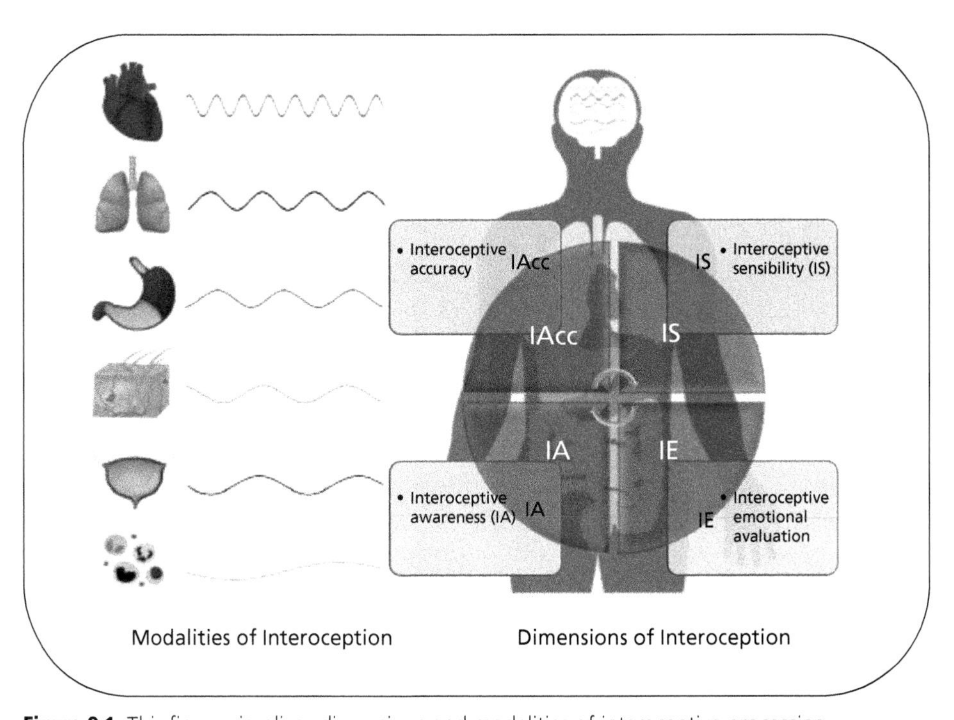

Figure 9.1 This figure visualizes dimensions and modalities of interoceptive processing.

reaction towards food, and interoceptive signals of, for example, hunger and fullness, as well as in typical distortion of body image—are part of the core symptoms in ED.

The relevance of emotional evaluation of interoceptive (and other bodily) signals as an independent process is also supported by Smith and Lane's multi-hierarchical model of emotion processing (Smith & Lane, 2015), suggesting a multi-stage interoceptive/somatosensory process by which distinct body state patterns (discrete body features that are represented in somatosensory cortices, posterior insula, nucleus of the tractus solitarii, hypothalamic nuclei, and the parabrachial nucleus; whole-body patterns that are represented in the mid and anterior insula) are detected and assigned conceptual emotional meaning. Emotional concepts are suggested to occur by appraisal mechanisms involving other brain regions such as the anterior cingulate and the medial prefrontal cortices that refer to this mapping of the body state. These assumptions are in accordance with studies showing that the insular cortex and anterior cingulate cortex (ACC) play crucial roles in connecting interoceptive processes and emotions (Pollatos, Gramann, & Schandry, 2007).

There is evidence that certain dimensions of interoception do not overlap in healthy populations but represent dissociable measures (Garfinkel et al., 2015). However, IS and IAcc have been shown to be aligned in those individuals with high precision of interoceptive perception (IAcc) (Garfinkel et al., 2015), supporting the idea that IAcc might be the core ability within the construct of interoception underpinning other dimensions.

Dissociability of dimensions of interoception is suggested to have variable relevance for different clinical disorders and maladaptive functions (Garfinkel et al., 2016a; Herbert et al., 2012b; Murphy et al., 2016 and Chapter 7 in the present volume). Dissociation between objectively and subjectively quantified interoceptive indices has been suggested to reflect interoceptive (trait) prediction error and to be greater in individuals with lower IAcc (Garfinkel et al., 2016a). This divergence of dimensions has been evidenced to be large, for example in persons with Autism Spectrum Conditions (ASC) (Garfinkel et al., 2016b). We suggest that in ED there is larger dissociation of dimensions of interoception (e.g. IS and IAcc), that may reflect greater interoceptive (trait) prediction error (see section 9.5). The question of overlap of interoception across modalities has been discussed on the assumption that interoceptive information may be processed within a unity of nervous systems entities (Craig, 2009). There is some scope to conceptualize multimodal interoception either as individual coherence of crossmodal unity of interoceptive processing, or as fractionation of multimodal interoception, and/or both (Garfinkel et al., 2016a; Herbert et al., 2012a; Whitehead & Drescher, 1980; Pollatos et al., 2016). It has been suggested that this depends on dynamically changing environmental demands and corresponding physiological adaptations (Herbert et al., 2012a, 2012b).

With regard to the eating domain, relevant studies on interoception across modalities are sparse, reporting evidence for significant, but moderate, correlations of cardiac IAcc and intensity of gastric perception, as measured by adapted water-loading tests (WLT), using non-caloric water drinking and filling levels (Herbert et al., 2012a; Whitehead & Drescher, 1980 van Dyck et al., 2016) in healthy samples. Data suggest that in a controlled, baseline setting, there may be a trait-like overlap in perceiving cardiac signals accurately and in perceiving gastric signals of fullness more precisely, suggestive of individual differences. Heart and stomach have been also shown to have partially overlapping cortical representations within the interoceptive insula (Avery et al., 2015), suggesting that a unitary structure may exist in some modalities, especially in cardiovascular and gastric domains. This may be related to relevance of vagal afferents in both modalities. It has been shown that many of the signals relevant to satiety and food intake travel via the vagus nerve from the stomach to the brain, terminating in a unique region of the insula that subserves both monitoring the state of the body and the sense of taste (Bartoud, 2008). However, this multimodal unity may not exist in other modalities (e.g. cardiac and respiratory resistance perception; Garfinkel et al., 2016a), as well as in other populations or clinical disorders (e.g. autism; Garfinkel et al., 2015, 2016b). Moreover, multimodal interoception may not be continuous across situations, over development, or in neurodevelopmental and psychiatric conditions (Murphy et al., 2017) .

Dimensions of interoception in relation to adaptive or maladaptive eating behavior, obesity, or EDs have been mainly investigated by self-report, that is via questionnaire measures, primarily covering the IS dimension (Merwin et al., 2010). There are far fewer results focusing on objective performance measures of interoception in relation to eating behavior, body weight, and EDs. As in general interoception research, objective performance measures of IAcc primarily focused on the cardiac modality, that is, heartbeat perception tests. When investigating eating-related phenomena, it is obviously of interest to measure individual perception sensitivity of gastric functions, sensations of hunger, fullness, or satiety, that characterize relevant specific interoceptive symptoms of EDs and obesity. Up to now, there are sparse data on gastric interoceptive perception in relation to eating behavior and EDs, especially when non-invasive paradigms with high ecological validity are intended to be used (e.g. Geliebter & Hashim, 2001; Herbert et al., 2012a, 2012b; van Dyck et al., 2016; Beglinger & Degen, 2006).

Finally, extant investigation of dimensions and modalities of interoception has mainly focused on disorders of eating behavior, much more than on adaptive eating. Section 9.2 and 9.3 summarize some relevant findings in both domains.

9.2 Interoception and adaptive eating, body weight, and obesity

Adaptive behaviors, that is, regulation of behavior according to bodily needs and environmental demands, play an important role in maintaining somatic and mental health, and trait-like IAcc, as measured by heartbeat perception tasks, have been demonstrated to be positively connected with relevant aspects of adaptive behavior regulation (Herbert, Ulbrich, & Schandry, 2007; Herbert et al., 2013; Furman, 2013; Kirk, Doawnar, & Montague, 2011) and emotion regulation (Füstös et al., 2013).

Eating adaptively is of relevance for body-weight regulation, the brain's capability to balance food intake with energy needs, and finally for obesity, that results from persistent failure of this balance and ends in chronic energy surplus. In studies investigating adaptive eating behaviors in unrestrained eating and in eating disorders, adaptive eating has been primarily defined as the absence of eating disorder symptoms; however, adaptive eating obviously is more than just the absence of clinical symptoms. Although there are many factors that predispose individuals to weight gain and obesity (e.g. Cui, López, & Rahmouni, 2017), we focus here on how eating behavior and body weight may be influenced by sensitivity to interoceptive signals.

A possibly adaptive form of eating that has recently gained recognition is the construct of "intuitive eating" (Herbert et al., 2013). It has been defined as eating in response to internal physiological hunger and satiety cues rather than to emotional reasons, and relying on internal hunger and satiety cues to determine when and how much to eat. It includes the unconditional permission to eat when hungry and what food is desired (Tylka, 2006). This form of adaptive eating is commonly assessed via self-report such as the Intuitive Eating Scale (IES) (Tylka, 2006). There are supporting data that scoring high in intuitive eating is associated with self-reported eating according to physiological reasons and with reduced emotional eating, improved emotional well-being, less preoccupation with food choice, as well as less ED (Faith et al., 2004; Tylka, 2006). Accordingly, there is some evidence from cross-sectional studies showing lower/normal body weight in intuitive eaters, especially in early and mid-aged women (Madden et al., 2012).

Herbert, Blechert, Hautzinger, and colleagues (2013) examined the connection of facets defining intuitive eating as assessed by the IES and (trait) IAcc, as measured by heartbeat tracking, as well as IE (affective ratings during heartbeat perception) in 111 healthy, normal-weight women. Two key findings from that study highlighted the relevance of different interoceptive dimensions in shaping adaptive eating and body weight. First, IAcc was significantly positively related to those facets of self-reported intuitive eating that have been supposed to represent eating for physical rather than emotional reasons, as well as trusting and relying on internal hunger and satiety cues. Furthermore, IAcc mediated the negative relationship between the tendency to eat intuitively and lower body weight. However, IAcc was not related to self-reported "unconditional permission to eat when hungry." We proposed that this unrestricted eating reflects the influence of other external and internal factors that affect eating behavior, such as environmental pressure to be thin, others' acceptance of body shape, emphasis on body appearance, as well as aspects comprising cognitive inhibition of behavior, such as shows up, for example, in restrictive eating (Herbert et al., 2013; Kaye, Fudge, & Paulus, 2009). Thus, although more accurate interoceptive perception might represent a prerequisite for eating adaptively, the *permission* to eat without restrictions and to respond behaviorally accordingly, may involve further relevant factors such as top-down control, that have been shown to be impaired at one end, that is in obesity and BN, or that is dominating at the other end, that is in restrictive AN (Wierenga et al., 2014; Kaye et al., 2009). The second main finding of this study showed that the degree of negative evaluation of one's interoceptive signals (IE) during heartbeat tracking was negatively correlated to "eating for physical reasons rather than emotional cues" as well as significantly predicted higher BMI. IE and IAcc were not related. This highlights the independent roles of IAcc and of emotional evaluation of one's interoceptive cues (IE) as unpleasant in shaping body weight and those aspects of adaptive eating, that are related to successful emotion regulation.

The relevance of the IE dimension is also underscored by the prominence of both disturbed perception of interoceptive signals (Kaye et al., 2009; Lilenfeld et al., 2006; Pollatos et al., 2008) and aversive experience of visceral sensations during exposure to food or food-related stimuli (Kaye et al., 2009) or one's own or other's bodily cues (Vocks et al., 2010) in samples with disordered eating behavior (see section 9.3).

The role of IE as well as of higher-order top-down related cognitive control in shaping adaptive or maladaptive eating is supported by hypotheses on extremes of eating behavior. It is suggested that dysregulated eating, obesity, and EDs emerge from an altered balance of reward and inhibitory processing (see Wierenga et al., 2014). Altered activation within brain networks, including corticostriatal limbic and dorsal cognitive (control) neural circuitry (e.g. DLPFC), as well as anterior insula, has been observed in substance use disorders, obesity, and in ED (Wierenga et al., 2014). These limbic, cognitive, and salience circuits interact to valuate reward, assess future consequences of one's behavior, and integrate and evaluate reward prediction to guide decisions by using both interoceptive bottom-up signalling and top-down cognitive control. Altered reward appraisal (not only restricted to food cues and eating) has been demonstrated in obesity, as well as in ED, and is linked to emotional dysregulation, manifesting as exaggerated anxiety and sensitivity to punishment (Kaye et al., 2009; Wierenga et al., 2014). Inhibitory function is suggested to vary between different diagnoses (Kaye et al., 2009). In obesity and in BN there is evidence for deficits in cognitive control, proposed to increase instability and erratic responding to appetitive stimuli, whereas restrictive type of AN has been related to exaggerated cognitive control, suggested to be used for compensating for dysfunctional reward processing (Wierenga et al., 2014). Thus, maladaptive eating/overeating and obesity as well as EDs may represent a spectrum anchored by extremes of inhibition and dysregulation interacting with altered and dysfunctional interoception at its base.

Concerning obesity, there is evidence supporting attenuated cardiac IAcc in overweight and obese women and men that is associated with higher BMI in these samples (Herbert & Pollatos, 2014), suggesting that low IAcc impairs detection of bodily changes accompanying satiety.

This is complemented by findings by our findings (van Dyck et al., 2016), measuring gastric interoception by an adapted, standardized, non-invasive WLT protocol in a large healthy sample of 99 women. Results showed that BMI was positively associated with drunk water volume until feeling satiation as well as with maximum capacity of drunk water volume, suggesting attenuated gastric interoceptive sensitivity (IAcc dimension). Additionally, cardiac IAcc was positively correlated with a gastric sensitivity measure of drunk water volume until satiation in the whole sample, supporting earlier findings on cardiac and gastric crossmodal overlap within a similar protocol (Herbert et al., 2012a). Recent results based on another non-invasive WLT protocol (Arrouk et al., 2017) support the finding that obese children drink more water until sensing maximum fullness, suggesting abnormal satiety perception. Medical interventions using intragastric filling of the stomach mechanically by balloons that intend to stimulate gastric mechanoreceptors triggering short-acting vagal signals to interoceptive brain regions have been reported to help obese people lose weight, and may support the relevance of mechanoreceptor-driven interoceptive perception facilitating body-weight regulation (Tate & Geliebter, 2017). Taken together, this evidence supports a hypothesis of *in- or hyposensitivity* of interoceptive signals across gastric and cardiac modalities in obesity and overeating. Existent results on gastric sensitivity specifically suggest interoceptive *hyposensitivity for signals of satiety and fullness*.

However, for dysfunctional body-weight regulation (i.e. obesity), there might also exist another prediction regarding IAcc. Positive and negative alliesthesia for food cues (i.e. increase or decrease in reward value of a stimulus that is based on its potential to move the body's physiological state towards homeostasis) is basically driven by interoceptive processing of the body's state (e.g. glucose, insulin levels, visceral signals of fullness, hunger, etc.; Stice, Burger, & Yokum, 2013). Accordingly, it may be argued that greater sensitivity of interoceptive signals of hunger or bodily weakness, signalling energy depletion of the body, such as during food-deprivation, facilitates generation of behaviors in reaction to these signals (i.e. seeking food and eating). This mechanism is supported by increasing the motivational salience of food cues. Thus, positive alliesthesia might be supposed to facilitate obesity in interaction with interoceptive sensitivity.

Page, Seo, Belfort-DeAguiar, and colleagues (2011) demonstrated that obese adults exhibit greater activation of bilateral insula, hypothalamus, striatum, substantia nigra, and ventral tegmental area during hypoglycaemia which occurs during food-deprivation. Comparable to drug abuse, hypersensitivity to internal signals associated with hunger and other bodily states of energy loss might contribute to the experience of positive alliesthesia for food cues, and thereby may undermine attempts to lose weight. Until now there is only sparse evidence from behavioral studies resolving this idea (e.g. Stevenson, Mahmut, & Rooney, 2015). However, the findings may suggest that within this process, top-down inhibitory control as well as appraisal processes of interoceptive signals (IE) interact in steering final eating behavior: for example, less capability of behavioral inhibition (e.g. in BN and obesity) is suggested to support food consumption; negative evaluation of interoceptive cues (e.g. satiation) is assumed to restrict eating behavior in order to avoid negative sensations (e.g. in AN) (see section 9.3).

Eating adaptively according to the balance of interoceptive cues of hunger and satiety may be disrupted by early restrictive or monitoring feeding practices, external eating rules, or dietary restraint, that is, pressures that may induce a disconnection of internal (interoceptive multidimensional and multisensory) experience and food intake regulation. This disconnection has been reported to be related to the emergence of dieting, weight gain, and eating in the absence of hunger and in response to emotional and situational factors (e.g. Birch & Fisher, 2000; Galloway, Farrow, & Martz, 2010).

Dieting and fasting represent one of those interruptions that has been recognized as a major risk factor in triggering and maintaining disordered eating, obesity, and EDs (Hetherington, 2000). Acute, short-term fasting in healthy young women has been shown to alter cardiac IAcc and IE via differential psychophysiological, cardiodynamic, and vagal mechanisms which may shape functions of interoceptive brain regions by altered sensory feedback from visceral systems (Herbert et al., 2012b). This finding supports the relevance of fasting on interoceptive mechanisms of positive alliesthasia, with potential relevance for obesity. Acute fasting induced an increase in cardiac IAcc that was directly related to ongoing changes of sympathetic and parasympathetic activity and corresponding cardiodynamic alterations during the fasting period, thereby facilitating cardiac signal strength and improving IAcc. It is suggested that (frequent) short-term food deprivation involves visceral learning processes that may induce more intense processing of and a sensitization for visceral bodily signals, especially of hunger states, that depend on changes in autonomic activity and self-control. This may facilitate *hypersensitivity* for hunger-related interoceptive cues and thereby impact the development of obesity.

On the contrary, specific diets and specific food consumption may impair interoceptive perception accuracy of satiety, and thus facilitate *interoceptive hyposensitivity of fullness*. This idea is supported by recent evidence (Attuquayefio et al., 2017) showing that a Western-style diet (high in saturated fat and added sugar) compared to healthier food intake over four consecutive days induced impairment of cognitive functions (i.e. hippocampal-dependent learning and memory), as well as rated sensitivity and perception of hunger and fullness. In obesity, both factors, attempts of diets as well as intake of palatable, high-caloric food, often coexist, thereby potentially triggering specific interoceptive hypo- and hypersensitivity.

However, the findings mentioned earlier are primarily based on cross-sectional designs that do not allow us to draw firm conclusions regarding the causal directional relation between IAcc, other dimensions of interoception, and eating behavior and body weight. Furthermore, maladaptive eating behavior, obesity, as well as EDs, have developmental roots and early manifestations in childhood and youth. Hence, in order to improve our understanding of the interaction between interoception, eating behavior, body weight, and experience of the body it is necessary to investigate longitudinal processes of development in healthy and in pathological samples. There is one prospective study (Koch & Pollatos, 2014) with a large sample of 1657 children, aged between 6 and 11 years, that investigated development of cardiac IAcc over one year as well as its prospective association with food approach behaviors. The findings support interoceptive hyposensitivity in the cardiac domain (IAcc) in overweight compared to normal weight children. Only in overweight children was external and emotional eating behavior predictive of later IAcc, highlighting that existent eating behavior preceded low cardiac IAcc and not vice versa. This corroborates the reported findings in adults and demonstrates the impact of food and eating behavior in shaping interoception in children.

9.3 Interoception in eating disorders

Concerning developmental factors, physiological changes represent relevant disturbances challenging homeostasis and allostatic adaptation as well as requiring new and adaptive ways of reducing increased “prediction errors” (see Chapter 9.5) of all bodily sensory channels, including interoceptive signals. For example, cardiac IAcc has been shown to depend on individual differences of cardiodynamic mechanisms that either facilitate or dampen perception and processing of cardiac signals (Herbert et al., 2010). These physiological mechanisms may alter attention focus towards interoceptive sensations as well as visceral learning, thereby influencing development of IAcc. There is certainly no more profound metamorphosis of all bodily and physiological systems than in puberty, especially in girls and adolescent women. Therefore, it is not surprising that puberty in particular represents the critical period for first manifestation of disorders of EDs. We will focus here on AN and BN.

AN is the psychiatric disorder with the highest rate of mortality (Arcelus et al., 2011), the onset mainly occurring in adolescent girls and young women. AN is characterized by extremely low body weight and on obsessive fear of becoming fat, as well as abnormal experiences of the body interior, such as vague feelings of fullness or failure (American Psychiatric Association, 2013; Bruch, 1962, 1973). Bulimia nervosa (BN) is characterized by recurrent episodes of binge eating large amounts of food and self-induced vomiting or other compensatory behaviors for body-weight maintenance (American Psychiatric Association, 2013). Hilde Bruch summarized the outstanding interoceptive characteristic of EDs, as "disturbance in the accuracy of perception or cognitive interpretation of stimuli arising in the body, with failure to recognize signs of nutritional need as the most prominent deficiency of this type" (Bruch, 1962, p. 189). In addition to interoceptive deficits, clinical descriptions of EDs portray distorted "body image" (Bruch, 1973; Fairborn & Harrison, 2003). Body image refers to a diverse, multifaceted psychological construct that relies primarily on exteroceptive (here mostly visual) information and beyond perceptual and behavioral dimensions, and incorporates subjective evaluation; that is, whether an individual is satisfied or dissatisfied with his or her physical appearance (Emanuelsen, Drew, & Köteles, 2015).

Numerous empirical studies document severe distortions of all facets of body image in EDs, supporting clinical observations that AN patients perceive themselves as fat despite often severe state of emaciation, in combination with fundamental body dissatisfaction (Fairburn & Harrison, 2003). In contrast, study results on interoception in EDs are still sparse. At the self-report level, studies primarily used the Eating Disorders Inventory (EDI) subscale "interoceptive deficits" to assess subjectively rated identification of bodily signals, especially hunger or satiety, in AN and BN samples (see Klabunde, Collado, & Bohon, 2017; Merwin et al., 2010). Results have shown that interoceptive impairments predict risk for developing EDs (Clausen et al., 2011), as well as that patients with BN show problems in perception of bodily signals and its evaluation (Merwin et al., 2010). However, the EDI subscale refers to a mixture of self-reported bodily sensations and affective experiences, such as experiencing affective confusion and fear (a mixture of IS and IE) by asking for difficulties in identification and interpretation of internal, emotional signals as well as of interoceptive hunger and satiety cues (e.g. Merwin et al., 2010).

Beyond self-report, only a few, cross-sectional studies up to today demonstrated impaired IAcc in ED. Pollatos and colleagues (2008) found decreased IAcc, as measured by a heartbeat tracking task in female AN patients. EDI interoceptive deficiency was also impaired in AN, however IAcc was not correlated with EDI interoceptive deficits scores. This underscores that the subjective, evaluative interoceptive experience and IAcc do not overlap in AN. Acknowledging the fact that EDI interoception score is a mixed measure, this may explain this incoherence. However, this finding may be recognized as a deviation across interoceptive dimensions, that is as a mismatch of subjective expectation/prediction and sensory afferent perception accuracy that may result from an altered interoceptive prediction signal (see section 9.5). Accordingly, the findings may be interpreted as a rough estimate for elevated interoceptive (trait) prediction error in patients with AN (Garfinkel et al., 2016b).

These results may tentatively suggest that in AN patients with active illness there exists dampened IAcc that does not match self-perceived judgment of one's bodily states, suggesting a failure to integrate or minimize ongoing discrepancy of "prior" predictions (see section 9.5) about bodily states and afferent interoceptive prediction errors adaptively. Low trait-like IAcc might mediate this failure. This interpretation is consistent with results in healthy subjects demonstrating that dissociation between interoceptive dimensions is greatest in those individuals with lower in IAcc (Garfinkel et al., 2015), as well as in clinical conditions, such as autism spectrum disorders (Garfinkel et al., 2016b).

Whereas these results, based on measures of IAcc at rest, may reflect dampened interoceptive perception as a trait-like condition in AN, there are interesting findings reporting more intense interoceptive signal processing, especially during meal anticipation. Khalsa and colleagues (2015) investigated cardiorespiratory interoceptive processing in AN by disturbing autonomic nervous system afferent signalling by use of infusions of isoproterenol during meal anticipation and after consumption. In this critical food-related context, AN patients demonstrated exaggerated *interoceptive bias*; that is, patients with AN experienced cardiorespiratory sensations abnormally intensely, as well as exaggerated detection of symptoms even during control saline infusion, but only during meal anticipation. This suggests that AN patients perceive interoceptive symptoms in critical—arousing and aversive—food-anticipatory contexts more intensely, and not in a more dampened way. This finding provides more direct evidence that IAcc is varying in a context-specific way in AN. This also supports the idea that interoceptive prediction (anticipatory condition) signalling is distorted in AN (Khalsa et al., 2015), especially in a fear-related and self-referential context, which is important for these patients.

Complementing these findings there is ample evidence in ED for abnormal neural encoding of interoceptive signals in relevant neurocircuitry, involving insula, anterior cingulate, somatosensory cortices, and amygdala (see Khalsa & Lapidus, 2016). Interesting study results show more intense activation of insula and anterior cingulate cortex in recovered patients as well as those with acute AN during viewing food pictures (Cowdrey et al., 2011), or when confronted with aversive self-comparison or with desirable ideal body shape (Friederich et al., 2010). However, there is evidence for decreased insular cortex activation when food was actually tasted (Oberndorfer et al., 2013), or when confronted with self-body images (Gaudio & Quattrocchi, 2012). These results support the view that in critical situations that are intruding relevant symptom areas, interoceptive perception and signal processing is intensified in active AN. This speaks in favour of the hypothesis that—phasic—interoceptive hypersensitivity may be of relevance in AN (Zucker et al., 2017). Dampening of interoceptive brain activation, on the one hand, might be interpreted as downregulation of interoceptive perception as a possible coping strategy of aversive interoceptive signalling. On the other hand, when challenging stimuli or bodily sensations become overwhelming and/or top-down inhibition fails, interoceptive processing might break through.

The non-acceptance or aversive experience of affective and bodily signals may contribute to symptoms of disordered eating (e.g. Merwin et al., 2010). For instance, binge eating has been proposed to function as an escape from aversive self-awareness or feelings of dysphoria (Heatherton & Baumeister, 1991), and (long-term) dietary restraint has been suggested as a way to avoid internal sensations of fullness and/or feelings of guilt and shame (Schmidt & Treasure, 2006). Relief from negative affective states or bodily discomfort by the use of avoidance strategies or manipulations influencing these negative bodily sensations is suggested to be highly reinforcing for individuals with an ED, thus perpetuating ED symptoms (Kaye et al., 2009).

These mechanisms may be affected in both AN and BN, with potential differences in top-down cognitive control mediating this process. This interpretation is supported by the augmented proactive inhibitory motor control and delay of gratification in AN compared to BN and healthy controls (Bartholdy et al., 2017).

Findings of a paradoxical effect of self-focus (viewing one's own face) on cardiac IAcc in AN (Pollatos et al., 2016) as compared to healthy controls, who typically show an increased IAcc evoked by focusing on oneself (Ainley et al., 2012), support the idea that AN patients "shut down" interoceptive perception when confronted with highly salient, aversive exteroceptive processing of their body exterior. This atypical effect remained after cognitive-behavioral psychotherapy and questions the usefulness of direct body confrontation techniques for changing interoception in AN. Therefore, IAcc and other dimensions of interoceptive sensibility are not constant in EDs but may show variations depending on salient context, such as expecting food confrontation, or confrontation with the body.

Regarding BN, results are more heterogeneous, suggesting impaired cardiac IAcc (Klabunde et al., 2017) or no differences compared to healthy controls (Pollatos & Georgiou, 2016). However, reduced sensitivity of gastric perception has been reported in BN, as evidenced by increased gastric capacity compared to obese and normal-weight comparisons (Geliebter & Hashim, 2001), as well as lower responding to satiety signalling in a yoghurt consumption paradigm (Beglinger & Degen, 2006). This is in accord with our recent finding (van Dyck et al., 2016) that satiation volume, as assessed by an adapted standardized, non-invasive WLT paradigm and corrected to individual maximum fullness capacity, was significantly positively associated with bulimic symptoms in a non-clinical sample of young adults. Hence, individuals with bulimic symptoms (with binge-eating and purging behaviors) are less sensitive to gastric signals and therefore drink beyond the satiation threshold. Additionally, it has been demonstrated that BN patients show negative attribution style towards interoceptive sensations, suggesting more aversive perception of interoceptive signals, and thereby underscoring the relevance of IE (Morrison, Waller, & Lawson, 2006).

In accordance with our conceptualization of interoception and empirical findings (Tsakiris et al., 2017 Ainley & Tsakiris, 2013; Seth & Friston, 2016 Crucianelli et al., 2016), we assume dysfunctional interoception to lie at the core of maladaptive eating and EDs, of related dysfunctions of embodied cognition, as well as deficient unity and stability of an embodied self (Herbert & Pollatos, 2012; Tsakiris, 2017). The perception and knowledge of one's own body is due to co-perception and integration of the different sensory information (visual, tactile, proprioceptive, and interoceptive) that enables an individual to gain an accurate perception of one's own body (Tsakiris, 2017).

We suggest that in EDs, integrative multisensory processes, forming the self are basically disturbed, by this supporting what Hilde Bruch (1962, 1982) recognized: that at the root of EDs, especially and most deeply in AN, is fundamentally a deficit of the self.

9.4 Eating disorders as disorders of the self

The self may be considered as an integrative structure of the mind that organizes and coordinates affective, cognitive, social, sensorimotor, and vegetative functions with regard to interoceptive and exteroceptive stimuli from one's own body and the environment (Amianto et al., 2016). Recent accounts (Amianto et al., 2016; Gaete & Fuchs, 2016) suggest that the integrative function of the self (i.e. its ability to integrate cognitive, affective, and conative functions) as well as its diachronic function (i.e. the experience of a consistent self over time indicated by one's identity) is profoundly compromised in EDs. This implies problems in integrating one's own internal experiences within a meaningful narrative of the self as persisting across time, which results in an unstable sense of self that weakens related functions like self-esteem, emotion regulation, and interpersonal effectiveness (Amianto et al., 2016).

At the core of our self is the experience of our body, our bodily self. Embodied cognition approaches agree that the self is grounded in the body (Herbert & Pollatos, 2012; Fuchs & Schlimme, 2009) and that the body is the starting point for understanding self-awareness as well as social interactions.

The experience of our body as our own is fundamentally based on multimodal integration of signals from the whole body (e.g. Herbert & Pollatos, 2012; Tsakiris, 2017; Picard & Friston, 2014). Exteroceptive multisensory bodily sources and their percepts are related to concepts of body image—and associated with it—with fundamental dimensions of the bodily self such as the sense of body ownership (Tsakiris, 2017; Eshkevari et al., 2012). This refers to the special status of one's own body that is characterized by the feeling that my "body belongs to me." Hilde Bruch (1972) described individuals with AN as functioning with a "false-self," suggesting that they may not be able to discriminate between their own and their caregivers' or others' expectations and needs. Distinguishing "self" from "other" is of fundamental importance for self-awareness as well as for successful social interactions and has been demonstrated to depend on multisensory integration of exteroceptive and interoceptive bodily perceptions (see Tsakiris, 2017).

Research in healthy samples has used multisensory stimulation between "self" and "other" to induce controlled changes in the representation of one's identity (Tajadura-Jiménez & Tsakiris, 2014; Tajadura-Jimenez et al., 2014). This was examined by use of experimental paradigms that allow the quantification of the contribution of exteroceptive information on distinguishing between self and other, such as manipulation of self-face recognition ("enfacement illusion") and Rubber Hand Illusion paradigms (RHI). Beyond the known role of multisensory integration, it was shown that individuals with lower IAcc experienced more intense changes in body ownership and self-identification, suggestive of a dominance of perceiving the body from the outside, that is, a greater weighting of exteroceptive over interoceptive information in these individuals (Tsakiris et al., 2011; Tajadura-Jiménez & Tsakiris, 2014; see also Chapter 2 in the present volume).

Thus, higher interoceptive accuracy (precision) is suggested to be critical for ensuring psychophysiological stability of the organism and the bodily self as well as its embodied unity in a changing environment with alternating challenges (Herbert & Pollatos, 2012; Tsakiris, 2017). Furthermore, results in healthy samples (Ainley & Tsakiris, 2013) highlighted that individuals with lower cardiac IAcc show a greater tendency to consider their body as an object, suggesting that low IAcc facilitates this self-objectification tendency. Precisely this dysbalanced dominance of exteroceptive focus of body perception and of exaggerated self-objectification has been demonstrated in EDs. In accordance with reported impaired IAcc in EDs, there is evidence for more intense body-illusion effects, that is, greater plasticity of the bodily self (Eshkevari et al., 2012). This underscores an overreliance on exteroceptive information (i.e. vision), and a stronger focus on the body from the outside in EDs.

Self-objectification has been related to increasing number of EDs in the Western world, with the influence of media communicating images that convey ideals of beauty, especially of girls and women, that are unattainable for most persons. This has been reported to be of relevance for increasing body dissatisfaction in girls and women (Emanuelsen et al., 2015), and facilitating internalization of typical beauty ideal and produce objective body consciousness, the tendency towards body surveillance (watching oneself from the outside as an observer), as well as the appearance of control beliefs (believing that cultural body standards can be achieved if one tries hard enough) (McKinley, 1999). This is of major relevance in EDs.

We propose that perceptual and cognitive-affective body image disturbances in EDs may reflect an increased focus to mainly visually perceiving the body from the outside at the expense of sensing internal bodily states. Body focus varies dynamically in AN, depending on salient, aversively evaluated contexts (Khalsa et al., 2015). These shifts of body focus may depend on compromised coping resources in dealing with bodily sensations and with environmental demands. This supports considerations of Amianto,

Northoff, Abbate Daga, and colleagues (2016) proposing that in EDs, especially in AN, the experience of the *body* is not integrated into the self. The authors state:

> "even though patients with AN do not perceive their body as sharply extraneous, as sometimes happens in schizophrenia . . . they do appear to maintain an attitude of 'objectification' toward their body, as if their body does not pertain to their self. The body is no longer experienced in a subjective way as 'my' body, and thus as personal or self-related." (Amianto et al., 2016, p.2)

This is suggested to lead to pervasive weakness of the integrative functions of the self, which may explain why certain personality traits that are common to AN become rigid, such as high harm avoidance, low self-directedness, and perfectionism.

This view is in accord with Gaete and Fuchs (2016) who state that EDs may be characterized by an embodied defense, so that patients experience their own bodies primarily as objects, at the expense of the "subject body." This is based on a phenomenological approach of psychopathologies of embodiment by Fuchs and Schlimme (2009), who differentiate between the body that one "pre-reflectively" lives, the lived or "subject body" (implicit in one's ongoing experience), and the physical body (that appears as an object of conscious attention, and that one can perceive or that is perceived by others), the "object body." This means that the body has a double or ambiguous experiential status, with an ongoing oscillation between these bodily modes as a foundation of all experiences. It is to conclude, that an adaptive, healthy self emanates when we are able to integrate "subject" and "object body" fluctuations continuously in a balanced way, balancing the inner and outer self (e.g. Tajadura-Jiménez & Tsakiris, 2014).

The exaggerated self-objectification associated with greater malleability of sense of body-ownership that has been found in EDs, paired with aversive experience of the body and a "sense of ineffectiveness" (Bruch, 1962), fits with our hypothesis of a failure to balance the two modes of body experience, at the expense of the subject body. Accordingly, therapeutic interventions should focus on helping patients to recover in particular the subjective experience of their bodies, their lived body. Concentrating on interoceptive dimensions of relevance (e.g IAcc, IE, and eventual IA) should play a major role in strengthening the lived body.

The most outstanding symptoms in EDs, distortion of body image and dysfunctional interoception may be interpreted as failure to *balance* interoceptive and exteroceptive perception. We suggest that the lack of integration of interoceptive signals and exteroceptive sensory information results in an impoverished sense of self (as a single entity, distinct from others) and in social difficulties. Within this process, aversive affective experience of the body and interoceptive signals (IE) seem to play a major role in EDs (Gadsby, 2017).

Attachment insecurity during development has been described to result in self-deficits and failing processes of self/other differentiation (i.e. development of individuation) (Amianto et al., 2016) and it is suggested that early intersubjective interactions may be critical for the development of our ability to mentalize homeostatic interoceptive states (Fotopoulou & Tsakiris, 2017). Quattrocki and Friston (2014) suggest that infants associate interoceptive signals of warmth and satiety with their caregiver's face, which in turn drives attachment behavior and the development of endogenous social attention. The authors consider impaired integration of interoceptive signals with salient information from other sensory domains to hamper the infant in forming a higher representation of self, that allows feeling distinct from other, and that results in an impoverished sense of self.

9.5 Conceptualizing eating disorders within interoceptive predicting coding theories

How interoception, as well as multisensory integration of interoceptive, exteroceptive and proprioceptive bodily signals may construe a "sense of self" has been addressed by Bayesian predictive coding accounts (Apps & Tsakiris, 2014; Picard & Friston, 2014; Seth & Friston, 2017; see Chapter 2 in the present volume). Anatomical models have been proposed delineating cortico-cortical connections of limbic brain regions and the insular cortex, with anterior insula operating as an "error module" (Barrett & Simmons, 2015).

Instead of a linear translation from sensations to perceptions, these models state that incoming sensory data are compared with internal models, that is, with the brain's probabilistic predictions about the body and the environmental causes that affect the organism. This leads to bottom-up prediction errors (PE), that must be minimized, according to the "free energy principle" that warrants adaptive functioning of the organism (Seth & Friston, 2017; Picard & Friston, 2014). With respect to the body, PE arise when the actual state of the body does not match the predicted state. This may occur in each sensory system, and also within interoception. This means that exteroceptive and interoceptive perceptions are continuously constructed by the probabilistically computing brain, and thereby sensory perceptions, including interoceptive perceptions, may occur through an active, iterative inference process of comparing the brain's anticipation of sensations with incoming afferent input. Thus, also interoceptive experience reflects predictions about the state of the body.

With respect to multisensory integration of interoceptive, exteroceptive and proprioceptive sensory channels within self-processing, one's body is suggested to be processed in a probabilistic manner as the most likely to be "me" (Apps & Tsakiris, 2014). Accordingly, for a body to be represented as self, exteroceptive and interoceptive streams have to be integrated in order to minimize PEs across multisensory bodily systems (e.g. Tsakiris, 2016; Picard & Friston, 2014). As has been summarized, maladaptive eating and EDs are characterized by dysfunctional interoception as well as deficient multisensory interoceptive and exteroceptive integration that shows up in greater malleability of the sense of body-ownership. Especially, lower IAcc has been demonstrated in EDs, as well as in obesity, that may vary dynamically related to self-relevant context. We also summarized evidence for a basic exteroceptive/interoceptive imbalance in EDs with a dominant focus on the body from the outside, that is paired with body dissatisfaction, and an experience of an "object body" that is or has to be controlled.

Within interoceptive coding accounts higher IAcc should reflect less noisy information in this domain, that is, greater "precision" within the interoceptive system. This has been suggested to determine the dominance of the brain's weighing interoceptive predictions and PEs as more reliable (Ainley et al., 2016). This then supports resistance to exteroceptive multisensory conflicts, as shows up in less malleability to body illusions (see Tsakiris, 2017). This process might explain the emphasis on the body as object in patients with EDs, who seem to shut down interoceptive perceptions (e.g. not to sense hunger or unpleasant, fear-related bodily sensations) and in doing so they are able to control the "object body," that is, body weight and body shape by fasting, for example.

Additionally, large interoceptive PEs are suggested to occur in EDs, that is when incoming interoceptive information is discordant with interoceptive predictions. This is also reflected in massive body image distortion. We reported clues from very few studies up to now that investigated interaction of different dimensions of interoception to grasp the degree of mismatch of self-ascribed proficiency in interoceptive ability and actual capacity to perceive interoceptive signals accurately, which may serve as an estimate of "interoceptive (trait) prediction error" (Garfinkel et al., 2016b). In a sample of women with AN, greater mismatch of interoceptive dimensions has indeed been reported (Pollatos et al., 2008).

We suggest that larger PEs arise either by trait-like impaired IAcc and/or by externally and internally (physiologically) disturbing processes such as food-deprivation, rigid exercising, bingeing and purging (BN), as well as overeating and unhealthy food-consumption (obesity). Indeed, these clinical symptoms of EDs and features of obesity may obviously in turn influence dimensions of interoception and IAcc via physiological changes of autonomic nervous activity (see Herbert et al., 2012b). A noisy interoceptive (and/or a noisy, dynamically varying multisensory bodily) system may prompt the brain to find ways of reducing (interoceptive, as well as exteroceptive, proprioceptive) PEs either by (a) (selectively) attenuating processing of incoming sensory input; (b) by triggering changes in the body that resemble the expected input; or (c) by altering perceptual inferences about bodily states (Khalsa & Lapidus, 2016). In many ways the clinical symptoms of EDs as well as use of overeating or high-caloric food-choice in obesity can be characterized as ways of minimizing PEs within the interoceptive system as well as in other sensory systems, (i.e. coping with sensory and expected inconsistencies or challenges) in order to modulate the object body.

We assume that a core mechanism of all eating-related disorders is a history of learning during development that information from the body is not reliable. Thus, bodily signals cannot be adequately used to update prior predictions across multimodal bodily sensations in order to minimize PEs, that results in dysfunction of the self. Instead, eating, fasting, and other clinical symptoms characterizing obesity or EDs develop as (dysfunctional) strategies to cope with an "insufficient self" (Bruch, 1962).

9.6 Conclusion

Interoceptive deficits are major clinical characteristics in AN and BN, and interoception plays an important role in steering eating behavior according to hunger and satiety signals and bodily needs. We outlined the relevance of dimensions of interoception, including IAcc and IE, in shaping eating behavior. Eating according to interoceptive signals of hunger and satiety, undisturbed from external or emotional cues, has been shown to represent one way of adaptive eating that is associated with body weight in the normal range in healthy individuals.

We discussed evidence for *hyposensitivity* of interoceptive signals across gastric and cardiac modalities in obesity. However, we also proposed the view that *hypersensitivity* of interoceptive signals associated with hunger and bodily states of energy loss may contribute to the experience of positive alliesthesia for food cues in obesity, and thereby may undermine attempts to lose weight.

For EDs, dysfunctional IAcc lies at the core of clinical symptoms of AN and BN. In line with evidence showing context-dependent biased IAcc in AN, and together with the well-documented aversive evaluation of interoceptive cues and the negative appreciation of the body from the outside in EDs, we suggest that IAcc and other interoceptive dimensions may not be constantly dampenend in EDs but show variations depending on salient (aversively experienced and/or fear provoking) contexts, such as expecting food confrontation, or confrontation with the body. Aversive body appreciation and negative evaluation of interoceptive cues (IE) play a major role in shaping the process of shutting-down interoceptive sensations, and of dominantly focusing on the exteroceptive body, the "object body."

A major difference between AN and BN is supposed to be the capacity of top-down inhibitory function, that is greatest in AN, and is low in binge-eating BN. Maladaptive eating or overeating may represent a spectrum anchored by extremes of inhibition and dysregulation interacting with altered interoception at its base.

Going beyond its relevance for eating behavior, we highlight the importance of interoception in shaping dimensions of the self that is thought to be disordered in EDs. This shows up in perceptive and cognitive-affective body image distortion and "an overwhelming sense of ineffectiveness" (Bruch, 1962). The lack of integration of interoceptive signals and exteroceptive sensory information results in an impoverished sense of self. Within this process, aversive experience of the body and of interoceptive signals (IE) play a major role in EDs. We delineated that in EDs, long-term, dysfunctional strategies are used (e.g. fasting, exteroceptive body focus, bingeing, heavy exercising) in order to minimize existent large PEs within the interoceptive system, as well as in exteroceptive sensory systems, to control the body as an object. Clinical symptoms of EDs may reflect an insufficient self that is aimed to be stabilized by inadequate actions to minimize free energy. This may explain the persistence of clinical symptoms in ED that are so often resistant to therapy.

References

Ainley, V., **Tajadura-Jiménez, A.**, **Fotopoulou, A.**, and **Tsakiris, M.** (2012). Looking into myself: Changes in interoceptive sensitivity during mirror self-observation. *Psychophysiology*, *49*(11) 1672–6. doi:10.1111/j.1469-8986.2012.01468.x.

Ainley, V. and **Tsakiris, M.** (2013). Body conscious? Interoceptive awareness, measured by heartbeat perception, is negatively correlated with self-objectification. *PLoS One*, **8**(2) e55568. <http://dx.doi.org/10.1371%2Fjournal.pone.0055568>

Ainley, V., Apps, M. A. J., Fotopoulou, A., and **Tsakiris M.** (2016). "Bodily precision": A predictive coding account of individual differences in interoceptive accuracy. *Philosophical Transactions of the Royal Society of London B, 371*(1708), 20160003. doi:10.1098/rstb.2016.0003.

Apps, M. A. J. and **Tsakiris, M.** (2014). The free-energy self: A predictive coding account of self-recognition. *Neuroscience and Biobehavioral Reviews,* **41**, 85–97. doi:10.1016/j.neubiorev.2013.01.029.

Arrouk, R., Karpinski, A., Lavenbarg, T., Belmont, J., McCallum, R. W., and **Hyman, P.** (2017). Water load test in children with chronic abdominal pain or obesity compared with nonobese controls. *Southern Medical Journal, 110*(3), 168–71. doi:10.14423/SMJ.0000000000000612.

Amianto, F., Northoff, G., Abbate Daga, G., Fassino, S., and **Tasca, G.A.** (2016). Is anorexia nervosa a disorder of the self? A psychological approach. *Frontiers in Psychology,* 7, 849. <https://doi.org/10.3389/fpsyg.2016.00849>

American Psychiatric Association (2013). *Diagnostic and Statistical Manual of Mental Disorders,* 5th edn. Washington, DC: American Psychiatric Association.

Arcelus, J., Mitchell, A. J., Wales, J., and **Nielsen, S.** (2011). Mortality rates in patients with anorexia nervosa and other eating disorders: A meta-analysis of 36 studies. *Archives of General Psychiatry, 68*(7), 724–31. doi:10.1001/archgenpsychiatry.2011.74.

Attuquayefio, T., Stevenson, R. J., Oaten, M. J., and **Francis, H. M.** (2017). A four-day Western-style dietary intervention causes reductions in hippocampal-dependent learning and memory and interoceptive sensitivity. *PloS One, 12*(2), e0172645. doi:10.1371/journal.pone.0172645.

Avery, J. A., Kerr, K. L., Ingeholm, J. E., Burrows, K., Bodurka, J., and **Simmons, W. K.** (2015). A common gustatory and interoceptive representation in the human mid-insula. *Human Brain Mapping, 36*(8), 2996–3006. doi:10.1002/hbm.22823.

Barrett, L. and **Simmons, W.K.** 2015. Interoceptive predictions in the brain. *Nature Reviews Neuroscience, 16*(7) 419–29. <http://dx.doi.org/10.1038/nrn3950>

Bartholdy, S., Rennals, S. J., Jacques, C., Danby, H., Campbell, I. C., Schmidt, U., et al. (2017). Proactive and reactive inhibitory control in eating disorders. *Psychiatry Research,* **255**, 432–40. doi:10.1016/j.psychres.2017.06.073.

Beglinger, C. and **Degen, L.** (2006). Gastrointestinal satiety signals in humans—physiologic roles for GLP-1 and PYY? *Physiology & Behavior, 89*(4), 460–4. doi:10.1016/j.physbeh.2006.05.048.

Bertoud, H. R. (2008). The vagus nerve, food intake and obesity. *Regulatory Peptides, 149*(1), 15–25. doi:10.1016/j.regpep.2007.08.024.

Birch, L. L. and **Fisher, J. O.** (2000). Mothers' child-feeding practices influence daughters' eating and weight. *American Journal of Clinical Nutrition, 71*(5), 1054–61.

Bruch, H. (1962). Perceptual and conceptual disturbances in anorexia nervosa. *Psychosomatic Medicine, 24*(2), 187–94.

Bruch, H. (1973). *Eating Disorder: Obesity, Anorexia Nervosa and the Person Within.* New York, NY: Basic Books.

Clausen, L., Rosenvinge, J. H., Friborg, O., and **Rokkedal, K.** (2011). Validating the Eating Disorder Inventory-3 (EDI-3): A comparison between 561 female eating disorders patients and 878 females from the general population. *Journal of Psychopathology and Behavioral Assessment, 33*(1), 101–10. doi:10.1007/s10862-010-9207-4.

Cowdrey, F. A., Park, R. J., and **McCabe, C.** (2011). *Biological Psychiatry,* **15**, 736–43. doi:10.1016/j.biopsych.2011.05.028.

Craig, A. D. (2009). How do you feel—now? The anterior insula and human awareness. *Nature Reviews Neuroscience, 10*(1), 59–70. doi:10.1038/nrn2555.

Crucianelli, L., Cardi, V., Treasure, J., Jenkinson, P. M., and **Fotopoulou, A.** (2016). The perception of affective touch in anorexia nervosa. *Psychiatry Research,* **239**, 72–8. doi:10.1016/j.psychres.2016.01.078.

Cui, H., **López, M.**, and **Rahmouni, K.** (2017). The cellular and molecular bases of leptin and ghrelin resistance in obesity. *Nature Reviews Endocrinology*, *13*(6), 338–51. doi:10.1038/nrendo.2016.222.

Emanuelsen, L., **Drew, R.**, and **Köteles, F.** (2015). Interoceptive sensitivity, body image dissatisfaction, and body awareness in healthy indivdiuals. *Scandinavian Journal of Psychology*, *56*(2), 167–74. doi:10.1111/sjop.12183.

Eshkevari, E., **Rieger, E.**, **Longo, M. R.**, **Haggard, P.**, and **Treasure, J.** (2012). Increased plasticity of the bodily self in eating disorders. *Psychological Medicine*, *42*(4), 819–28. doi:10.1017/S0033291711002091.

Fairburn, C. G. and **Harrison, P. J.**, (2003). Eating disorders. *Lancet*, **361**(9355), 407–16.

Faith, M. S., **Scanlon, K. S.**, **Birch, L. L.**, **Francis, L. A.**, and **Sherry, B.** (2004). Parent–child feeding strategies and their relationships to child eating and weight status. *Obesity*, *12*(11), 1711–22. doi:10.1038/oby.2004.212.

Fotopoulou, A. and **Tsakiris, M.** (2017). Mentalizing homeostasis: The social origins of interoceptive inference. *Neuropsychoanalysis*, *19*(1), 3–28. doi:10.1080/15294145.2017.1294031.

Fuchs, T. and **Schlimme, J. E.** (2009). Embodiment and psychopathology: A phenomenological perspective. *Current opinion in Psychiatry*, *22*(6), 570–5. doi:10.1097/YCO.0b013e3283318e5c.

Furman, E. (2013). The theory of compromised eating behavior. *Research in Gerontological Nursing*, *7*(2), 78–86. doi:10.3928/19404921-20130930-01.

Füstös, J., **Gramann, K.**, **Herbert, B. M.**, and **Pollatos, O.** (2013). On the embodiment of emotion regulation: Interoceptive awareness facilitates reappraisal. *Social Cognitive and Affective Neuroscience*, *8*(8), 911–17. doi:10.1093/scan/nss089.

Friederich, H.C., **Brooks, S.**, **Uher, R.**, **Campbell, I.C.**, **Giampietro, V.**, **Brammer, M.**, et al. (2010). Neural corelates of body dissatisfaction in anorexia nervosa. *Neuropsychologia*, **48**, 2878–85. doi:10.1016/j.neuropsychologia.2010.04.036.

Gadsby, S. (2017). Distorted body representations in anorexia nervosa. *Consciousness and Cognition*, *51*, 17–33. doi:10.1016/j.concog.2017.02.015.

Gaete, M. I. and **Fuchs, T.** (2016). From body image to emotional bodily experience in eating disorders. *Journal of Phenomenological Psychology*, **47**(1), 17–40. doi:10.1163/15691624-12341303.

Garfinkel, S. N., **Seth, A. K.**, **Barrett, A. B.**, **Suzuki, K.**, and **Critchley, H. D.** (2015). Knowing your own heart: Distinguishing interoceptive accuracy from interoceptive awareness. *Biological Psychology*, **104**, (0) 65–74. doi:10.1016/j.biopsycho.2014.11.004.

Garfinkel, S. N., **Manassei, M. F.**, **Hamilton-Fletcher, G.**, **den Bosch, Y. I.**, **Critchley, H. D.**, and **Engels, M.** (2016a). Interoceptive dimensions across cardiac and respiratory axes. *Philosophical Transactions of the Royal Society B*, *371*,1708, 20160014. doi:10.1098/rstb.2016.0014.

Garfinkel, S. N., **Tiley, C.**, **O'Keeffe, S.**, **Harrison, N. A.**, **Seth, A. K.**, and **Critchley, H. D.** (2016b). Discrepancies between dimensions of interoception in autism: Implications for emotion and anxiety. *Biological Psychology*, *114*, 117–26. doi:10.1016/j.biopsycho.2015.12.003.

Galloway, A. T., **Farrow, C. V.**, and **Martz, D. M.** (2010). Retrospective reports of child feeding practices, current eating behaviors, and BMI in college students. *Obesity*, *18*(7), 1330–5. doi:10.1038/oby.2009.393.

Gaudio, S. and **Quattrocki, C.C.** (2012). Neural basis of multimodal model of body image distortion in anorexia nervosa, *Neuroscience and Biobehavioral Reviews*, **36**(8), 1839–47. doi:10.1016/j.neubiorev.2012.05.003.

Geliebter, A. and **Hashim, S. A.** (2001). Gastric capacity in normal, obese, and bulimic women. *Physiology & Behavior*, *74*(4), 743–6. doi:10.1016/S0031-9384(01)00619-9.

Heatherton, T. F. and **Baumeister, R. F.** (1991). Binge eating as escape from self-awareness. *Psychological Bulletin*, *110*(1), 86. doi:10.1037/0033-2909.110.1.86.

Herbert, B. M., **Ulbrich, P.**, and **Schandry, R.** (2007). Interoceptive sensitivity and physical effort: Implications for the self-control of physical in everyday life. *Psychophysiology*, **44**, 194–202. doi:10.1111/j.1469-8986.2007.00493.x.

Herbert, B.M., **Pollatos, O.**, **Flor, H.**, **Enck, P.**, and **Schandry, R.** (2010). Cardiac awareness and autonomic cardiac rseactivity during emotional picture viewing and mental stress. *Psychophysiology*, **47**, 342–54. doi:10.1111/j.1469-8986.2009.00931.x.

Herbert, B. M. and **Pollatos, O.** (2012). The body in the mind: On the relationship between interoception and embodiment. *Topics in Cognitive Science*, **4**, 692–704. doi:10.1111/j.1756-8765.2012.01189.x.

Herbert, B. M., **Muth, E. R.**, **Pollatos, O.**, and **Herbert, C.** (2012a). Interoception across modalities: On the relationship between cardiac awareness and the sensitivity for gastric functions. *PloS One*, *7*(5), e36646. doi:10.1371/journal.pone.0036646.

Herbert, B. M., **Herbert, C.**, **Pollatos, O.**, **Weimer, K.**, **Enck, P.**, **Sauer, H.**, and **Zipfel, S.** (2012b). Effects of short-term food deprivation on interoceptive awareness, feelings and autonomic cardiac activity. *Biological Psychology*, *89*(1), 71–9. doi:10.1016/j.biopsycho.2011.09.004.

Herbert, B. M., **Blechert, J.**, **Hautzinger, M.**, **Matthias, E.**, and **Herbert, C.** (2013). Intuitive eating is associated with interoceptive sensitivity. Effects on body mass index. *Appetite*, *70*, 22–30. doi:10.1016/j.appet.2013.06.082.

Hetherington, M. M. (2000). Eating disorders: Diagnosis, etiology, and prevention. *Nutrition*, **16** (7–8), 547–51.

Khalsa, S. S., **Craske, M. G.**, **Li, W.**, **Vangala, S.**, **Strober, M.**, and **Feusner, J. D.** (2015). Altered interoceptive awareness in anorexia nervosa: Effects of meal anticipation, consumption and bodily arousal. *International Journal of Eating Disorders*, *48*(7), 889–97. doi:10.1002/eat.22387.

Khalsa, S. S. and **Lapidus, R. C.** (2016). Can interoception improve the pragmatic search for biomarkers in psychiatry?. *Frontiers in Psychiatry*, *7*. doi:10.3389/fpsyt.2016.00121.

Kaye, W. H., **Fudge, J. L.**, and **Paulus, M.** (2009). New insights into symptoms and neurocircuit function of anorexia nervosa. *Nature Reviews Neuroscience*, *10*(8), 573–84. doi:10.1038/nrn2682.

Kirk, U., **Downar, J.**, and **Montague, P. R.** (2011). Interoception drives increased rational decision-making in meditators playing the ultimatum game. *Frontiers in Neuroscience*, *5*. doi:10.3389/fnins.2011.00049.

Klabunde, M., **Collado, D.**, and **Bohon, C.** (2017). An interoceptive model of bulimia nervosa: A neurobiological review. *Journal of Psychiatric Research*, **94**, 36–46. <https://doi.org/10.1016/J.JPSYCHIRES.2017.06.009>

Koch, A. and **Pollatos, O.** (2014). Interoceptive sensitivity, body weight and eating behavior in children: A prospective study. *Frontiers in Psychology*, *5*. doi:10.3389/fpsyg.2014.01003.

Lilenfeld, L. R., **Wonderlich, S.**, **Riso, L. P.**, **Crosby, R.**, and **Mitchell, J.** (2006). Eating disorders and personality: A methodological and empirical review. *Clinical PsychologyRreview*, *26*(3), 299–320. doi:0.1016/j.cpr.2005.10.003.

Madden, C. E., **Leong, S. L.**, **Gray, A.**, and **Horwath, C. C.** (2012). Eating in response to hunger and satiety signals is related to BMI in a nationwide sample of 1601 mid-age New Zealand women. *Public Health Nutrition*, *15*(12), 2272–9. doi:10.1017/S1368980012000882.

McKinley, N. M. (1999). Women and objectified body consciousness: Mothers' and daughters' body experience in cultural, developmental, and familial context. *Developmental Psychology*, *35*, 760–9.

Merwin, R. M., **Zucker, N. L.**, **Lacy, J. L.**, and **Elliott, C. A.** (2010). Interoceptive awareness in eating disorders: Distinguishing lack of clarity from non-acceptance of internal experience. *Cognition and Emotion*, *24*(5), 892–902. doi:10.1080/02699930902985845.

Morrison, T., **Waller, G.**, and **Lawson, R.** (2006). Attributional style in the eating disorders. *Journal of Nervous and Mental Disease*, *194*(4), 303–5. doi:10.1097/01.nmd.0000208114.79179.7e.

Murphy, J., **Brewer, R.**, **Catmur, C.**, and **Bird, G.** (2017). Interoception and psychopathology: A developmental neuroscience perspective. *Developmental Cognitive Neuroscience*, *23*, 45–56. doi:10.1016/j.dcn.2016.12.006.

Page, K. A., Seo, D., Belfort-DeAguiar, R., Lacadie, C., Dzuira, J., Naik, S., et al. (2011). Circulating glucose levels modulate neural control of desire for high-calorie foods in humans. *Journal of Clinical Investigation*, *121*(10), 4161. doi:10.1172/JCI57873.

Picard, F. and **Friston, K.** (2014). Predictions, perception, and a sense of self. *Neurology*, *83*(12), 1112–18. doi:10.1212/WNL.0000000000000798.

Pollatos, O., Gramann, K., and **Schandry, R.** (2007). Neural systems connecting interoceptive awareness and feelings. *Human Brain Mapping*, *28*(1), 9–18. doi:10.1002/hbm.20258.

Pollatos, O., Kurz, A. L., Albrecht, J., Schreder, T., Kleemann, A. M., Schöpf, V., et al. (2008). Reduced perception of bodily signals in anorexia nervosa. *Eating Behaviors*, *9*(4), 381–8. doi:10.1016/j.eatbeh.2008.02.001.

Pollatos, O., and **Georgiou, E.** (2016). Normal interoceptive accuracy in women with bulimia nervosa. *Psychiatry Research*, **240**, 328–32. doi:10.1016/j.psychres.2016.04.072.

Pollatos, O., Herbert, B.M., Mai, S., and **Kammer, T.** (2016). Changes in interoceptive processes following brain stimulation. *Philosophical Transactions of the Royal Society B*, **371**, 1708. doi:10.1098/rstb.2016.0016.

Quattrocki, E. and **Friston, K.** 2014. Autism, oxytocin and interoception. *Neuroscience and Biobehavioral Reviews*, **47**, 410–30. <http://www.sciencedirect.com/science/article/pii/S0149763414002395>

Schmidt, U. and **Treasure, J.** (2006). Anorexia nervosa: Valued and visible. A cognitive-interpersonal maintenance model and its implications for research and practice. *British Journal of Clinical Psychology*, *45*(3), 343–66. doi:10.1348/014466505X53902.

Seth, A. K. and **Friston, K. J.** (2016). Active interoceptive inference and the emotional brain. *Philosophical Transactions of the Royal Society B*, **371**, 20160007. doi:10.1098/rstb.2016.0007.

Smith, R. and **Lane, R. D.** (2015). The neural basis of one's own conscious and unconscious emotional states. *Neuroscience and Biobehavioral Reviews*, *57*, 1–29. doi:10.1016/j.neubiorev.2015.08.003.

Stevenson, R. J., Mahmut, M., and **Rooney, K.** (2015). Individual differences in the interoceptive states of hunger, fullness and thirst. *Appetite*, *95*, 44–57. doi:10.1016/j.appet.2015.06.008.

Stice, E., Burger, K. S., and **Yokum, S.** (2013). Relative ability of fat and sugar tastes to activate reward, gustatory, and somatosensory regions. *American Journal of Clinical Nutrition*, *98*(6), 1377–84. doi:10.3945/ajcn.113.069443.

Tajadura-Jiménez, A. and **Tsakiris, M.** (2014). Balancing the 'inner' and the 'outer' self: Interoceptive sensitivity modulates self–other boundaries. *Journal of Experimental Psychology: General*, *143*(2), 736. doi:10.1037/a0033171.

Tate, C. M. and **Geliebter, A.** (2017). Intragastric balloon treatment for obesity: Review of recent studies. *Advances in Therapy*, 1–17. doi:10.1007/s12325-017-0562-3.

Tsakiris, M., Tajadura-Jiménez, A., and **Costantini, M.** (2011). Just a heartbeat away from one's body: Interoceptive sensitivity predicts malleability of body-representations. *Proceedings of the Royal Society of London B*, *278*(1717), 2470–6. doi:10.1098/rspb.2010.2547.

Tsakiris, M. (2017). The multisensory basis of the self: From body to identity to others. *Quarterly Journal of Experimental Psychology*, **70**, 597–609. doi:10.1080/17470218.2016.1181768.

Tylka, T. L. (2006). Development and psychometric evaluation of a measure of intuitive eating. *Journal of Counselling Psychology*, *53*(2), 226. doi:10.1037/0022-0167.53.2.226.

Whitehead, W. E. and **Drescher, V. M.** (1980). Perception of gastric contractions and self-control of gastric motility. *Psychophysiology*, *17*(6), 552–8. doi:10.1111/j.1469-8986.1980.tb02296.x.

Wierenga, C. E., Ely, A., Bischoff-Grethe, A., Bailer, U. F., Simmons, A. N., and **Kaye, W. H.** (2014). Are extremes of consumption in eating disorders related to an altered balance between reward and inhibition? *Frontiers in Behavioral Neuroscience*, *8*. doi:10.3389/fnbeh.2014.00410.

Van Dyck, Z., Vögele, C., Blechert, J., Lutz, A. P., Schulz, A., and **Herbert, B. M.** (2016). The water load test as a measure of gastric interoception: Development of a two-stage protocol and application to a healthy female population. *PloS One*, *11*(9), e0163574. doi:10.1371/journal.pone.0163574.

Vocks, S., Busch, M., Grönemeyer, D., Schulte, D., Herpertz, S., and **Suchan, B.** (2010). Neural correlates of viewing photographs of one's body and another woman's body in anorexia and bulimia nervosa: An fMRI study. *Journal of Psychiatry and Neuroscience*, **35**, 163–76. doi:10.1503/jpn.090048.

Zucker, N. L., Kragel, P. A., Wagner, H. R., Keeling, L., Mayer, E., Wang, J., et al. (2017). The clinical significance of posterior insular volume in adolescent anorexia nervosa. *Psychosomatic Medicine*, *79*(9), 1025–35. doi:10.1097/PSY.0000000000000510.

Chapter 10

Cardiac interoception in neurological conditions and its relevance for dimensional approaches

Adrián Yoris, Adolfo M. García, Paula Celeste Salamone, Lucas Sedeño, Indira García-Cordero, and Agustín Ibáñez

10.1 Interoception as a new dimensional and transdiagnostic framework for neurology

Mental disorders have been classically defined in terms of mutually exclusive sets of discrete symptoms, yet they can be fruitfully reconceptualized along *dimensions* of normal and abnormal behavior. Building on the Research Domain Criteria (Insel et al., 2010), this perspective has already afforded breakthroughs concerning phenomenological, cognitive, and neural alterations in psychopathological conditions. Its application to neurological diseases, however, remains comparatively limited (Ibanez et al., 2016b; Ibanez et al., 2014), despite accruing evidence that cognitive, emotional, behavioral, and autonomic neurological impairments may affect (or predict) dimensionally different clinical conditions (Kling et al., 2013).

As shown by recent research on psychiatric populations (Muller et al., 2015; Yoris et al., 2017), informative dimensional insights into mental disorders can be gained by assessing interoception (Khalsa & Lapidus, 2016), a complex construct subsuming multiple forms of visceral signal processing (Craig, 2009). Though somewhat more incipiently, studies on neurological disorders also suggest that specific dimensions of interoception may be differentially compromised across pathologies (Garcia-Cordero et al., 2016). Thus, more classical approaches focused on externally triggered neurocognitive processes (e.g. perception, recognition or classification of outer stimuli) could be fruitfully complemented by assessments of neurocognitive processes triggered by internal cues (e.g. heartbeats, respiration changes, visceral sensations).

In this sense, cardiac interoception (the ability to monitor one's own heartbeats) emerges as a potential transdiagnostic and dimensional biomarker for neurological disorders. Research on healthy and brain-damaged individuals (Couto et al., 2015; Garcia-Cordero et al., 2016) shows that heartbeat detection (HBD) and heartbeat discrimination tasks shed light on several key phenomena. First, they can tap into different dimensions of interoception (as defined in (Garfinkel et al., 2015; see also Chapter 7 in the present volume), including interoceptive accuracy (the ability to monitor each heartbeat correctly), interoceptive sensitivity (the subjective perception of one's interoceptive performance), interoceptive awareness or metacognition (the association between confidence about one's own performance and the actual performance), and a measure developed by our group termed interoceptive learning, that reflects the improvement of interoceptive accuracy after auditory feedback of one's own heartbeats (Garcia-Cordero et al., 2016; Garfinkel et al., 2015) (details in Table 10.1). Second, these tasks and dimensions allow us to investigate the functions of different interoceptive pathways, such as the vagal and the somatosensory pathways (Khalsa et al., 2009a). Finally, they illuminate the relations between interoception and emotional or social cognition processes (Adolfi et al., 2016), among others. Thus, the cardiac interoception paradigm represents a validated, promising approach to explore how various functions in the brain–body interface are compromised across neurological conditions.

Here we deploy this proposal considering behavioral, neuroanatomical, and brain functional evidence in the context of experimental and clinical settings. We also evaluate the potential role of interoception as (a) predictor of clinical outcomes, (b) marker of neurocognitive deficits in neuropsychiatric diseases, and (c) general source of insights for breakthroughs in the treatment and prevention of multiple disorders.

Table 10.1 Interoceptive dimensions addressed through our group's HBD task.

Dimension	Definition	Instruction	Observations
Accuracy	Behavioral precision in tracking one's own heartbeat via finger taps	"Tap the keyboard with the middle finger of your dominant hand when you feel or think about your heart beats"	Accuracy index is obtained by comparing the temporal proximity between the subject's ECG signal and his/her finger taps.[1]
Learning	Behavioral precision after receiving external feedback of one's own heartbeats	"Now, after feedback, tap the keyboard each time you feel or think about your heart beats"	Learning is calculated exactly as done for the accuracy index, but after the subject was exposed to his/her own heartbeats through a stethoscope during a so-called feedback condition.
Awareness	Subject's confidence in his/her own behavioral performance is controlled in base of his/her accuracy performance in HBD	"Rate your confidence in your performance from 1 (not confident at all) to 9 (fully confident)"	Awareness index is obtained normalizing scores of self-confidence with the accuracy performance. Higher awareness scores appear close to zero.

[1] Note that the calculation of accuracy is similar to Schandry's, although the actual formula differs.

10.2 Disruptions of interoceptive mechanisms in neurological disorders

Recent research on interoceptive deficits in neurological disorders has focused on ischemic stroke (IS), Alzheimer's disease (AD), behavioral variant fronto-temporal dementia (bvFTD), multiple sclerosis (MS), Parkinson's disease (PD), functional motor disorders (FMDs), and chronic pain (CP). The key brain areas, neural pathways, and interoceptive dimensions compromised in each case, considering behavioral, electrophysiological, neuroanatomical, and functional imaging findings, are presented in Table 10.2.

10.2.1 Stroke

Cardiovascular lesions in the brain are often caused by ischemic stroke (IS). While hemorrhagic stroke refers to burst blood vessels, IS constitutes a pervasive condition caused by the block of a blood vessel (e.g. a blood clot) (Sacco et al., 2013). IS involves high levels of mortality and disability, burdening health systems worldwide. Research into its associated cognitive, behavioral, and affective changes has long yielded theoretical and clinical insights into the human brain (Ibanez, Gleichgerrcht, & Manes, 2010). As shown below, assessments of interoception in this condition may also afford conceptual and translational breakthroughs.

In a pioneering study, Khalsa, Rudrauf, Feinstein, and colleagues (Khalsa et al., 2009a) examined the contributions of two complementary interoceptive pathways (vagal and somatosensory) in a patient with bilateral damage to two critical interoceptive regions (the insula and the anterior cingulate cortex (ACC), closely related with cardiac activity) (Critchley et al., 2004) alongside full preservation of his somatosensory cortex. The patient was asked to turn a dial to track his ongoing experience of the overall intensity of heartbeat sensations in a baseline condition and during pharmacologically induced tachycardia (details in (Khalsa et al., 2009a)). While interoceptive perception was reduced at baseline, it proved normal during pharmacological condition. Poor performance would reflect damage to the insula and the ACC, with pharmacological restoration apparently acted on preserved somatosensory structures. These patterns suggest a differential participation of the vagal and the somatosensory pathways during interoception, such that both internal (e.g. cardiac) and external (e.g. skin) afferents can contribute to this domain.

Further insights into the neural bases of such pathways were offered by Couto, Adolfi, Sedeno, and colleagues (Couto et al., 2015). They assessed interoceptive accuracy through a multidimensional HBD task tapping into interoceptive accuracy (behavioral precision in tracking one's own heartbeat via finger taps), and exteroceptive skills (a control condition measuring behavioral precision in following an auditorily presented heartbeat (for details see Couto et al., 2015). Also, additional somatosensory domains (e.g. taste, pain, and smell recognition) were measured to examine alternative afferent mechanisms relying on regions and pathways different from those engaged by interoception. Two patients were recruited, one with grey matter compromise in the right insula and another one with white matter damage in the subcortical tracts connecting fronto-temporal

Table 10.2 Studies on interoception in neurological disorders.

Authors	Disorders, samples	Tasks, dimensions	Results	Implications
Couto et al., 2015	**IS** (N = 2, insular lesion and subcortical lesion); frontal lesion (N = 5) and HC (N = 7).	- *HBD task* **(accuracy)** -Taste, smell, and pain recognition tasks **(somatosensory perception)**	**BVL:** The insular lesion patient showed impaired internal signal processing (interoception), while the subcortical lesion patient exhibited external perception deficits (smell, taste, and pain). Such selective deficits remained even when comparing each patient with controls and frontal patients.	Results indicate that two patients presenting selective damage to different areas of the insular body-sensing network, share a differential pattern of disruption of internal and external perception.
García-Cordero et al., 2016	**bvFTD), AD and FIS** bvFTD (N = 18); AD (N = 21); non-hemorrhagic FIS (N = 18) and HC (N = 42).	- *HBD task* **(accuracy, awareness, learning)**	**BVL:** Accuracy was impaired in all patient groups, associated with insular damage, connectivity alterations, and abnormal HEP modulations. Learning was differentially impaired in AD patients. Awareness results showed that bvFTD and AD patients overestimated their performance. **EEG:** Relative to the three patient groups, controls exhibited more negative HEP modulations during the accuracy condition. **MRI**: Impairments were associated with frontal-temporo-insular damage and widespread connectivity abnormalities.	Damage to specific fronto-temporo-insular hubs differentially compromises interoceptive dimensions.
Seeley, 2010	**bvFTD** (Review of image studies)	Review	**MRI/fMRI:** BvFTD involves both ventral and dorsal anterior insula by the time of early clinical presentation. An early-stage fronto-insular that leaves patients unable to model the emotional impact of their own actions or inactions.	The search for bvFTD treatments will depend on a rich understanding of insular biology and could help clarify specialized human language, social, and emotional functions.
Ricciardi et al., 2016	**PD** (N = 20) and HC (N = 20)	- *HBD* **(accuracy)**	**BVL:** PD patients showed reduced accuracy and higher levels of depression, anhedonia, and apathy. Accuracy did not correlate with motor, non-motor, affective, and emotion symptoms.	Lower interoceptive accuracy in PD might be related to insular degeneration, irrespective of multiple symptom types.
Criaud, 2016	**PD** Meta-analysis: 132 insular foci from 96 published experiments. PD patients.	Meta-analysis	**MRI/fMRI:** Significant convergence of activation maxima related to PD in different insular regions including anterior and posterior regions bilaterally. PD patients medicated showed a more physiological involvement of bilateral anterior insula.	The insula should be considered a region of interest studying cognitive and behavioral changes, as well as disruptions in viscerosensory or somatosensory processes in PD.

Christopher, 2014	**PD** (image studies)	Review	**MRI/fMRI:** The insula processes cognitive, affective and interoceptive information in uncertain conditions and subjective feeling or state of awareness. Its disruption may alter the subjective state and ultimately behavior in patients with PD.	Mid and posterior insular cortex serve a crucial role in interoceptive sensation and behavior, and seems related to neurobehavioral disturbances in PD.
Ricciardi et al., 2016	**FMD** FMD (*N* = 16) and HC (*N* = 17)	- *HBD task*: **(accuracy and awareness)**	**BVL:** FMD patients have lower accuracy, predicting their depressive symptoms and their tendency to focus on external bodily features.	FMD patients have interoceptive deficits which may be predictive of their depressive symptoms, as well as their tendency to focus on the external features of their body.
Xie et al., 2012	**MCI** MCI (*N* = 30) and HC (*N* = 26)	Resting-state	**MRI/fMRI:** Patients showed reduced right posterior insula volumes, cognitive deficits and disrupted intrinsic connectivity of insular networks. The latter pattern was associated with EM deficits only in the patients.	The disrupted insula network connectivity would significantly contribute to EM impairment in aMCI patients. The disturbance of emotional awareness regulation in aMCI patients will have a negative impact on the process of cognition, and ultimately lead to cognitive decline.
Di Lernia et al., 2016	**CP** 8 studies.	Systematic review: - *MAIA questionnaire* **(awareness)** - *Heartbeat perception task* **(accuracy)**	**BVL:** Chronic pain subjects present low accuracy. Accuracy negatively correlates with symptoms severity in specific disorders. Data were inconclusive for interoceptive awareness.	Different patterns across pain disorders was observed. That indicates interoceptive dimensions could explain differentially pain disorders in a dimensional approach.
Duscheck et al., 2016	**FMS** FMS (*N* = 45) and HC (*N* = 31)	- *Heartbeat perception task* **(accuracy)**	**BVL:** Patients exhibited reduced heartbeat perception. Moreover, there was an inverse relationship between awareness and FMS symptom severity.	Poor access to bodily signals may restrict patients′ ability to integrate these signals during emotional processing, which, by extension, may preclude optimal emotional self-regulation.

aMCI: amnestic mild cognitive impairment; **aPFC**: anterior prefrontal cortex; **AD**: Alzheimer disease; **bvFTD**: behavioral variant fronto temporal dementia; **BVL**: behavioral; **DMN**: default mode network: **EEG**: electroencephalogram; **EM**: episodic memory; **FIS**: fronto-insular stroke; **FMD**: functional motor disorders; **FMS**: fibromyalgia syndrome; **FTD**: fronto temporal dementia; **HBD**: heartbeat detection; **HEP**: heart-evoked potential; **HC**: healthy controls; **Accuracy**: interoceptive accuracy; **Awareness**: interoceptive awareness; **MCI**: mild cognitive impairment; **MRI/fMRI**: image results; **PD**: Parkinson disease; **pDMN**: posterior default mode network; **RSNs**: resting state networks; **vmPFC**: ventromedial prefrontal cortex; **vSN**: ventral salience network.

areas (right putamen and claustrum, and the white matter of the external capsule, see Figure 10.1). Relative to healthy controls and control patients with lesions in other areas, the stroke patients exhibited a double dissociation: while the former showed interoceptive impairments with good somatosensory performance, the latter showed the opposite pattern. These results suggest the existence of distinct and dissociable streams for body-signal processing: a purely interoceptive one, affording low-level processing of autonomic inputs; and a somatosensory one, subserving high-level integration of external signals involving other areas and networks.

More recently, interoceptive accuracy, awareness, and learning were assessed in frontal IS patients relative to healthy controls and subjects with neurodegenerative conditions (AD and bvFTD) (Garcia-Cordero et al., 2016). Participants completed an HBD task with ongoing EEG recordings (aimed at examining the heart-evoked potential (HEP)), and they underwent resting functional magnetic resonance imaging (fMRI) measurements for connectivity analysis. All patient groups presented deficits in interoceptive accuracy as indexed by HBD, accompanied by reduced HEP modulations and insular damage. Interoceptive awareness (based on a measure that associates a self-report questionnaire of the confidence about one's performance and the actual performance) remained intact in IS, but it proved altered in neurodegenerative conditions. Finally, interoceptive learning (indexed as behavioral performance after exposure to heartbeat feedback via a stethoscope) remained intact in IS in contrast to neurodegenerative diseases. Thus, this study showed that these three dimensions are subserved by partially distinct neural mechanisms, suggesting that distinguishable patterns of neurological damage may be associated with recognizable interoceptive profiles. In particular, the selective compromise of interoceptive accuracy in IS, with preserved functioning of the awareness and learning dimensions, could have important implications to guide therapeutic interventions (see section 10.3.1).

Finally, another study (Adolfi et al., 2016) explored the convergence of aberrant interoception with affective impairments in IS patients with fronto-insular-temporal lesions and healthy controls. All subjects performed an HBD task tapping interoceptive accuracy, a complementary exteroceptive task assessing tracking of an auditorily presented heartbeat, and tests assessing emotion recognition, verbal prosody, and theory of mind (ToM). The patients were selectively impaired in cardiac interoception, emotion recognition, and ToM (Figure 10.2). Such first direct evidence highlights the fronto-insular-temporal networks as critical hubs for the integration of internal sensations with emotional and social information.

In sum, studies on patients with IS have revealed key aspects of interoceptive deficits following brain damage (Ibanez et al., 2010), such as the dimensional specializations of specific regions and pathways, the complementary participation of cortical and subcortical substrates in the integration of internal and external information, and the role of specific interoceptive hubs for the convergence of visceral and socio-emotional processes.

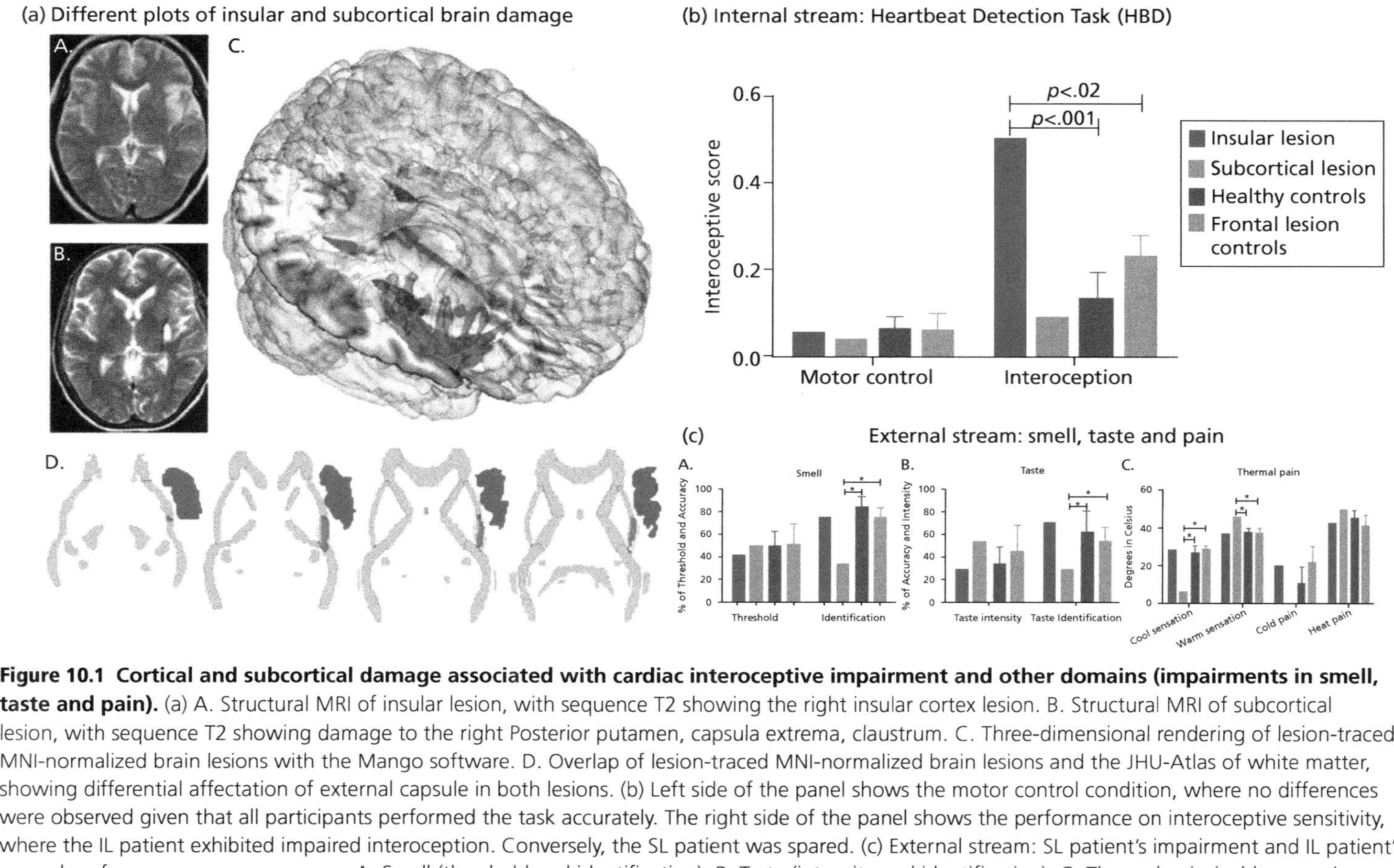

Figure 10.1 Cortical and subcortical damage associated with cardiac interoceptive impairment and other domains (impairments in smell, taste and pain). (a) A. Structural MRI of insular lesion, with sequence T2 showing the right insular cortex lesion. B. Structural MRI of subcortical lesion, with sequence T2 showing damage to the right Posterior putamen, capsula extrema, claustrum. C. Three-dimensional rendering of lesion-traced MNI-normalized brain lesions with the Mango software. D. Overlap of lesion-traced MNI-normalized brain lesions and the JHU-Atlas of white matter, showing differential affectation of external capsule in both lesions. (b) Left side of the panel shows the motor control condition, where no differences were observed given that all participants performed the task accurately. The right side of the panel shows the performance on interoceptive sensitivity, where the IL patient exhibited impaired interoception. Conversely, the SL patient was spared. (c) External stream: SL patient's impairment and IL patient's normal performance across measures. A. Smell (threshold and identification). B. Taste (intensity and identification). C. Thermal pain (cold perception, warm perception, cold pain, heat pain).

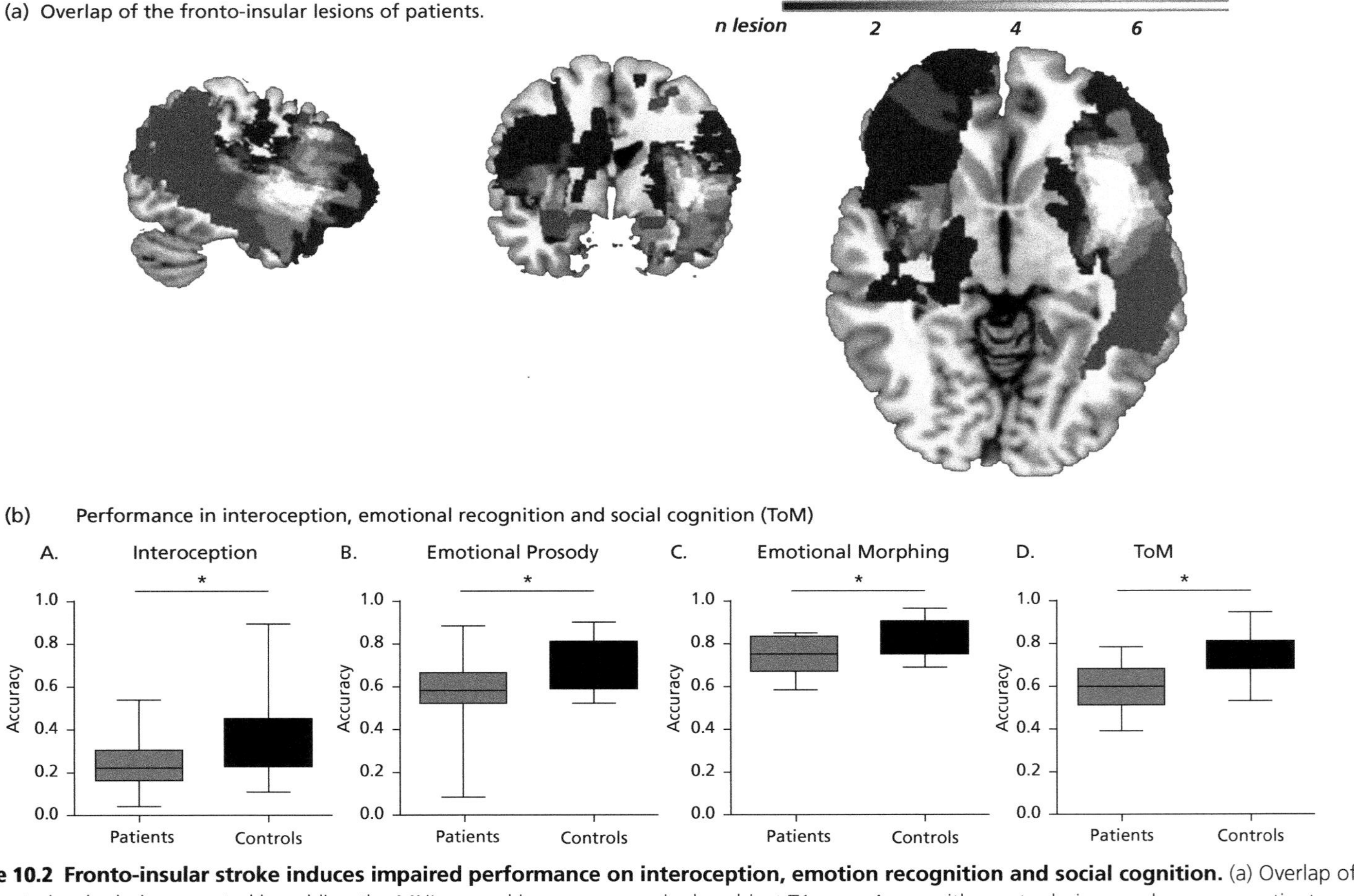

Figure 10.2 Fronto-insular stroke induces impaired performance on interoception, emotion recognition and social cognition. (a) Overlap of the fronto-insular lesions created by adding the MNI warped images over a single-subject T1 scan. Areas with greater lesion overlap across patients are shown brighter. (b) Box-plot diagram shows significantly worse performance in patients (grey) than controls (black) in all three domains.

10.2.2 Alzheimer's disease

In addition to cognitive and emotional changes, healthy aging also seems to disrupt interoceptive mechanisms. Indeed, a study with 59 participants ranging from 22 to 63 years old (Khalsa et al., 2009) revealed that interoceptive accuracy decreased as age increased. This pattern could reflect reduced sensitivity of central nervous system (and, more precisely, bodily receptors) due to aging, or a higher incidence of cardiac impairments in elder than younger subjects (Khalsa, Rudrauf, & Tranel, 2009). Additional insights come from pathological aging models. For instance, patients with MCI—a subtle form of non-demential cognitive impairment intermediate between healthy age-related decline and AD (Teipel & Grothe, 2015)—can present atrophy and reduced intrinsic and extrinsic connectivity of the insula, a key interoceptive hub (Xie et al., 2012). While such evidence remains indirect, specific links between interoceptive deficits and brain deterioration can be found in AD research.

AD, the most prevalent age-related neurodegenerative disease worldwide, involves progressive cognitive, behavioral, and functional abnormalities (Dubois et al., 2014). While such deficits are mainly related with temporo-posterior network damage (Buckner et al., 2009), recent studies indicate that key interoceptive areas (insula, ACC) and related functional networks could be affected in AD (Moon et al., 2014). Moreover, AD patients exhibit delayed modulations of the vagal evoked potential (VSEP), triggered by stimulation of the vagal pathway (Polak et al., 2014). Importantly, this same pattern has been reported in MCI (Metzger et al., 2012) and MS (Polak et al., 2013) but not in other psychiatric conditions (Polak et al., 2014), which underscores the relevance of selective interoceptive mechanisms as potential transdiagnostic markers for neurological diseases. Moreover, AD has been linked with reduced cardiovascular capacity (Jin et al., 2017), which could imply higher susceptibility to strokes and related autonomic disruptions. This suggests that at least some dimensions of cardiac interoception could be systematically affected in AD.

This hypothesis was tested in a multi-group study assessing interoceptive dimensions via behavioral, electrophysiological, neuroanatomical and functional imaging methods (Garcia-Cordero et al., 2016). Similar to IS and bvFTD patients, AD patients showed impaired interoceptive accuracy, as indexed by poor precision in tracking their own heartbeats via fingertaps. However, they differed from the former in showing interoceptive learning deficits (revealed by a negligible enhancement of performance after interoceptive feedback) and awareness (indexed by the association between a self-report questionnaire of the confidence about one's performance and the actual performance). For AD, performance on the latter two dimensions was associated with the structural integrity of temporal and fronto-temporal areas, respectively, and both were functionally related to fronto-temporal hubs (see Figure 10.3). Additionally, interoceptive awareness was associated to cingulate, prefrontal, and fronto-temporal cortices involved in self-awareness and error monitoring processes (Shany-Ur et al., 2014). These results reinforce role of fronto-temporo-insular networks across interoceptive dimensions.

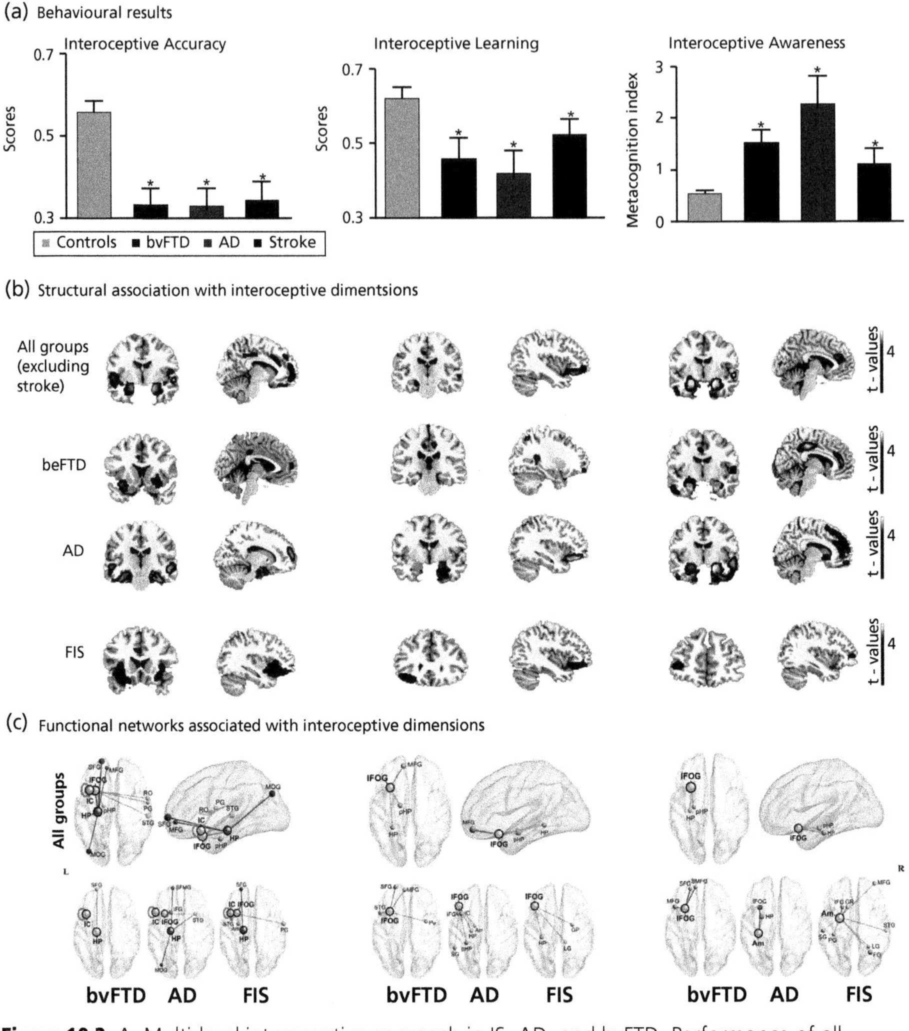

Figure 10.3 A. Multi-level interoceptive approach in IS, AD, and bvFTD. Performance of all four groups in each interoceptive dimension. Interoceptive (accuracy and learning) scores vary between 0 and 1, with higher scores indicating better performance. For awareness, scores nearer zero mean better metacognition. (b) Structural association with interoceptive dimensions. Accuracy was positively associated with the volume of temporal, hippocampus, and frontal regions. Interoceptive learning was associated with the temporal pole and the para-hippocampal together with the inferior frontal gyrus, superior and middle temporal gyrus; and the regions associated with awareness included the para-hippocampus, temporal pole, inferior-frontal gyrus, pre-frontal cortex, supplementary motor area, ACC, and inferior temporal gyrus. (c) Functional networks associated with interoceptive dimensions shows insular cortex, inferior and superior frontal gyri, temporal pole and middle occipital gyrus, were associated to interoceptive accuracy; inferior-frontal gyrus, hippocampus, amygdala, para-hippocampus, insular cortex and supramarginal gyrus with interoceptive learning; and hippocampus, amygdala, and IFG for interoceptive awareness).

In sum, critical regions subserving specific interoceptive dimensions can become compromised in AD. Moreover, imaging findings from MCI suggest that these disruptions might appear even in pre-demented stages of cognitive decline, although direct testing of interoception in such a condition is still wanting.

10.2.3 Behavioral variant fronto-temporal dementia

BvFTD, the second most prevalent type of dementia after AD, is associated with changes in personality, behavior, executive functions (Ibanez & Manes, 2012), and social cognition (Báez et al., 2016a, 2016b). Though predominantly frontal, early neurodegeneration in this condition also affects core interoceptive hubs (in particular, the ventral and dorsal anterior insula), disrupting their dynamic interactions with medial cingulo-frontal, frontopolar, orbitofrontal, striatal, and other subcortical sites (Seeley, 2010). Predictably, such patterns involve abnormalities in some interoceptive dimensions, such as accuracy and awareness (Garcia-Cordero et al., 2016).

In the above-cited study by García-Cordero, Sedeno, de la Fuente, and colleagues (Garcia-Cordero et al., 2016), bvFTD patients showed impairments of interoceptive accuracy and awareness (with higher interoceptive learning but poor interoceptive accuracy, as compared to controls). Structurally, accuracy deficits positively correlated with the volume of the insula and the medial cingulate cortex, whereas awareness results were associated with the medial cingulate cortex, the para-hippocampus, the amygdala, and temporal and parietal regions. Functionally, accuracy results were positively associated with connectivity within the insular cortex, the superior frontal gyrus, and the hypothalamus, while awareness positively correlated with connectivity within the inferior, middle, and superior frontal gyri. Fronto-temporo-insular areas, considered key nodes of metacognition, could be responsible for the construction of subjective feeling states and their disruption could explain the impairments in patients' awareness (see Figure 10.3).

Compatibly, indirect evidence further suggests that daily behavioral alterations in bvFTD may be related to interoceptive deficits. For example, neuroimaging evidence suggests that binge-eating tendencies and altered satiety awareness in this condition are associated with atrophy in a network linking the right insula with other subcortical targets of neurodegeneration (Woolley et al., 2007). This finding aligns with previous results to suggest that altered processing of visceral signals (such as those coming from the heart or the stomach) could lie at the core of the patients' daily behavioral abnormalities.

10.2.4 Multiple sclerosis

MS is a neurodegenerative condition affecting young (mainly female) adults (Ron, 2016). Its varied symptomatology includes deficits in smell, taste, and temperature perception, alongside pain and fatigue symptoms. Considering that these impairments are related to abnormal body-signal processing, a recent proposal suggests that they may all be related to core interoceptive dysfunctions (Salamone et al., accepted). To test this hypothesis, Salamone and colleagues conducted the first assessment of cardiac interoception in two neuroscientific studies.

First, they showed that, relative to controls, MS patients did not show the expected HEP modulations during the interoceptive condition of an HBD task, accompanied by significant atrophy in the bilateral insula and the left ACC. While task-related HEP results in controls were associated with these key interoceptive areas, in patients they only correlated with the somatosensory cortex. The second study relied on fMRI to examine functional connectivity during two resting-state conditions: mind-wandering (thinking about nothing in particular) and interoception (directing attention to one's own heartbeats or respiration). Results showed that the patients' interoceptive network, unlike that of controls, was not differentially engaged by the above states (see Figure 10.4). Taken together, these findings suggest that multidimensional disruptions of interoceptive mechanisms may be hallmark of abnormal body-signal processing in MS.

10.2.5 **Parkinson's disease**

PD is a neurodegenerative disorder mainly characterized by movement abnormalities. However, cognitive and autonomic symptoms can actually precede motor dysfunction (Hanağası, Bilgiç, & Emre, 2016). While this condition is typically linked with cortico-striatal degeneration, atrophy can also compromise interoceptive hubs, such as the insula (Christopher et al., 2014).

In fact, insular disruptions in PD can impair the integration of interoceptive, cognitive, and affective processes, eventually altering subjective states (Christopher et al., 2014). Compatibly, meta-analytical evidence (Criaud et al., 2016) points to the bilateral insula as a convergence hub cutting across multiple symptoms, including disturbances of bodily awareness and autonomic function, sensorimotor systems, and cognitive, affective, and behavioral domains. Whereas such convergences were maximal in dorsal posterior insular regions for unmedicated patients, they mainly involved anterior portions in medicated patients. Insular disruptions, then, seem to lie at the core of viscerosensory or somatosensory processes in PD (Criaud et al., 2016).

More particularly, direct assessment of cardiac interoception via an HBD task revealed significant deficits in PD patients (Ricciardi et al., 2016b). Of note, such dysfunctions emerged irrespective of the severity of motor and non-motor (including affective) symptoms, highlighting their sensitivity as potential early biomarkers of PD. These findings open new opportunities for translational research fine-grained interoceptive dimensions in this condition.

10.2.6 **Functional motor disorders**

Within the broad spectrum of movement diseases, FMDs are characterized by neurological symptoms like motor weakness, epileptic-type attacks, and sensory disturbances, although body-part function is preserved beyond clinical assessment. In a behavioral study, Ricciardi, Demartini, Crucianelli, and colleagues (Ricciardi et al., 2016a) compared FMD patients with a control sample in interoceptive accuracy via an HBD task. FMD patients had poorer interoceptive accuracy, and this pattern was predictive of their depressive symptoms as well as their tendency to focus on the external features of their

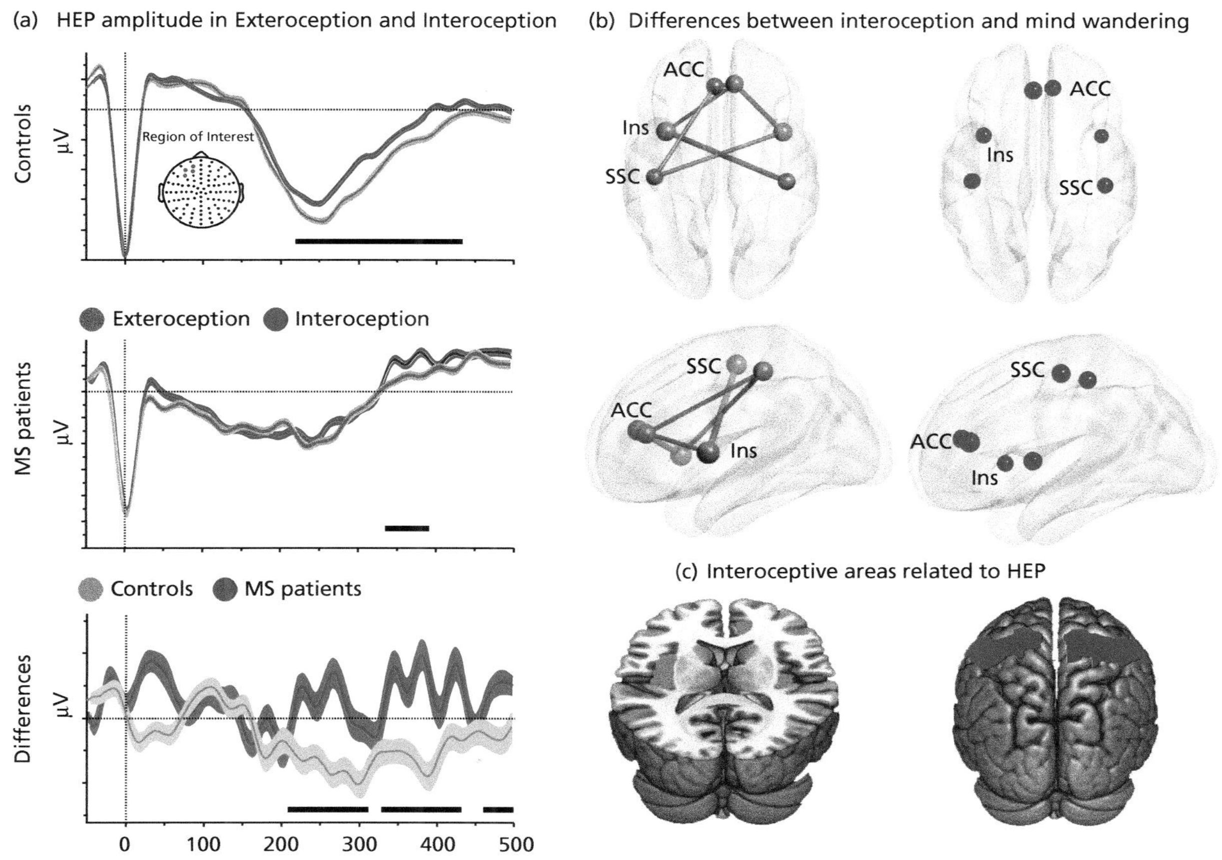

Figure 10.4 Electrophysiological (HEP) and neuroimaging (MRI and functional connectivity) correlates of interoception in MS. (a) No HEP modulation in MS shows neurodegenerative effect in cortical signals. Red lines indicate interoceptive condition and black ones exteroceptive condition. Horizontal shadows lines show statistically significant differences (at $p < .05$ for a minimum extension of five consecutive points of difference. (b) No functional association of interoceptive areas in MS reveals interoceptive network impairment. (c) The bilateral insula and the right ACC were significantly associated with HEP subtraction results in the control sample. HEP amplitude is associated with the somatosensory cortex in MS.

body (self-objectification). On the contrary, interoceptive accuracy was not predictive of alexithymia (Watters et al., 2016). Thus, this particular interoceptive dimension is not only compromised following motor dysfunction but it also seems to underlie concomitant psychiatric manifestations. This reinforces the notion that interoceptive mechanisms are intimately linked with affective domains.

10.2.7 **Chronic pain**

CP is a condition in which signals triggered by aversive stimuli and/or damaged tissue persist over time, beyond their normal duration. The varied epidemiology of CP overlaps with musculoskeletal disorders (arthritis, osteoarthritis), oncologic diseases, and neuropathies like MS, PD, and AD (Di Lernia, Serino, & Riva, 2016). Acute pain in this condition seems to engage specific neural areas (e.g. somatosensory cortex, insula, and mid-cingulate cortex) and networks (e.g. the default mode, the salience, the sensorimotor, and the fronto-parietal networks (Farmer, Baliki, & Apkarian, 2012)).

Classical descriptions of pain (Craig, 2003) mechanisms highlight the role of vagal and somatosensory pathways subserving interoceptive processing (Khalsa et al., 2009a). Moreover, the interoceptive network (comprising the insular cortex, the ACC, and the somatosensory cortex) (Critchley et al., 2004) is associated with subjective anticipation, perception, and generation of pain. Indeed, such circuitry exhibits distinct activity patterns in subjects with CP (Kupers, Gybels, & Gjedde, 2000).

A systematic review (Di Lernia et al., 2016) shows that different interoceptive dimensions (accuracy, metacognition, and awareness) have been experimentally evaluated in various pathologies involving CP. Patients with fibromyalgia exhibit reduced interoceptive accuracy and an inverse association with symptom severity (Duschek, Montoro, & Reyes del Paso, 2016), as well as normal performance in interoceptive metacognition (Borg et al., 2015). Reduced interoceptive accuracy has also been reported in somatoform disorders, together with an association between pain sensitivity and pain symptoms (Pollatos et al., 2011). Deficits in interoceptive accuracy, with poor interoceptive awareness and high attention to bodily symptoms, have also been reported in patients with chronic low back pain (Mehling et al., 2013). The former domain is also affected in patients with migraine and temporomandibular pain disorder (for details see Di Lernia et al., 2016). In sum, the systematicity of interoceptive deficits (especially in the accuracy dimension) across such varied conditions highlights their relevance as a potential transdiagnostic marker for the field of neurology.

10.3 **Discussion**

As seen by the previous discussion, several neurocognitive mechanisms underlying interoceptive skills are dimensionally and transdiagnostically affected in neurological disorders. Building on these findings, we now discuss (a) the relevance of neurological lesion models to study interoception, (b) the relationship between this domain and socio-emotional processes, (c) the specific roles of different interoceptive pathways across disorders, and (d) the future of cardiac interoception research in health and neuroscience.

10.3.1 Neurological disorders as key models to characterize interoceptive mechanisms

As reviewed earlier, interoceptive processes rely on neurocognitive mechanisms that are affected in numerous neurological disorders. This growing empirical corpus informs interoceptive research by providing critical lesion models, revealing fine-grained links between interoceptive disruptions and other disease symptoms, and yielding insights on plastic mechanisms which could prove relevant for recovery in specific disorders (e.g. IS).

First, the relatively specific patterns of brain damage of each condition shed light on the neurocognitive organization of interoceptive mechanisms. For example, fronto-cingulo-insular lesions following frontal IS seem to compromise interoceptive accuracy without affecting interoceptive awareness and learning, which highlights the relative dissociation between all three dimensions and the dependence of the latter two on posterior regions (Garcia-Cordero et al., 2016). Also, evidence from focal strokes suggests that while interoception would be mainly subserved by the right insula, such a region would not be so critical for sensing body-external stimuli (Couto et al., 2015). Furthermore, evidence from MS indicates that interoceptive deficits can become manifest upon atrophy of the insula and the ACC even if the somatosensory cortex is preserved, which highlights the secondary role of the latter structure (Salamone et al., accepted). Additional clinical evidence shows that a wide network linking the insula with frontal and temporal structures integrates interoceptive functions with emotional and social cognition processes (Adolfi et al., 2016). As exemplified by these findings, neurological lesion models offer crucial data to understand the neurocognitive basis of interoception.

Indeed, such models can complement the insights yielded by research on psychiatric disorders. For example, interoceptive accuracy reveals variable patterns across psychiatric diseases (e.g. it is enhanced in obsessive–compulsive and panic disorders but disturbed in depression, depersonalization, bipolar disorder, borderline personality disorder, and anorexia) (Dunn et al., 2007; Khalsa et al., 2015; Muller et al., 2015; Sedeno et al., 2014; Yoris et al., 2015; Yoris et al., 2017). However, this dimension is consistently impaired in neurological conditions, thus emerging as a potentially robust and more predictable transdiagnostic marker. Also, whereas interoceptive awareness or metacognitive estimations of cardiac interoception appear to be impaired in highly disabling psychiatric disorders but not in subclinical cases of anxiety or social phobia (Yoris et al., 2015), this domain seems compromised in early stages of neurological conditions, such as AD, bvFTD (Garcia-Cordero et al., 2016), and CP (Di Lernia et al., 2016). Thus, this dimension may prove particularly relevant for early (and, ideally, preclinical) characterization of neurological, as opposed to psychiatric, disorders. Moreover, specific dissociations across neurological conditions underscore the usefulness of teasing apart interoceptive skills into identifiable dimensions. Indeed, interoceptive learning seems specifically related to the physiopathology of AD, given that neither focal nor neurodegenerative damage to fronto-insular damage seems to disrupt it (Garcia-Cordero et al., 2016) (see findings summarized in Figure 10.5).

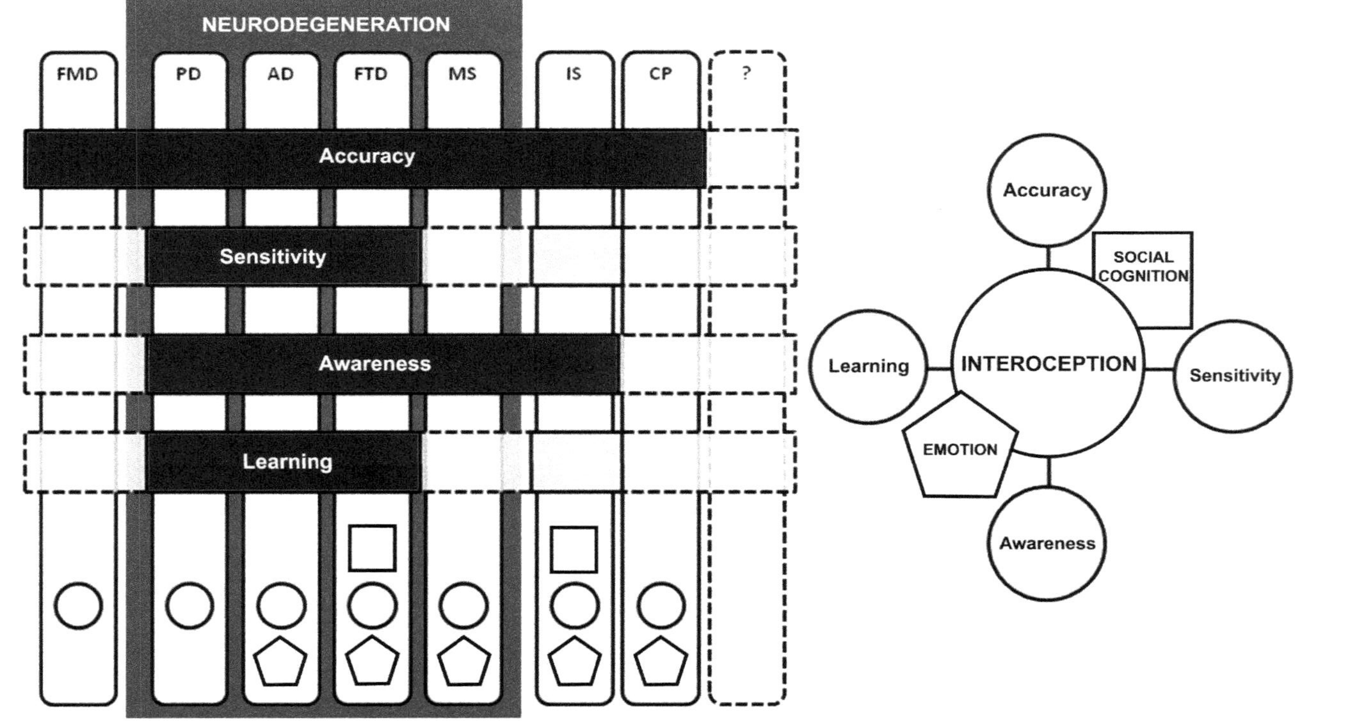

Figure 10.5 Representative schema of main results: interoceptive dimensions, emotion and social cognition across neurologic diseases. Left: Columns represent categorical diagnostics in neurology where the interoception was studied. Pointed lines represent categories not yet explored. Rows show principal interoceptive dimensions explored. Black areas indicate disorders where those dimensions were explored, whereas white pointed lines areas those unexplored. Neurodegenerative disorders are emplaced over a shadow block. **Above:** Boxes represent social cognition. Circles represent interoception. Pentagons represent emotion. **Right:** Diagram that represents the relationship of interoception (and its different dimensions) with the domains of emotion and social cognition.

In addition, these models can reveal links between high and low levels of interoceptive dimensions and differential symptomatology. In particular, systematic cognitive dysfunctions may be more readily identifiable in specific neurological conditions than in psychiatric disorders. Thus, the detection of distinctive interoceptive deficits in the former may illuminate the interaction between viscerosensory and exteroceptive processing beyond the contributions of more diffuse conditions. Indeed, disruptions of interoceptive learning and awareness have been linked to specific metacognitive and memory deficits in neurodegenerative diseases (Garcia-Cordero et al., 2016).

Finally, neurological disorders may reveal subtle plastic mechanisms acting on interoceptive networks post-morbidly. For example, cognitive decline has been linked to insular atrophy in MCI (Xie et al., 2012), whereas memory and interoceptive learning deficits seem to rely on extended insulo-temporal damage in AD (Garcia-Cordero et al., 2016). This perspective opens new opportunities to explore both the role of interoceptive areas in overall cognitive performance across disorder types. Indeed, in PD, insular damage increases as the disease progresses, which could partially explain the development of several non-motor symptoms (Christopher et al., 2014).

Neurological disorders also allow us to explore the recruitment of alternative circuits for possible functional compensation. For example, while HEP modulations during cardiac interoception are associated with the main interoceptive hubs (the insula and the ACC) in controls, in MS patients they only correlated with a complementary interoceptive area (the somatosensory cortex) (Salamone et al., accepted). Useful insights could also be gained by assessing plastic changes in stroke patients. Speculatively, interoceptive dimensions which are specifically affected by focal fronto-insular lesions could eventually become (optimally or suboptimally) subserved by perilesional or homologous contralateral structures. Beyond neurological conditions, hitherto unexplored forms of plasticity involving interoceptive mechanisms could be revealed by studying patients who undergo heart transplants. Indeed, ongoing work by our team seeks to examine the timing and effectiveness of the vagal re-innervation and its impact on interoceptive and related domains (e.g. emotion processing) by comparing relevant behavioral and neurocognitive markers before and after surgery. These possibilities pave the way for a promising agenda in the field of interoception.

10.3.2 Interactions between interoceptive dimensions and socio-emotional processes

Visceral-interoceptive signals seem to interact with emotional and socio-cognitive mechanisms (Adolfi et al., 2016). Such an interaction likely reflects the neural overlap between both domains in the anterior insular cortex and the ACC (Adolfi et al., 2016), but it also seems to involve more extended neural networks. Indeed, several neurological conditions leading to interoceptive deficits (see section 10.2) are also linked with impaired emotional processing. In AD, for example, facial emotion recognition (particularly in the domain of negative emotions) is disturbed in line with the progression of dementia. Similar deficits have also been reported in IS, MCI, bvFTD, and MS, as well as in other conditions in which interoception has not been studied so far, like Huntington's disease (for a review see Ibanez et al., 2016b).

Similarly, several disorders linked with interoceptive abnormalities are known to affect social cognition skills (Adolfi et al., 2016), including empathy, theory of mind (ToM), moral judgment, among others (Adolphs, 1999). For example, pervasive ToM deficits have been documented in PD. This domain is also compromised in bvFTD and related neurodegenerative conditions, which also impairs empathy processes, moral judgment, and social emotions (Báez et al., 2014; Báez et al., 2016a; Báez et al., 2016b; Báez et al., 2017; Báez et al., 2016c; Ibanez et al., 2016a; Melloni et al., 2016; Melloni, Lopez, & Ibanez, 2013; Sedeno et al., 2016).

While the above associations are indirect, meta-analytic evidence from more than 4,500 neuroimaging studies revealed a robust overlap among regions supporting interoceptive, emotional, and social cognition processes (Adolfi et al., 2016). Convergences between the three domains were maximal in the right anterior insula, a core interoceptive hub. However, ignificant overlaps were also found in the left anterior insula, the right ACC, and the right temporal pole. Thus, although most research on interoception in neurological disorders has not empirically examined linked with socio-emotional mechanisms (but see Figure 10.6 and Adolfi et al., 2016), this evidence strongly suggests that all three domains may be rooted in partially shared fronto-insulo-temporal networks whose hubs are affected by multiple brain diseases.

Future studies should explore these relationships via multilevel designs tapping different interoceptive dimensions. In particular, the available evidence invites new questions on as yet unexamined issues, including the potential role of cardiac interoception or vagal stimulation as facilitators or inhibitors of emotion recognition, or the relationship between interoceptive performance and emotional regulation. Research along these lines could broaden our current understanding of interoception and the overarching impact of its disruption in neurological conditions.

10.3.3 Ascertaining the roles of different interoceptive pathways

Beyond the evidence afforded by lesion models (Khalsa et al., 2009a), little is known about how different interoceptive pathways are affected by pharmacological interventions and cardiovascular impairments. This limitation could be overcome by replicating extant designs in neurological samples. For example, enhancements of the somatosensory pathway via bolus isoproterenol infusion (Khalsa et al., 2009b) could reveal which interoceptive dimensions (accuracy, awareness, and learning) are more critically dependent on secondary interoceptive regions. Likewise, evidence that peripheral cardiac dysfunction in hypertensive subjects impairs neurocognitive interoceptive mechanisms (Yoris et al., 2018) suggests that the vagal signalling may play a causal role in the neural dynamics on this domain. Thus, vagal stimulation, a therapeutic intervention in CP (Goadsby et al., 2014) and other conditions, could constitute a promising option for experimental research and clinical interventions in neurological disorders.

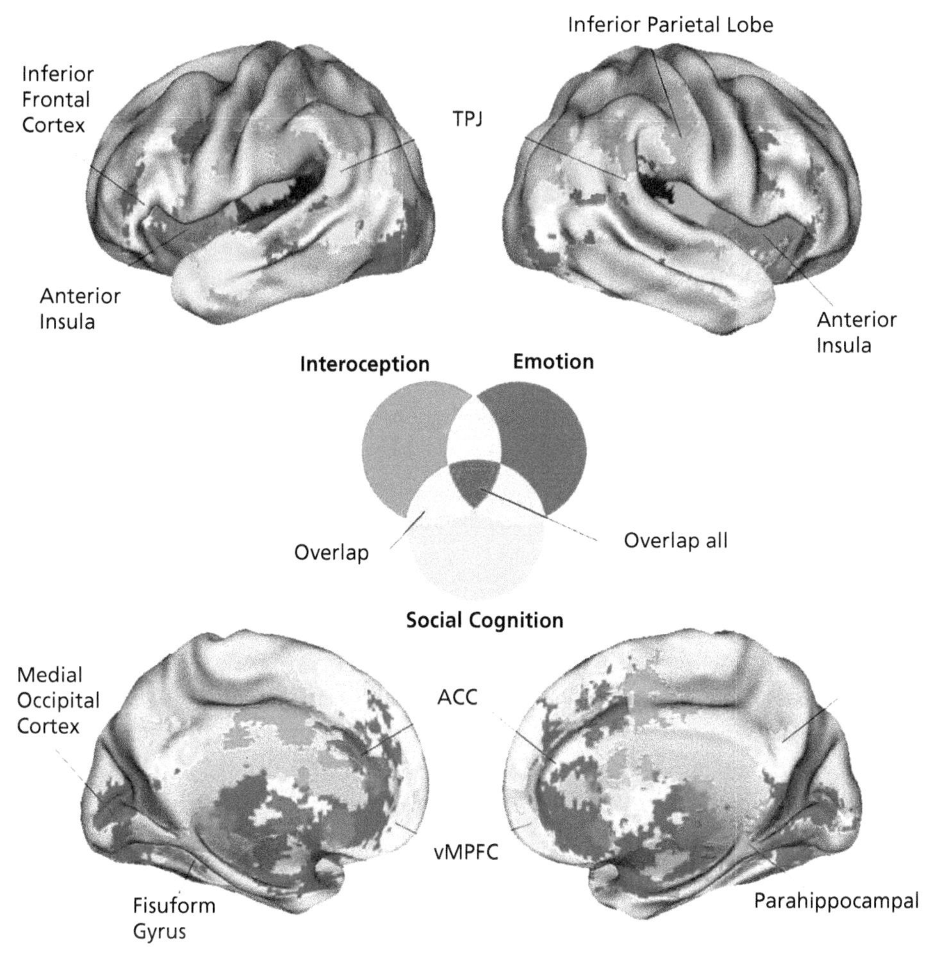

Figure 10.6 Meta-analytic evidence (fMRI) of convergence across interoception, emotion, and social cognition. Meta-analyses of cortical overlap (red). Significantly activated (meeting height- or extent-based threshold at $p < 0.05$, FWE corrected) clusters from studies of interoception (sky blue), emotion recognition, perception (violet), and social cognition (green). A conjunction analysis performed revealed common activations throughout an insular-frontotemporal network: the right anterior insula, the ACC, the bilateral para-hippocampal gyrus, the hippocampus, the right amygdala, the inferior frontal gyrus, and the right globus pallidus ($p < .001$, FWE corrected)).

10.3.4 The future of cardiac interoception research in health and neuroscience

The considerations covered could improve clinical assessment and the description and prognosis of signs and symptoms across multiple brain diseases. In particular, dimensional approaches like the Research Domain Criteria offer new opportunities to integrate clinical knowledge with genes, tissues, anatomy and physiology, electrophysiology, observable behavior, measurable laboratory behavior, and self-report data. Under this framework, the study of interoception can be segmented into multiple levels of analysis (from accuracy to awareness; Garfinkel et al., 2015), so that common and specific dimensional symptoms can be identified within the broad spectrum of neurological diseases. Likewise, this approach would permit connecting contributions from research on language, memory, decision-making, learning, and embodied cognition, while revealing cross-domain interactions between the brain, the heart, and the rest of the organism.

The evidence reviewed above suggests that alterations in interoceptive accuracy might emerge as either primary or secondary deficits, depending on the condition. The initial atrophy pattern of bvFTD affects putative interoceptive hubs, such as the insular cortex and the ACC, among other frontal structures (Seeley, 2010). Moreover, these areas are comprised by the salience network, a resting-state network which is also affected in this disease (Ibanez & Manes, 2012). Although further research is needed, interoceptive alterations in bvFTD patients might constitute primary deficits. Be that as it may, little is known about the relation between such impairments and socio-emotional deficits typical of bvFTD, which are also related to fronto-insular disruptions (Van den Stock & Kumfor, 2017). Interoceptive deficits may also prove primary in PD, given the evidence highlighting the critical role of the insula across many of its symptoms (e.g. disturbances of bodily awareness and autonomic functions, sensorimotor systems) (Christopher et al., 2014).

Alterations of interoceptive accuracy in the broad spectrum of CP conditions might be related to the overlap between interoceptive hubs and the activation of the pain matrix network (e.g. somatosensory cortex, insula, and mid-cingulate cortex). However, given the lack of a clear and systematic cortical damage across forms of CP, it remains unclear whether the deficits in question represent primary or secondary symptoms. Although the scenario is also heterogeneous for MS, some studies have reported cortical alterations in the insula and the ACC in this pathology. Also, MS patients present deficits related to the sensing of physiological body signals (e.g. olfaction, taste, temperature, fatigue) that have recently been proposed as related to core interoceptive dysfunctions (Salamone et al., accepted). However, further research is needed to determine the nature of interoceptive impairments in such a disorder.

The situation seems to be different in the case of AD. Although interoceptive accuracy deficits have been reported in this disease (Garcia-Cordero et al., 2016), its atrophy pattern involves temporo-parietal regions (Du et al., 2007). As such damage is consistently associated with impairments in memory mechanisms, it has been suggested that interoceptive deficits are secondary in AD given that they may be epiphenomenal to memory deficits (Garcia-Cordero et al., 2016).

Relative to awareness or learning, it is difficult to determinate whether they are primary or secondary affectations in these conditions. First, most studies focused merely on accuracy. This is the case of learning that has only been explored one work in neurological diseases (Garcia-Cordero et al., 2016). It has been suggested that in AD this dimension might be considered as a manifestation of its impairment in more basic memory mechanisms (Garcia-Cordero et al., 2016). However, further research in this and other conditions is needed to disentangle the relation between interoceptive learning and other memory dimensions. Second, dimensions such as interoceptive sensibility and awareness are suggested to depend on widespread anatomical networks and not on core interoceptive areas, as shown by the preservation of interoceptive awareness in fronto-insular strokes (Garcia-Cordero et al., 2016). In this way, their disruption might be secondary to the alteration of extended brain damage instead of being circumscribed to specific hubs (Garcia-Cordero et al., 2016).

Be that as it may, future efforts in this line of research should strive to integrate cognitive, autonomic, behavioral, neuroimaging, and electrophysiological data via designs which combine measures of interoception, emotion, and social cognition. This prospective agenda should particularly emphasize (a) the systematic operationalization of specific dimensions, (b) the development of more sensitive and specific measurements to such an end, (c) the search for common and differential disturbances across conditions, and (d) the conduction of longitudinal studies to measure relevant plastic changes and associated behavioral adaptations. Thereupon, possible lines of innovation might be forged, including the development of new pharmacologic therapies that reduce the negative impact on other areas of health; prevention programmes focusing on nutrition, physical activity, and stress reduction; and activities of high impact on health, such as meditation and interventions based on well-being, among others. In sum, the interoception framework may pave the way for fruitful breakthroughs towards the consolidation of a dimensional and transdiagnostic approach for neurological research.

10.4 Conclusion

The study of interoceptive domains in neurology offers new possibilities for experimental research and clinical interventions in cognitive neuroscience. Here we showed that neurological disorders present deficits in diverse interoceptive domains, evidencing a disrupted interplay between neurocognitive and autonomic processes. These findings highlight the potential of dimensional and transdiagnostic approaches to better characterize the manifold manifestations of cerebral damage. New experimental studies could afford important breakthroughs in this direction, and eventually inspire new forms of testing and intervention in clinical settings.

Acknowledgments

This work has been partially supported by the CONICET, the INECO foundation and projects of CONICYT/FONDECYT Regular (1170010); FONCyT-PICT (2012-0412 and 2012-1309), and FONDAP (15150012).

References

Adolfi, F., Couto, B., Richter, F., Decety, J., Lopez, J., Sigman, M., et al. (2016). Convergence of interoception, emotion, and social cognition: A twofold fMRI meta-analysis and lesion approach. *Cortex*, *88*, 124–42. doi:10.1016/j.cortex.2016.12.019.

Adolphs, R. (1999). Social cognition and the human brain. *Trends in Cognitive Sciences, 3*(12), 469–79. doi:S1364-6613(99)01399-6 [pii].

Báez, S., Couto, B., Torralva, T., Sposato, L. A., Huepe, D., Montañes, P., et al. (2014). Comparing moral judgments of patients with frontotemporal dementia and frontal stroke. *JAMA Neurology*, doi:10.1001/jamaneurol.2014.347.

Báez, S., Kanske, P., Matallana, D., Montanes, P., Reyes, P., Slachevsky, A., et al. (2016a). Integration of intention and outcome for moral judgment in frontotemporal dementia: Brain structural signatures. *Neurodegenerative Diseases, 16*(3–4), 206–17.

Báez, S., Morales, J. P., Slachevsky, A., Torralva, T., Matus, C., Manes, F., et al. (2016b). Orbitofrontal and limbic signatures of empathic concern and intentional harm in the behavioral variant frontotemporal dementia. *Cortex, 75*, 20–32. doi:10.1016/j.cortex.2015.11.007.

Báez, S., Santamaría-García, H., Orozco, J., Fittipaldi, S., García, A., Pino, M., et al. (2016c). Your misery is no longer my pleasure: Reduced *Schadenfreude* in Huntington's disease families. *Cortex*. <http://dx.doi.org/10.1016/j.cortex.2016.07.009>

Báez, S., Pino, M., Berrío, M., Santamaría-García, H., Sedeño, L., García, A., et al. (2017). Corticostriatal signatures of *Schadenfreude*: Evidence from Huntington's disease. *Journal of Neurology, Neurosurgery & Psychiatry*, **1**, *89*(1), 112–16.

Borg, C., Emond, F. C., Colson, D., Laurent, B., and **Michael, G. A.** (2015). Attentional focus on subjective interoceptive experience in patients with fibromyalgia. *Brain and Cognition, 101*, 35–43.

Buckner, R. L., Sepulcre, J., Talukdar, T., Krienen, F. M., Liu, H., Hedden, T., et al. (2009). Cortical hubs revealed by intrinsic functional connectivity: Mapping, assessment of stability, and relation to Alzheimer's disease. *Journal of Neuroscience, 29*(6), 1860–73.

Couto, B., Adolfi, F., Sedeno, L., Salles, A., Canales-Johnson, A., Alvarez-Abut, P., et al. (2015). Disentangling interoception: Insights from focal strokes affecting the perception of external and internal milieus. *Frontiers in Psychology, 6*, 503. doi:10.3389/fpsyg.2015.00503.

Craig, A. D. (2003). Pain mechanisms: Labeled lines versus convergence in central processing. *Annual Reviews in Neuroscience, 26*, 1–30. doi:10.1146/annurev.neuro.26.041002.131022.

Craig, A. D. (2009). How do you feel—now? The anterior insula and human awareness. (Research Support, Non-U.S. Gov't). *Nature Reviews Neuroscience, 10*(1), 59–70. doi:10.1038/nrn2555.

Criaud, M., Christopher, L., Boulinguez, P., Ballanger, B., Lang, A. E., Cho, S. S., et al. (2016). Contribution of insula in Parkinson's disease: A quantitative meta-analysis study. *Human Brain Mapping*, April 1, *37*(4), 1375–92.

Critchley, H. D., Wiens, S., Rotshtein, P., Ohman, A., and **Dolan, R. J.** (2004). Neural systems supporting interoceptive awareness. (Research Support, Non-U.S. Gov't). *Nature Neurosciences, 7*(2), 189–95. doi:10.1038/nn1176.

Christopher, L., Koshimori, Y., Lang, A. E., Criaud, M., and **Strafella, A. P.** (2014). Uncovering the role of the insula in non-motor symptoms of Parkinson's disease. *Brain, 137*(8), 2143–54.

Di Lernia, D., Serino, S., and **Riva, G.** (2016). Pain in the body. Altered interoception in chronic pain conditions: A systematic review. *Neuroscience and Biobehavioral Reviews, 71*, 328–41.

Du, A.-T., Schuff, N., Kramer, J. H., Rosen, H. J., Gorno-Tempini, M. L., Rankin, K., et al. (2007). Different regional patterns of cortical thinning in Alzheimer's disease and frontotemporal dementia. *Brain, 130*(4), 1159–66.

Dubois, B., Feldman, H. H., Jacova, C., Hampel, H., Molinuevo, J. L., Blennow, K., et al. (2014). Advancing research diagnostic criteria for Alzheimer's disease: The IWG-2 criteria. *Lancet Neurology, 13*(6), 614–29.

Dunn, B. D., Dalgleish, T., Ogilvie, A. D., and **Lawrence, A. D.** (2007). Heartbeat perception in depression. (Research Support, Non-U.S. Gov't). *Behavioral Research Therapy, 45*(8), 1921–30. doi:10.1016/j.brat.2006.09.008.

Duschek, S., **Montoro, C. I.**, and **Reyes del Paso, G. A.** (2016). Diminished interoceptive awareness in fibromyalgia syndrome. *Behavioral Medicine*, 1–8. *17*(S), 723.

Farmer, M. A., **Baliki, M. N.**, and **Apkarian, A. V.** (2012). A dynamic network perspective of chronic pain. *Neuroscience Letters*, *520*(2), 197–203.

Garcia-Cordero, I., **Sedeno, L.**, **de la Fuente, L.**, **Slachevsky, A.**, **Forno, G.**, **Klein, F.**, et al. (2016). Feeling, learning from and being aware of inner states: Interoceptive dimensions in neurodegeneration and stroke. *Philosophical Transactions of the Royal Society of London B*, *371*(1708). doi:10.1098/rstb.2016.0006.

Garfinkel, S. N., **Seth, A. K.**, **Barrett, A. B.**, **Suzuki, K.**, and **Critchley, H. D.** (2015). Knowing your own heart: Distinguishing interoceptive accuracy from interoceptive awareness. (Research Support, Non-U.S. Gov't). *Biological Psychology*, *104*, 65–74. doi:10.1016/j.biopsycho.2014.11.004.

Goadsby, P., **Grosberg, B.**, **Mauskop, A.**, **Cady, R.**, and **Simmons, K.** (2014). Effect of noninvasive vagus nerve stimulation on acute migraine: An open-label pilot study. *Cephalalgia*, *34*(12), 986–93.

Hanağası, H. A., **Bilgiç, B.**, and **Emre, M.** (2016). Dementia with Lewy bodies and Parkinson's disease dementia. In: M. Husain and J. M. Schott (eds), *Oxford Textbook of Cognitive Neurology and Dementia*. Oxford: Oxford University Press, pp. 399–412.

Ibanez, A., **Gleichgerrcht, E.**, and **Manes, F.** (2010). Clinical effects of insular damage in humans. (Review). *Brain Structure and Function*, *214*(5-6), 397–410. doi:10.1007/s00429-010-0256-y.

Ibanez, A. and **Manes, F.** (2012). Contextual social cognition and the behavioral variant of frontotemporal dementia. *Neurology*, *78*(17), 1354–62. doi:10.1212/WNL.0b013e3182518375.

Ibanez, A., **Kuljis, R. O.**, **Matallana, D.**, and **Manes, F.** (2014). Bridging psychiatry and neurology through social neuroscience. *World Psychiatry*, *13*(2), 148–9. doi: 10.1002/wps.20125

Ibanez, A., **Billeke, P.**, **de la Fuente, L.**, **Salamone, P.**, **Garcia, A. M.**, and **Melloni, M.** (2016a). Reply: Towards a neurocomputational account of social dysfunction in neurodegenerative disease. *Brain*, doi:10.1093/brain/aww316.

Ibanez, A., **Garcia, A. M.**, **Esteves, S.**, **Yoris, A.**, **Munoz, E.**, **Reynaldo, L.**, et al. (2016b). Social neuroscience: Undoing the schism between neurology and psychiatry. *Society Neuroscience*, doi:10.1080/17470919.2016.1245214.

Insel, T., **Cuthbert, B.**, **Garvey, M.**, **Heinssen, R.**, **Pine, D. S.**, **Quinn, K.**, et al. (2010). Research domain criteria (RDoC): Toward a new classification framework for research on mental disorders: American Psychiatric Association. *American Journal of Psychiatry*, *167*(7), 748–51.

Jin, W., **Bu, X.**, **Wang, Y.**, **Li, L.**, **Li, W.**, **Liu, Y.**, et al. (2017). Reduced Cardiovascular Functions in Patients with Alzheimer's Disease. *Journal of Alzheimer's Disease*, *58*(3), 919–25.

Khalsa, S. S., **Rudrauf, D.**, **Feinstein, J. S.**, and **Tranel, D.** (2009a). The pathways of interoceptive awareness. (Research Support, N.I.H., Extramural). *Nature Neuroscience*, *12*(12), 1494–6. doi:10.1038/nn.2411.

Khalsa, S. S., **Rudrauf, D.**, **Sandesara, C.**, **Olshansky, B.**, and **Tranel, D.** (2009b). Bolus isoproterenol infusions provide a reliable method for assessing interoceptive awareness. (Randomized Controlled Trial Khalsa, S. S., Craske, M. G., Li, W., Vangala, S., Strober, M., and Feusner, J. D. (2015). Altered interoceptive awareness in anorexia nervosa: Effects of meal anticipation, consumption and bodily arousal. (Research Support, N.I.H., Extramural). *International Journal of Eating Disorders*, *48*(7), 889–97. doi:10.1002/eat.22387.

Khalsa, S. S. and **Lapidus, R. C.** (2016). Can interoception improve the pragmatic search for biomarkers in psychiatry? [Review]. *Frontiers in Psychiatry*, *7*, 121. doi:10.3389/fpsyt.2016.00121.

Research Support, N.I.H., Extramural). *International Journal of Psychophysiology*, *72*(1), 34–45. doi:10.1016/j.ijpsycho.2008.08.010.

Khalsa, S. S., **Rudrauf, D.**, and **Tranel, D.** (2009). Interoceptive awareness declines with age. (Research Support, N.I.H., Extramural). *Psychophysiology*, *46*(6), 1130–6. doi:10.1111/j.1469-8986.2009.00859.x.

Kling, M. A., Trojanowski, J. Q., Wolk, D. A., Lee, V. M., and **Arnold, S. E.** (2013). Vascular disease and dementias: Paradigm shifts to drive research in new directions. *Alzheimer's & Dementia*, *9*(1), 76–92.

Kupers, R. C., Gybels, J. M., and **Gjedde, A.** (2000). Positron emission tomography study of a chronic pain patient successfully treated with somatosensory thalamic stimulation. *Pain*, *87*(3), 295–302.

Mehling, W. E., Daubenmier, J., Price, C. J., Acree, M., Bartmess, E., and **Stewart, A. L.** (2013). Self-reported interoceptive awareness in primary care patients with past or current low back pain. *Journal of Pain Research*, 6,403, 403–18.

Melloni, M., Lopez, V., and **Ibanez, A.** (2013). Empathy and contextual social cognition. *Cognitive and Affective Behavioral Neuroscience*. doi:10.3758/s13415-013-0205-3.

Melloni, M., Billeke, P., Báez, S., Hesse, E., de la Fuente, L., Forno, G., et al. (2016). Your perspective and my benefit: Multiple lesion models of self-other integration strategies during social bargaining. *Brain*. <http://dx.doi.org/10.1093/brain/aww1231. doi: 10.1093/brain/aww231>

Metzger, F. G., Polak, T., Aghazadeh, Y., Ehlis, A.-C., Hagen, K., and **Fallgatter, A. J.** (2012). Vagus somatosensory evoked potentials: A possibility for diagnostic improvement in patients with mild cognitive impairment? *Dementia and Geriatric Cognitive Disorders*, *33*(5), 289–96.

Moon, Y., Moon, W.-J., Kim, H., and **Han, S.-H.** (2014). Regional atrophy of the insular cortex is associated with neuropsychiatric symptoms in Alzheimer's disease patients. *European Neurology*, *71*(5–6), 223–9.

Muller, L. E., Schulz, A., Andermann, M., Gabel, A., Gescher, D. M., Spohn, A., et al. (2015). Cortical representation of afferent bodily signals in borderline personality disorder: Neural correlates and relationship to emotional dysregulation. (Research Support, Non-U.S. Gov't). *JAMA Psychiatry*, *72*(11), 1077–86. doi:10.1001/jamapsychiatry.2015.1252.

Polak, T., Zeller, D., Fallgatter, A. J., and **Metzger, F. G.** (2013). Vagus somatosensory-evoked potentials are prolonged in patients with multiple sclerosis with brainstem involvement. *Neuroreport*, *24*(5), 251–3.

Polak, T., Dresler, T., Zeller, J. B., Warrings, B., Scheuerpflug, P., Fallgatter, A. J., et al. (2014). Vagus somatosensory evoked potentials are delayed in Alzheimer's disease, but not in major depression. *European Archives of Psychiatry and Clinical Neuroscience*, *264*(3), 263–7.

Pollatos, O., Herbert, B. M., Wankner, S., Dietel, A., Wachsmuth, C., Henningsen, P., et al. (2011). Autonomic imbalance is associated with reduced facial recognition in somatoform disorders. *Journal of Psychosomatic Research*, *71*(4), 232–9.

Ricciardi, L., Demartini, B., Crucianelli, L., Krahé, C., Edwards, M. J., and **Fotopoulou, A.** (2016a). Interoceptive awareness in patients with functional neurological symptoms. *Biological Psychology*, *113*, 68–74.

Ricciardi, L., Ferrazzano, G., Demartini, B., Morgante, F., Erro, R., Ganos, C., et al. (2016b). Know thyself: Exploring interoceptive sensitivity in Parkinson's disease. *Journal of Neurological Sciences*, *364*, 110–15.

Ron, M. A. (2016). Cognition in multiple sclerosis. In: M. Husain and J. M. Schott, (eds), *Oxford Textbook of Cognitive Neurology and Dementia*. Oxford: Oxford University Press, pp. 123–76.

Sacco, R. L., Kasner, S. E., Broderick, J. P., Caplan, L. R., Culebras, A., Elkind, M. S., et al. (2013). An updated definition of stroke for the 21st century. *Stroke*, *44*(7), 2064–89.

Salamone, P., Esteves, S., Sinay, V., Garcia-Cordero, I., Abrevaya, S., Couto, B., et al. (accepted). Altered neural signatures of interoception in multiple sclerosis. *Human Brain Mapping*.

Sedeno, L., Couto, B., Melloni, M., Canales-Johnson, A., Yoris, A., Báez, S., et al. (2014). How do you feel when you can't feel your body? Interoception, functional connectivity and emotional processing in depersonalization-derealization disorder. *PLoS One*, *9*(6), e98769. doi:10.1371/journal.pone.0098769.

Sedeno, L., Couto, B., Garcia-Cordero, I., Melloni, M., Báez, S., Morales Sepulveda, J. P., et al. (2016). Brain network organization and social executive performance in frontotemporal dementia. *Journal of the International Neuropsychology Society*, *22*(2), 250–62. doi:10.1017/S1355617715000703.

Seeley, W. W. (2010). Anterior insula degeneration in frontotemporal dementia. *Brain Structure and Function*, *214*(5-6), 465–75.

Shany-Ur, T., Lin, N., Rosen, H. J., Sollberger, M., Miller, B. L., and **Rankin, K. P.** (2014). Self-awareness in neurodegenerative disease relies on neural structures mediating reward-driven attention. *Brain*, *137*(8), 2368–81.

Teipel, S. J., and **Grothe, M. J.** (2015). The relative importance of imaging markers for the prediction of Alzheimer's disease dementia in mild cognitive impairment: The curse of dimensionality. *Alzheimer's & Dementia*, *11*(7), P10–P11.

Van den Stock, J. and **Kumfor, F.** (2017). Behavioural-variant frontotemporal dementia: At the interface of interoception, emotion and social cognition? *Cortex*. In Press. <https://doi.org/10.1016/j.cortex.2017.08.013>

Watters, C. A., Taylor, G. J., Quilty, L. C., and **Bagby, R. M.** (2016). An examination of the topology and measurement of the alexithymia construct using network analysis. *Journal of Personality Assessment*, *98*(6), 649–59.

Woolley, J. D., Gorno-Tempini, M. L., Seeley, W. W., Rankin, K., Lee, S. S., Matthews, B. R., and **Miller, B. L.** (2007). Binge eating is associated with right orbitofrontal-insular-striatal atrophy in frontotemporal dementia. (Case Reports Research Support, N.I.H., Extramural). *Neurology*, *69*(14), 1424–33. doi:10.1212/01.wnl.0000277461.06713.23.

Xie, C., Bai, F., Yu, H., Shi, Y., Yuan, Y., Chen, G., et al. (2012). Abnormal insula functional network is associated with episodic memory decline in amnestic mild cognitive impairment. *Neuroimage*, *63*(1), 320–7.

Yoris, A., Esteves, S., Couto, B., Melloni, M., Kichic, R., Cetkovich, M., et al. (2015). The roles of interoceptive sensitivity and metacognitive interoception in panic. *Behavioural and Brain Functions*, *11*, 14. doi:10.1186/s12993-015-0058-8.

Yoris, A., García, A., Traiber, L., Santamaría-García, H., Martorell, M., Alifano, F., et al. (2017). The inner world of overactive monitoring: Neural markers of interoception in obsessive–compulsive disorder. *Psychological Medicine*, *47*(11), 1–14.

Yoris, A., Abrevaya, S., Esteves, S., Salamone, P., Lori, N., Martorell, et al. (2018). Multilevel convergence of interoceptive impairments in hypertension: New evidence of disrupted body–brain interactions. *Human Brain Mapping*, *39*(4) 39, 1563–81.

Chapter 11

Interoception, categorization, and symptom perception

Omer Van den Bergh, Nadia Zacharioudakis, and Sibylle Petersen

11.1 Introduction

Although the body is always immediately present, it seems to be a most elusive perceptual object (Leder, 1990; Chapter 17 in the present volume). Recent years have seen a growing interest in interoception and the perception of bodily sensations which has raised different opinions about which signals are interoceptive: signals emerging from the viscera only (Dworkin, 2000), or also proprio- and somatoceptive signals generated by the muscles, joints, and surface of the body (Craig, 2004) or, more broadly, all the information contributing to a mental meta-representation of the body as distinct from the outer world (Moseley, Gallace, & Spence, 2012). Also, different aspects of interoception have been distinguished such as interoceptive sensibility (i.e. the disposition to focus on bodily processes), interoceptive accuracy/sensitivity (i.e. the ability to detect internal bodily processes accurately), and interoceptive awareness (i.e. the metacognitive awareness of being accurate; Garfinkel et al., 2015). Interoception is thought to influence a vast array of psycho(physio)logical phenomena, ranging from eating and drinking, over emotion and emotional disorders, to time perception, decision-making, the sense of self in a spatiotemporal context, and several other domains (Ceunen, Vlaeyen, & Van Diest, 2016).

In this chapter, we focus on the relationship between interoception and symptom perception. We consider interoception rather broadly as the perception of both visceral and somatic sensations that, conjointly with external contextual information, produces a sense of the state of the body. Interoception seems a precondition for symptom perception, yet symptom perception is also more than that: it implies classifying (a pattern of) sensations into meaningful categories with behavioral relevance, indicating a non-normative state of the body that can vary from transient and rather vague (not well) to a life-threatening specific disease (cancer).

Here, we will not review empirical findings documenting how psychological factors impact symptom perception (see Van den Bergh, Bogaerts, & Van Diest, 2015) but will instead elaborate on a number of fundamental assumptions underlying symptom perception in medical practice.

11.2 Accuracy of symptom perception

Traditionally, a key interest of the research on symptom perception is *accuracy*. This research domain assumes that individuals are able to perceive their internal state and non-normative changes therein accurately. Accurate symptom perception implies that symptom reports closely reflect some physiological dysfunction and that the latter directly *causes* the experience of symptoms. The interest in accuracy of symptom perception has a clear rationale in line with the basic assumptions of a traditional disease model: if there is a close correspondence between the conscious experience of symptoms and the underlying physiological cause, symptoms are a valid source of diagnostic information and can be used as a readout of the underlying cause. In addition, it follows that remedying the underlying cause removes the symptoms.

Although it is acknowledged that psychological factors can bias symptom reports, either as overperception or underperception (Van den Bergh et al., 2015), the accuracy assumption in medical practice represents a fundamental implicit contract among the patient, the physician, and the healthcare system. First, the subjective experience of symptoms is considered a valid reason, typically the primary one, for a patient to consult a physician, to take medication, or undertake other actions to maintain or restore physical health. Second, the experience of symptoms is a major source of information for physicians to guide decisions on further medical examinations, on specific therapeutic interventions, and to assess the effectiveness of their interventions. Third, the healthcare system supports the patient–physician interaction resulting from this implicit contract by providing a wide range of technical and logistic facilities and financial compensations.

Fortunately, the accuracy assumption seems to hold quite well when physiological dysfunction generates rather intense and specific interoceptive sensations that are low in complexity, are clearly localized, and have clear on/off boundaries, such as with acute pain (Price, Riley, & Wade, 2001). However, for more systemic changes in the body and/or for chronic multisymptomatic conditions, the correspondence between symptoms and objective parameters indicating disease severity becomes highly variable and is only accurate under some conditions (Janssens et al., 2009; Van den Bergh et al., 2015, 2017a). The experience of breathlessness, for example, relies upon the integration by the brain of signals from up to 16 different afferent systems, such as stretch receptors in the chest, chemoreceptors in the brainstem, muscle afferents, and many others (Parshall et al., 2012). In addition, breathlessness is a highly distressing emotional experience involving a variety of attentional, cognitive, and behavioral responses that influence perception and reporting of symptoms. Poor correspondence between objective disease indicators and symptom reports is therefore rather common in a wide range of chronic respiratory conditions. For example, correlations between physiological measures of disease severity and self-reported dyspnea in patients with asthma or Chronic Obstructive Pulmonary Disease (COPD) are moderate at best (COPD: $r = 0.36$ in Agusti et al., 2010; $r = 0.28$ in Müllerová et al., 2014; see also Janssens et al., 2009). Correspondence between physiological test results and symptom reports is similarly low for symptoms of cardiovascular diseases (Barsky, 2001) or diabetes (Frankum & Ogden, 2005).

Failure to perceive and interpret symptoms accurately may have life threatening consequences for the patient (e.g. Banzett et al., 2000). Nevertheless, as long as critical disease processes can be assessed and described in a set of measurable variables, poor symptom perception in objectively defined diseases typically does not undermine the shared accuracy assumption, nor the implicit contract represented by the disease model. Medicine is focused on objective variables and is rarely interested in how, exactly, the experience of symptoms comes about, nor in systematically assessing the relationship between the experience of symptoms and physiological dysfunction.

The situation is more dramatic when symptoms are experienced in the absence of established physiological dysfunction after repeated medical examinations, leading to the conclusion that "nothing is wrong." Symptoms of that type are often called psychosomatic symptoms, medically unexplained symptoms (MUS), and functional symptoms, and patterns of them are the core of functional somatic syndromes, bodily distress syndrome, somatization disorder, etc. (Creed et al., 2010).[1] In such cases, the implicit contract is fundamentally violated and all parties are in problems. For patients, it often leads to perseverative needs to justify a symptom as legitimate and to consult more and other doctors. For the physician, it leads to ever more clinical and laboratory investigations to find the physiological dysfunctions and/or to exclude others. Eventually, it results in an erosion of trust in the relationship between patient and doctor and frustration on both sides which in turn has detrimental effects on the development and treatment of symptoms (Nettleton, 2006). For the healthcare system, an excessive use of technical facilities and of expert time, and an important financial burden for society ensues.

Despite these important consequences for the prevailing disease model, MUS are highly prevalent. Research reports that 40–50% of all *symptoms* presented in primary care are not, or not sufficiently, explained by physiological dysfunction (Haller et al., 2015). About 23% of the *patients* in general practice consult with such symptoms (one year prevalence; Steinbrecher et al., 2011) and this prevalence amounts to one-third to one-half of the patients referred to outpatient clinics for further investigation (Nimnuan, Hotopf, & Wessely, 2001). Interestingly, the occurrence of MUS is more likely in persons reporting elevated negative affectivity (Watson & Pennebaker, 1989) and mood and anxiety disorders (Wessely, Nimnuan, & Sharpe, 1999), and evidence shows that perceptual-cognitive mechanisms play an important and, most likely, a causal role (Van den Bergh et al., 2017a). The high prevalence of symptoms unrelated to observable physiological dysfunction constitutes a major theoretical, clinical, and socio-economical challenge.

[1] Although the concept of MUS is plagued by empirical and (meta-)theoretical problems reminding one of Cartesianism, alternatives are not less problematic (Creed et al., 2010). We will therefore use MUS in this text for the sake of convenience.

11.3 Traditional views on medically unexplained symptoms

Traditionally, the problem of how to understand symptoms that are poorly or unrelated to physiological dysfunction is typically addressed in two ways, both of which preserve the accuracy assumption. The first way assumes that the critical physiological dysfunction causing the symptoms is not yet found. A large array of potential etiological and pathogenic mechanisms is being investigated, such as autonomic, neuro-endocrine, inflammatory, infectious, and (auto-)immune responses. In general, the conclusion reached by Rief and Barsky (2005) still holds that physiological abnormalities are often not found in association with diagnostic categories of such symptoms, and if some are found, the associations are not strong, are inconsistently found, and lack specificity. In addition, a major problem is the causal status of these associations. The absence of convincing evidence for a critical dysfunction in peripheral physiology prompts an increasing tendency in researchers to search for abnormalities in central mechanisms of interoceptive information processing as an explanation for the symptoms (e.g. central sensitization).

The second way assumes that there are no distinct illness-related physiological dysfunctions but that bodily sensations associated with stress-related arousal are transformed into symptoms by psychological mechanisms. First, interoceptive hypervigilance is assumed to lower the perceptual threshold leading to perceiving bodily sensations. Second, negative interpretation biases toward perceived bodily sensations will result in illness-related interpretations and attributions of these sensations (e.g. an erratic heartbeat may be interpreted as a sign of impending heart attack). The absence of a clear medical explanation may further enhance interoceptive hypervigilance, while personality and contextual factors may further prompt negative interpretations of sensations lacking a clear explanation. This results in a positive feedback loop, eventually leading to a wide range of symptoms and a seriously disabling condition. Variations of this model tilt the balance between the role of stress-related bodily sensations on the one hand and of perceptual-cognitive mechanisms on the other hand more toward one of these interacting factors. The bottom-line, however, preserves the accuracy assumption, in that "the perception of physical symptoms is generally preceded by peripheral, physiological changes" (Kolk et al., 2003, p. 2344).

A review of the evidence related to latter perspective on MUS is beyond the scope of this chapter, but a recent critical analysis of the research findings concluded that the overall evidence is unconvincing that symptoms unrelated to physiological dysfunction "result from dysregulated peripheral (stress) physiology, hypervigilance for bodily sensations, heightened interoceptive accuracy, or misinterpretations of bodily sensations" (Van den Bergh et al., 2017a, p. 190; 2017b). Conversely, there is compelling experimental evidence that symptom experiences can be induced unrelated to physiological dysfunction. For example, in a series of conditioning studies creating experience-based expectations, we showed that repeated symptom inductions, either through hypercapnia from breathing of CO_2-enriched air or through hypocapnia from voluntary hyperventilation in association with a harmless odor, results in elevated symptom reports upon presenting the harmless odor only (see Van den Bergh et al., 2017b, and Table 11.1 for an overview of findings). A vast literature provides strong evidence that also (social) context-induced and instruction-based expectations can cause bodily symptoms (Webster, Weinman, & Rubin, 2016; Petersen et al., 2014). These nocebo effects show up as adverse side effects of placebo drugs or as symptoms attributed to modern technological triggers such as environmental chemicals, electromagnetic fields, windmills, and the like, for which there is no evidence that they are physiologically harmful (Van den Bergh et al., 2017b).

Nocebo effects violate the accuracy assumption and suggest that the idea that we first perceive a bodily sensation that is subsequently interpreted in a stepwise unidirectional bottom-up process may not be the proper way to look at symptom perception. However, this raises the fundamental question of how we can experience symptoms in the absence of distinct peripheral physiological dysfunction. We propose that symptoms unrelated to bodily dysfunction are not just an aberrant phenomenon that is at odds with "normal" symptom perception in standard medical practice, but are critically revealing basic mechanisms of symptom perception in a similar way as visual illusions reveal basic functional characteristics of the visual system.

Table 11.1 Differences in the definition of accuracy, bias, and error between traditional criterion approaches to validity of the perception of bodily sensations and Bayesian approaches emphasizing construct validity

	Criterion validity	**Construct validity**
Aim of perception	Assessment of the world in close correspondence to physiology or physical stimulus magnitude.	Initiating adaptive behavior.
Bias	◆ A lack of correspondence between perception and an external criterion. ◆ Is irrational.	◆ A directed hypothesis that optimizes perception. ◆ Rational if data is ambiguous. ◆ Rational if two (or more) competing hypotheses are not equally likely (base rates) and if costs and benefits of misses and false alarms are not equal.
Error	◆ Intra-individual variation in the perception of the same stimulus is error variance. ◆ Errors are mistakes.	◆ Intra-individual variation (IIV) in the perception of the same stimulus is a tool that helps to keep generative models of the body in the world up to date. ◆ IIV that corresponds with stimulus ambiguity is information that helps to navigate in dynamic environments.
Ways to optimize perception	◆ Avoid mistakes and minimize bias.	◆ Creating perceptual IIV (in response to ambiguity) to assess error feedback and to produce an adaptive (rational) bias.

11.4 Symptom perception as adaptive sense making

Psychology and philosophy have identified different types of "truth" such as criterion versus construct validity (Cronbach & Meehl, 1955) or correspondence versus pragmatic accuracy (Kruglanski, 1989; Petersen, von Leupoldt, & Van den Bergh, 2015).

11.4.1 Criterion validity

The accuracy assumption of symptom reports resembles criterion validity in test psychology: it refers to the correspondence of a test value (e.g. a participant reporting moderate breathlessness on a scale) with an external criterion such as a physiological measurement (e.g. a lung function test). Taking a correspondence approach to the perception of bodily sensations, symptoms that seem to be disproportional or unrelated to the objective state of the body appear to be "wrong". However, poor symptom perception is not necessarily "wrong" in a pragmatic sense: criterion validity of symptoms can be low while the predictive validity of symptom reports for morbidity, mortality, or development of comorbidities can still be high. In respiratory and cardiovascular disease, for example, the perception of dyspnea is a better predictor of mortality than objective physiological measures (Nishimura et al., 2002). One reason for a high predictive validity is that perceived symptoms rather than objective physiological impairment are related to avoidance of exercise, sedentary lifestyle, mood disorder, and further physiological deterioration (Prince et al., 2007). Thus, poor symptom perception can be valid in a pragmatic sense.

11.4.2 Construct validity

Aristotle's illusion is a tactile illusion that occurs when we close our eyes and cross two fingers while another person touches the space between the two fingertips with a cylindrical object, for example, a pencil. Aristotle (384–322 BC) first described that in these circumstances we perceive that we touch two objects instead of one. In everyday life, simultaneous stimulation of the left side of the index finger and the right side of the middle finger of the right hand nearly always involves two objects. Thus, the brain selects the most likely hypothesis, ignoring part of the sensory evidence. Aristotle's illusion illustrates that perception is based as much on prior beliefs about the world and the body as it is based on sensory information. Conceptualizing perception of bodily sensations as a series of tests, construct validity is the degree to which a percept is consistent within a network of other percepts and useful for inferring its causes and consequences. From this perspective, percepts need to make sense within a given context and enable adaptive behavior rather than to adhere to an objective truth (Petersen, von Leupoldt, & Van den Bergh, 2015b; Seth, Suzuki, & Critchley, 2011). Internal consistency is therefore more relevant for the brain than (unattainable) criterion accuracy (e.g. Kruglanski, 1989; Petersen et al., 2015b) and an external criterion is not necessary for this type of validation.

The latter conclusion is also exemplified in a recent (meta)theoretical account of brain functioning, known as predictive coding (Friston, 2005; Hohwy, 2012). This account starts from the observation that the brain has no direct access to the (outside or inside) world and that it only has its own neural activity to make sense of, or in other words, to make a model of the world that is useful and adaptive. A major task of the brain is then (a) to find statistical regularities in stimulation, (b) to formulate hypotheses about causes and consequences of stimulation, and (c) to integrate error feedback to increase precision of inferences. For symptom perception, the brain has to come up with a model that represents the internal state with reference to a normative versus non-normative state (e.g. from unwell to illness) and settle on a particular illness-related category that accounts for most of the information that is generated by somatic input. This perspective considers symptom perception as somatic decision-making, replacing the notion of (accurately) perceiving an absolute reality with an idea of perception as the creation of categorical meaning. From a predictive coding perspective, this is done in a Bayesian way; that is, taking benefit from previous experience as it is represented in the brain as an estimate of the likelihood that a specific illness category applies. Predictive coding approaches (Friston, 2005) also emphasize the importance of action for perception, implying that somatic decision-making is based on the active sampling of evidence via physiological activation and behavior. The relevance of behavior for perception underlines the importance of perception being adequate for a specific context rather than perception having some context-independent truth.

11.5 Symptom perception as categorical decision-making

Teachers of Bayesian statistics often use a simple example to explain Bayesian decision-making and learning: an experimenter draws poker chips from a bag one by one. Initially, the observers only know that these items can be one of two colours; for example, red or blue. The task of the observers is to guess the percentage of red items. At the start, the observers have no prior knowledge and formulate a random starting point. After each guess, another item is drawn from the bag resulting in accumulating observations that allow observers to update their cognitive representation of the unknown contents. A hypothesis based on robust and consistent evidence will act as a precise prior, creating a strong expectation of what is going to happen.

Modelling the perception of bodily sensations along this example, the body is a highly complex bag and the sensory information forwarded to the brain is like poker chips characterized by an infinite number of subtle variations, possibly having ambiguous meaning, or gaining meaning only when present together with other chips. As the brain draws samples of sensory input, initially random hypotheses become more reliable or precise as evidence is collected. Reliability expectations (precision) are weighing factors that play an important role in determining the relative impact of priors and sensory evidence on the eventual model. The process of evidence sampling, error detection, and updating of hypotheses is hierarchically organized in the brain and involves a bi-directional flow of information with increasing abstraction at higher levels of the hierarchy (Barrett & Simmons, 2015). Importantly, this process of hypothesis testing and updating is a fast, automatic, and unconscious inferential process that eventually promotes a categorical meaning with the maximum expected utility or likelihood. For example, the abstracted representation in the brain of (seeing) a chair acts as a categorical prior that allows us to see a new chair as a chair, automatically and compellingly, despite the huge variety of sensory stimuli that possibly can represent a chair. This implies that an inferential process is used to arrive at this specific meaningful percept (Geisler & Kersten, 2002).

Illness-related bodily sensations often have no clear onset or offset, are systemic (i.e. have multiple afferent sources), are unspecific regarding their cause, and are embedded in constant background noise (Petersen et al., 2011). Thus, the brain needs to generalize and apply rules established in prior experiences to create categorical meaning out of ambiguous, incomplete, and inconsistent information. These prior experiences act as a bias (or directed hypothesis) representing the likelihoods of competing causal explanations, for example, whether it is more likely that somatic input from an erratic heart rate is experienced as a panic attack or as cardiac failure.

Optimal decision-making requires a perceptual system that finds a balance between sensitivity for stimulation and the use of bias (Hahn & Harris, 2014). A perfectly sensitive system that responds to every single variation in stimulation would be unable to generalize and to learn from prior experience (Shepard, 1987), while a completely biased perceptual system would be oblivious to or unaffected by sensory information, and hold on to a priori beliefs about the state of the body without processing error feedback. So, optimal decisions take into account the likelihoods of competing hypotheses (base rates) and costs and benefits that arise from following one interpretation instead of another that have been established in prior, similar sensory events. The majority of perceptual "mistakes" and biases are rational and useful (e.g. Lynn & Barrett, 2014). Mathematical models suggest that the best perceptual performance will be obtained by a learner who has "a bias suitable to the problem at hand" (Hahn & Harris, 2014, p. 62). Table 11.1 lists the differences in perspective on accuracy and bias between a model based on the accuracy or correspondence assumption and the view on how the brain "makes sense" of interoceptive stimulation to enhance usefulness and adaptivity (for more background see Lynn & Barret, 2014; Hahn & Harris, 2014).

The overwhelming majority of studies on interoception take a correspondence approach to accuracy and correlate objective stimulation with self-reported perception (e.g. heartbeat tracking tasks, Domschke et al., 2010). Studies that test somatic decision-making are less common. However, the benefit of having categorical expectations as a directed hypothesis is that it reduces the amount of evidence that needs to be processed before a decision is made, suggesting that priming categories to perceive the internal state changes the way in which somatic information is processed. This is shown in a study with (healthy) persons scoring high or low on symptom reporting in daily life in which we calculated the within-subject correlation between respiratory changes induced by inhalation of CO_2-enriched air and moment-by-moment self-reports thereof. In one condition, participants rated sensations using a neutral category (faster/deeper breathing), whereas in another condition they used a symptom category (breathlessness). The within-subject correlation was equal for both groups when using a neutral category, but dropped significantly for the symptom category, but only in the high symptom reporting group (Bogaerts et al., 2008). In other studies, we used the Interoceptive Classification Task (Petersen et al., 2014). This task implies collecting ratings of inspiratory resistances that differed in magnitude by a constant factor. Presenting them in two different categories, A and B, compared to presenting them in one single category changed the intensity perception, affective ratings, and breathing behavior in the same way: differences within category diminished, whereas differences between categories increased. These examples show that (priming) categorical priors changes the impact of peripheral somatic input in a rather pervasive way and fits with the assumption that the experience of a symptom reflects the generative model of the state of the body that results from a continuous hierarchical interplay between prior hypotheses and sensory evidence, and their associated reliabilities (precision). Because precision expectations are context-dependent, it means that the relationship between experienced symptoms and input from physiological dysfunction is variable within and between persons and contexts. The conditions determining the relative impact of priors versus sensory evidence are extensively described elsewhere (Van den Bergh et al., 2017a).

11.6 **Another look at medically unexplained symptoms**

The above perspective underlies recent predictive coding models of nociception (Büchel et al., 2014) and MUS (Edwards et al., 2012; Van den Bergh et al., 2017a). These models suggest that the experience of a symptom is the result of an automatic inferential process across several hierarchical levels in which the brain interprets interoceptive sensations, informed by "predictions" (priors) about the cause of the sensations. The resulting prediction errors are propagated through the system in an error minimization process, eventually leading to a posterior model representing the conscious experience of a symptom. Both priors and prediction errors should be conceptualized as neural distributions with a variance (statistical confidence) or its inverse, precision, representing the reliability of the prior and prediction errors. Because more reliable distributions are given more weight, the experienced symptom may be more determined by prior expectations or by somatic prediction errors depending on their relative precision. Contextual cues, characteristics of the person, and their interactions may further influence the relative precisions and, consequently, the balance between priors and prediction errors in the eventual symptom experience, such as attention, affective states, memory processes, and personality traits. This perspective allows us to understand that the relationship between peripheral physiological dysfunction and the conscious experience of symptoms may vary between and within persons.

The categorical experience of a symptom can thus be seen as a posterior model of the state of the body, but it will also act as a categorical prior with a specific likelihood to apply in a given context, generating automatic feedforward hypotheses to represent the state of the body. If priors are regularly updated in the light of new evidence, being biased will lead to better decisions. However, somatic decision-making may become maladaptive if the assessment of base rates and costs and benefits is unrealistic because error feedback is not constantly incorporated in generative models. Several phenomena may interfere with optimization of perception by error feedback, such as the inertia effect (Peterson & Miller, 1965), confirmation bias (Nickerson, 1998), or the inferential leap effect (Van den Bergh et al., 2017a). A person can, for example, show inertia in updating perceptual hypotheses and avoid distress caused by ambiguity (Proulx, Inzlicht, & Harmon-Jones, 2012), or jump to conclusions that a symptom is present or absent without sufficiently detailed sensory-perceptual processing (Petersen et al., 2015a, b). According to Hahn and Harris (2014), the common causes for these maladaptive biases are misperceiving the diagnostic value of new evidence and underestimating variability in existing evidence.

In general, we propose that MUS arise when prediction errors from somatic input have low precision. This may occur when input is little intense, more widespread (systemic), and characterized by poor on/off boundaries, when a little detailed sampling strategy is used, or when sensitivity at the level of interoceptive signaling is reduced. In those conditions, a highly precise prior as resulting from contextual or learning factors will shift the experience of a symptom more toward the prior and make it less determined by somatic input (see Van den Bergh et al., 2017a). MUS can therefore be conceived as instances at the extreme end of the continuum representing the relationship between experienced symptoms and peripheral physiological dysfunction.

In order to understand the mechanism more clearly, it may be interesting to look at how risk factors may contribute to such symptoms. For example, a well-known vulnerability factor in the development of such symptoms is high trait negative affectivity. This trait is associated with an overreactive evaluative system and less efficient inhibitory systems to counteract negative affect (Hariri, 2009). Because somatic input generates both a sensory-perceptual and an affective-motivational aspect that are intuitively integrated into a unified symptom experience, enhanced affective responding to somatic stimulation may contribute to more elevated symptom reports found in this group (Van den Bergh & Walentynowicz, 2016).

However, enhanced affective-motivational responding may occur at the expense of detailed sensory-perceptual processing, resulting in augmented but imprecise prediction errors that largely overlap with prediction errors representing an emotional state (see Van den Bergh et al., 2017a, p. 196, for further elaboration). Reduced detail in sensory-perceptual processing of somatic input is suggested by a number of findings. First, in persons with high negative affect, with elevated habitual symptom reports, and in patients with somatoform disorders, self-reported symptoms are less strongly related with induced physiological changes, especially when put in a negative affective context (Bogaerts et al., 2008, 2010). Second, these persons, unlike healthy controls, do not exhibit a peak-end memory bias after an experimentally induced somatic episode despite identical physiological responses (Bogaerts et al., 2012; Walentynowicz et al., 2015). Apparently, patients' retrospective memory of the symptom episode is minimally affected by the actual sensory-perceptual changes during that somatic episode. Third, patients with somatoform disorder exhibit reduced health-related autobiographical memory specificity, suggesting that they process and encode sensory-perceptual aspects of symptom episodes in a broad-brush manner (Walentynowicz et al., 2017).

If somatic prediction errors are imprecise and largely overlapping with affective prediction errors, priors prompted by negative emotions and health concerns may easily come to dominate the posterior model of the somatic state. This is shown in studies that simply induce a negative affective state through picture viewing followed by a symptom questionnaire to assess somatic state: elevated symptom reports emerge in these persons, independent of physiological arousal during picture viewing and regardless whether the pictures are health-related or not (Constantinou et al., 2013). Interestingly, this symptom induction effect is particularly strong in persons who have difficulties in identifying feelings and tend to become absorbed in experiences (Bogaerts et al., 2015). The overall pattern of results suggests that offering a strong symptom-related prior while inducing a negative affective state prompts a symptom experience, because somatic input from affective states is insufficiently distinguished by these individuals from input produced by physiological dysfunction (see Van den Bergh et al., 2017a, for an elaboration on other risk factors).

Predictive coding approaches (Friston, 2005) also emphasize the role of active inference in the process of error minimization. In persons with symptoms unrelated to physiological dysfunction, this is evidenced by chronic scanning of their bodies for the signs of illness that are consistent with pre-existing illness beliefs. If there is little differentiation between somatic and affective prediction errors, chronic activation of illness-related priors and its associated scanning process will easily lead to confirming its own predictions, creating a vicious circle. Recent theorizing (Seth & Friston, 2016, p. 2) takes the idea of interoceptive inference one step further by assuming that "generative models of interoceptive signals should be geared toward control or regulation of physiological variables, rather than toward accurate representation of some extracranial state-of-affairs." In other words, it is assumed that interoceptive predictions about homeostatic setpoints and goal-directed allostatic behavior generate autonomic and other physiological responses to minimize prediction errors as a way of adaptive regulation. It is not clear, however, whether the latter kind of interoceptive inference contributes to symptoms unrelated to physiological dysfunction.

11.7 **Conclusion**

Bayesian approaches underlying a predictive coding model of the brain are promising in bridging the gap between epistemology and mechanistic common sense approaches by eliminating the idea of a homunculus in the mind (that does the perceiving) and replacing it with statistical processes of predictions based on likelihood estimation. These models discard the notion of error as mistake (i.e. as lack of correlation between percept and criterion), and instead attribute to error and bias the role of driving forces in maintaining adaptive perception and behavior (Hohwy, 2012).

This perspective fundamentally challenges the accuracy assumption underlying the traditional disease model and advocates a rather radical view by stating that peripheral physiological dysfunction is neither necessary nor sufficient for symptoms to be experienced. It implies that at the process level there is no categorical difference between symptoms closely related to physiological dysfunction and those that are not, and that all symptoms are characterized by an equally compelling experience of being "real" or "true" regardless whether there is a strong, weak, or absent relationship with peripheral dysfunction. It further accommodates empirical evidence that this relationship is variable both between and within persons, depending on both the precision of the sensory input and of prior expectations. It also recognizes that contextual variables and the person's learning history modulates this relationship.

Patients reporting symptoms unrelated to physiological dysfunction are considered to apply a useful, that is, rational bias. Therefore, instead of branding some patients as "poor" perceivers, or even malingering, or to label their symptoms as "unfounded," it is more useful to understand when and under which conditions it is the most rational choice of the brain to perceive a symptom to be present. This perspective may eliminate the need in these patients for exhausting and futile attempts to prove the validity of their symptoms as following from a perspective that takes accuracy as the validity criterion. In addition, further analysis of the underlying mechanisms of symptoms unrelated to physiological dysfunction may suggest therapeutic interventions. Conscious awareness of processes underlying perceptual inferences, however, is highly limited and replacing maladaptive perceptual biases that may have been established by the brain over years is a challenge. One way to go, as suggested earlier by the analysis of the role of negative affectivity for symptoms unrelated to physiological dysfunction, is "interoceptive differentiation training" (Van den Bergh et al., 2017a). This could help the individual to process sensory-perceptual aspects of the somatic input more closely and to differentiate them from affective sensations, and might be a promising way to treat patients with symptoms violating the traditional disease model. However, given the relative nature of perception of the body as somatic decision-making, a closer correspondence between a physiological criterion and perception cannot be the primary goal in such treatment. Rather, the goal should be to establish more adaptive biases in the perception of the body. While in some cases this might result in a higher criterion validity, the rationale behind these two approaches is fundamentally different.

References

Agusti, A., Calverley, P. M., Celli, B., Coxson, H. O., Edwards, L. D., Lomas, D. A., et al. (2010). Characterisation of COPD heterogeneity in the ECLIPSE cohort. *Respiratory Research, 11*(1), 122. doi:10.1186/1465-9921-11-122.

Banzett, R. B., Dempsey, J. A., O'Donnell, D. E., and **Wamboldt, M. Z.** (2000). Symptom perception and respiratory sensation in asthma. *American Journal of Respiratory and Critical Care Medicine, 162*(3), 1178–82. doi:10.1164/ajrccm.162.3.9909112.

Barrett, L. F., and **Simmons, W. K.** (2015) Interoceptive predictions in the brain. *Nature Reviews Neurosciences, 16*(7), 419–29. doi:10.1038/nrn3950.

Barsky, A. J. (2001). Palpitations, arrhythmias, and awareness of cardiac activity. *Annals of Internal Medicine, 134*(9 Pt 2), 832–37. doi:10.7326/0003-4819-134-9_Part_2-200105011-00006.

Bogaerts, K., Millen, A., Li, W., De Peuter, S., Van Diest, I., Vlemincx, E., et al. (2008). High symptom reporters are less interoceptively accurate in a symptom-related context. *Journal of Psychosomatic Research, 65*(5), 417–24. doi:10.1016/j.jpsychores.2008.03.019.

Bogaerts, K., Van Eylen, L., Wan, L., Bresseleers, J., Van Diest, I., Stans, L., et al. (2010). Distorted symptom perception in patients with medically unexplained symptoms. *Journal of Abnormal Psychology, 119*(1), 226–34. doi:10.1037/a0017780.

Bogaerts, K., Wan, L., Van Diest, I., Stans, L., Decramer, M., and **Van den Bergh, O.** (2012). Peak-end memory bias in laboratory-induced dyspnea: A comparison of patients with medically unexplained symptoms and healthy controls. *Psychosomatic Medicine, 74*(9), 974–81. doi:10.1097/PSY.0b013e318273099c.

Bogaerts, K., Rayen, L., Lavrysen, A., Van Diest, I., Janssens, T., Schruers, K., et al. (2015). Unraveling the relationship between trait negative affectivity and habitual symptom reporting. *PLoS One, 10*(1), e0115748. doi:10.1371/journal.pone.0115748.

Büchel, C., Geuter, S., Sprenger, C., and **Eippert, F.** (2014). Placebo analgesia: A predictive coding perspective. *Neuron, 81*(6), 1223–39. doi:10.1016/j.neuron.2014.02.042.

Ceunen, E., Vlaeyen, J. W., and **Van Diest, I.** (2016). On the origin of interoception. *Frontiers in Psychology, 7*, 743. doi:10.3389/fpsyg.2016.00743.

Constantinou, E., Bogaerts, K., Van Diest, I., and **Van den Bergh, O.** (2013). Inducing symptoms in high symptom reporters via emotional pictures: The interactive effects of valence and arousal. *Journal of Psychosomatic Research, 74*(3), 191–6. doi:10.1016/j.jpsychores.2012.12.015.

Creed, F., Guthrie, E., Fink, P., Henningsen, P., Rief, W., Sharpe, M., et al. (2010). Is there a better term than "medically unexplained symptoms"? *Journal of Psychosomatic Research, 68*(1), 5–8. doi:10.1016/j.jpsychores.2009.09.004.

Cronbach, L. J., and **Meehl, P. E.** (1955). Construct validity in psychological tests. *Psychological Bulletin, 52*(4), 281–302. doi:10.1037/h0040957.

Craig, A. D. (2004). Human feelings: Why are some more aware than others? *Trends in Cognitive Sciences, 8*(6), 239–41. doi:10.1016/j.tics.2004.04.004.

Domschke, K., Stevens, S., Pfleiderer, B., and **Gerlach, A. L.** (2010). Interoceptive sensitivity in anxiety and anxiety disorders: An overview and integration of neurobiological findings. *Clinical Psychological Review, 30*(1), 1–11. doi.org/10.1016/j.cpr.2009.08.008.

Dworkin, B. R. (2000). Interoception. In: Cacioppo, J. T., Tassinary, L. G., and Berntson, G. G. (Eds.), *Handbook of Psychophysiology* (2nd ed.) (pp. 482–506). Cambridge: Cambridge University Press.

Edwards, M. J., Adams, R. A., Brown, H., Pareés, I., and **Friston, K. J.** (2012). A Bayesian account of "hysteria". *Brain, 135*(11), 3495–512. doi.org/10.1093/brain/aws129.

Frankum, S., and **Ogden, J.** (2005). Estimation of blood glucose levels by people with diabetes: A cross-sectional study. *British Journal of General Practice, 55*(521), 944–8.

Friston, K. (2005). A theory of cortical responses. *Philosophical Transactions of the Royal Society B, 360*(1456), 815–36. doi:10.1098/rstb.2005.1622.

Garfinkel, S. N., Seth, A. K., Barrett, A. B., Suzuki, K., and **Critchley, H. D.** (2015). Knowing your own heart: Distinguishing interoceptive accuracy from interoceptive awareness. *Biological Psychology, 104*, 65–74. doi:10.1016/j.biopsycho.2014.11.004.

Geisler, W. S., and **Kersten, D.** (2002). Illusions, perception and Bayes. *Nature Neurosciences, 5*(6), 508–10. doi:10.1038/nn0602-508.

Hahn, U., and **Harris, A. J.** (2014). What does it mean to be biased: Motivated reasoning and rationality. *Psychology of Learning and Motivation, 61*, 41–102. doi:10.1016/B978-0-12-800283-4.00002-2.

Haller, H., Cramer, H., Lauche, R., and Dobos, G. (2015). Somatoform disorders and medically unexplained symptoms in primary care. *Deutsches Ärzteblatt International, 112*(16), 279–87. doi:10.3238/arztebl.2015.0279.

Hariri, A. R. (2009). The neurobiology of individual differences in complex behavioral traits. *Annual Review of Neurosciences, 32*, 225–47. doi:10.1146/annurev.neuro.051508.135335.

Hohwy, J. (2012). Attention and conscious perception in the hypothesis testing brain. *Frontiers in Psychology, 3*, 96. doi:10.3389/fpsyg.2012.00096.

Janssens, T., Verleden, G., De Peuter, S., Van Diest, I., and **Van den Bergh, O.** (2009). Inaccurate perception of asthma symptoms: A cognitive–affective framework and implications for asthma treatment. *Clinical Psychological Review, 29*(4), 317–27. doi:10.1016/j.cpr.2009.02.006.

Kruglanski, A. W. (1989). The psychology of being "right": The problem of accuracy in social perception and cognition. *Psychological Bulletin, 106*(3), 395–409. doi:10.1037/0033-2909.106.3.395.

Kolk, A. M., Hanewald, G. J., Schagen, S., and **van Wijk, C. M. G.** (2003). A symptom perception approach to common physical symptoms. *Social Sciences & Medicine, 57*(12), 2343–54. doi:10.1016/S0277-9536(02)00451-3.

Leder, D. (1990). *The Absent Body*. Chicago, IL: Chicago University Press.

Lynn, S. K. and **Barrett, L. F.** (2014). "Utilizing" signal detection theory. *Psychological Science, 25*(9), 1663–73. doi:10.1177/0956797614541991.

Moseley, G. L., Gallace, A., and **Spence, C.** (2012). Bodily illusions in health and disease: Physiological and clinical perspectives and the concept of a cortical "body matrix". *Neurosciences & Biobehavioral Reviews, 36*(1), 34–46. doi:10.1016/j.neubiorev.2011.03.013.

Müllerová, H., Lu, C., Li, H., and **Tabberer, M.** (2014). Prevalence and burden of breathlessness in patients with chronic obstructive pulmonary disease managed in primary care. *PloS One, 9(1)*, e85540. doi:10.1371/journal.pone.0085540.

Nettleton, S. (2006). "I just want permission to be ill": Towards a sociology of medically unexplained symptoms. *Social Sciences and Medicine, 62*(5), 1167–78. doi:10.1016/j.socscimed.2005.07.030.

Nickerson, R. S. (1998). Confirmation bias: A ubiquitous phenomenon in many guises. *Review of General Psychology, 2*(2), 175–220. doi:10.1037/1089-2680.2.2.175.

Nishimura, K., Izumi, T., Tsukino, M., and **Oga, T.** (2002). Dyspnea is a better predictor of 5-year survival than airway obstruction in patients with COPD. *Chest, 121*(5), 1434–40. doi:10.1378/chest.121.5.1434.

Nimnuan, C., Hotopf, M., and **Wessely, S.** (2001). Medically unexplained symptoms: An epidemiological study in seven specialities. *Journal Psychosomatic Research, 51*(1), 361–7. doi:10.1016/S0022-3999(01)00223-9.

Parshall, M. B., Schwartzstein, R. M., Adams, L., Banzett, R. B., Manning, H. L., Bourbeau, J., et al. (2012). An official American Thoracic Society statement: Update on the mechanisms, assessment, and management of dyspnea. *American Journal of Respiratory and Critical Care Medicine, 185*(4), 435–52. doi:10.1164/rccm.201111-2042ST.

Petersen, S., van den Berg, R., Janssens, T., and **Van den Bergh, O.** (2011). Illness and symptom perception: A theoretical approach towards an integrative measurement model. *Clinical Psychological Review, 31*(3), 428–39. doi:10.1016/j.cpr.2010.11.002.

Petersen, G. L., Finnerup, N. B., Colloca, L., Amanzio, M., Price, D. D., Jensen, T. S., et al. (2014). The magnitude of nocebo effects in pain: A meta-analysis. *Pain, 155*(8), 1426–34. doi:10.1016/j.pain.2014.04.016.

Petersen, S., Schroijen, M., Mölders, C., Zenker, S., and **Van den Bergh, O.** (2014). Categorical interoception: Perceptual organization of sensations from inside. *Psychological Science, 25*(5), 1059–66. doi:10.1177/0956797613519110.

Petersen, S., Van Staeyen, K., Vögele, C., von Leupoldt, A., and **Van den Bergh, O.** (2015a). Interoception and symptom reporting: Disentangling accuracy and bias. *Frontiers in Psychology, 6*(732). doi:10.3389/fpsyg.2015.00732.

Petersen, S., Von Leupoldt, A., and **Van den Bergh, O.** (2015b). Interoception and the uneasiness of the mind: Affect as perceptual style. *Frontiers in Psychology, 6*(1408). doi:10.3389/fpsyg.2015.01408.

Peterson, C., and **Miller, A.** (1965). Sensitivity of subjective probability revision. *Journal of Experimental Psychology, 70*(1), 117–21. doi:10.1037/h0022023.

Price, D. D., Riley, J. L., and **Wade, J. B.** (2001). Psychophysical approaches to measurement of the dimensions and stages of pain. In: D. C. Turk and R. Melzack (Eds.), *Handbook of Pain Assessment* (2nd ed.) (pp. 53–75). New York, NY: Guilford Press.

Prince, M., Patel, V., Saxena, S., Maj, M., Maselko, J., Phillips, M. R., et al. (2007). No health without mental health. *Lancet, 370*(9590), 859–77. doi:10.1016/S0140-6736(07)61238-0.

Proulx, T., Inzlicht, M., and **Harmon-Jones, E.** (2012). Understanding all inconsistency compensation as a palliative response to violated expectations. *Trends in Cognitive Sciences, 16*(5), 285–91. doi:10.1016/j.tics.2012.04.002.

Rief, W., and **Barsky, A. J.** (2005). Psychobiological perspectives on somatoform disorders. *Psychoneuroendocrinology, 30*(10), 996–1002. doi:10.1016/j.psyneuen.2005.03.018.

Seth, A. K., Suzuki, K., and **Critchley, H. D.** (2011). An interoceptive predictive coding model of conscious presence. *Frontiers in Psychology, 2*(395). doi:10.3389/fpsyg.2011.00395.

Seth, A. K., and **Friston, K. J.** (2016). Active interoceptive inference and the emotional brain. *Philosophical Transactions of the Royal Society B, 371*(1708), 20160007. doi:10.1098/rstb.2016.0007.

Shepard, R. N. (1987). Toward a universal law of generalization for psychological science. *Science, 237*(4820), 1317–23. doi:10.1126/science.3629243.

Steinbrecher, N., Koerber, S., Frieser, D., and **Hiller, W.** (2011). The prevalence of medically unexplained symptoms in primary care. *Psychosomatics, 52*(3), 263–71. doi:10.1016/j.psym.2011.01.007.

Van den Bergh, O., Bogaerts, K., and **Van Diest, I.** (2015). Symptom perception, awareness and interpretation. In: Wright, J. D. (Ed.), *International Encyclopedia of the Social & Behavioral Sciences* (2nd ed.) (pp. 866–72). Oxford: Elsevier.

Van den Bergh, O., and **Walentynowicz, M.** (2016). Accuracy and bias in retrospective symptom reporting. *Current Opinion in Psychiatry, 29*(5), 302–8. doi:10.1097/YCO.0000000000000267.

Van den Bergh, O., Witthöft, M., Petersen, S., and **Brown, R. W.** (2017a). Symptoms and the body: Taking the inferential leap. *Neurosciences & Biobehavioral Reviews, 74*(Pt A), 185–203. doi:10.1016/j.neubiorev.2017.01.015.

Van den Bergh, O., Brown, R. J., Petersen, S., and **Witthöft, M.** (2017b). Idiopathic environmental illnesses: A comprehensive model. *Clinical Psychological Science, 5*(3), 551–67. doi:10.1177/2167702617693327.

Walentynowicz, M., Bogaerts, K., Van Diest, I., Raes, F., and **Van den Bergh, O.** (2015). Was it so bad? The role of retrospective memory in symptom overreporting. *Health Psychology, 34*(12), 1166–74. doi:10.1037/hea0000222.

Walentynowicz, M., Raes, F., Van Diest, I., and **Van den Bergh, O.** (2017). The specificity of health-related autobiographical memories in patients with somatic symptom disorder. *Psychosomatic Medicine, 79*(1), 43–9. doi:10.1097/PSY.0000000000000357.

Watson, D., and **Pennebaker, J. W.** (1989). Health complaints, stress, and distress: Exploring the central role of negative affectivity. *Psychological Review, 96*(2), 234. doi:10.1037//0033-295X.96.2.234.

Webster, R.K., Weinman, J., and **Rubin, G. J.** (2016). A systematic review of factors that contribute to nocebo effects. *Health Psychology, 35*(12), 1334–55. doi:10.1037/hea0000416.

Wessely, S., Nimnuan, C., and **Sharpe, M.** (1999). Functional somatic syndromes: One or many? *Lancet, 354*(9182), 936–9. doi:10.1016/S0140-6736(98)08320-2.

Chapter 12

Interoceptive appraisal and mental health

Norman A. S. Farb and Kyle Logie

12.1 Introduction

Interoception is the sense of the internal state of the body (Craig, 2002). This sense is informed by the reception, representation, and appraisal of ascending autonomic signals that indicate changes in physiological arousal (Farb et al., 2015). Interoceptive signals play a vital role in homeostasis via the autonomic nervous system (Craig, 2003), and it is assumed that most of these signals do not reach conscious awareness. However, salient interoceptive signals seem to support the conscious experience of an embodied self (Seth & Friston, 2016) and influence cognition, feelings, and behavior (Critchley & Garfinkel, 2017; Katkin, Wiens, & Öhman, 2001; Dunn et al., 2012).

Awareness across sensory modalities is often discussed in terms of crossing a threshold, wherein stimulus perception requires a certain intensity to trigger conscious representation (Rouder & Morey, 2009). In interoception, such representation occurs in the form of subjective feeling states such as pain, itch, hunger, and thirst (Craig, 2002; Craig, 2003). These feeling states are described as "homeostatic emotions" (Craig, 2003; Strigo & Craig, 2016), which most likely evolved as a survival mechanism to allow for behavioral regulation to correct for physiological imbalances (Damasio & Carvalho, 2013). In addition to these feeling states, subjective experience of interoceptive signals can be appraised as a more generalized state of physiological arousal. This subjective experience of arousal is well documented as playing an important role in emotional experience (Schachter & Singer, 1962), such as feelings of attraction towards romantic partners (White, Fishbein, & Rutsein, 1981) and other aspects of cognition such as speed in decision-making (Hackley & Valle-Inclán, 1999).

As Leder discusses in Chapter 17 in the present volume, one feature of interoceptive experience is that particular interoceptive signals are often diffuse and difficult to differentiate from the integrated whole that characterizes our embodied experience in the world, yet despite the ambiguity of myriad competing signals, interoception often manifests within consciousness as a subjective gestalt. Changes in physiology can therefore contribute to interoceptive experience without being directly and distinctly perceived. Interoceptive appraisal is the process of integrating these diffuse physiological changes into a coherent feeling state.

We define interoceptive appraisal as the process of making sense of consciously detected physiological change, regardless of whether there is awareness of the appraisal process itself. We suggest that conscious detection of physiological change provokes interoceptive appraisal, whereas physiological change without awareness provides no basis for appraisal. We readily acknowledge that physiological change can influence cognition and behavior following implicit or unconscious pathways. However, unconscious responses to physiological change are not interoceptive appraisals because they do not, by definition, integrate physiological changes into subjective feeling states. Interoceptive appraisals determine the impact that physiological changes have on our sense of self, even if we are not always aware of how such integration occurs.

If interoceptive appraisal is provoked by awareness of physiological change, the ability to detect interoceptive change influences when appraisals are made. Interoceptive accuracy, the ability to reliably detect interoceptive signals, varies across individuals, and is often measured by evaluating accuracy in tasks involving heartbeat detection (Critchley et al., 2004; Ainley & Tsakiris, 2013) or perception of respiratory resistance (Harver, Katkin, & Bloch, 1993; Davenport & Kifle, 2001). To operationalize these terms, Garfinkel, Seth, Barrett, and colleagues (2015) define interoceptive awareness as the correlation between accuracy—objective performance on an interoceptive task, and sensibility—self-evaluated confidence ratings of task performance. However, interoceptive accuracy and sensibility are dissociable and only weakly correlated in the general population (Garfinkel et al., 2015), suggesting that appraisals of interoceptive change can vary independently from objectively observable physiological changes. Thus, while interoceptive appraisal is provoked by the detection of interoceptive signals, interoceptive signals need not be accurate representations of the body to provoke appraisal. Given this independence between interoceptive accuracy and appraisal, it is appraisal that is therefore most consistently determinant of subjective well-being, while interoceptive accuracy determines the extent to which such appraisals are provoked by real physiological changes.

Research supports the idea that appraisal tendency is a central determinant of well-being. Greater accuracy of heartbeat detection has been associated with greater reactivity to emotionally provocative stimuli but it does not determine the affective tone of such reactivity (Barrett, et al., 2004; Herbert, Pollatos et al., 2007). Indeed, emotional reactivity is agnostic with respect to well-being, an ambiguity clarified only through interoceptive appraisal. For example, an accurately perceived stirring in one's chest could just as easily be appraised as excitement or anxiety, depending on one's appraisal tendencies. When low interoceptive accuracy interacts with strong interoceptive appraisal biases, it provides a framework for unfettered appraisal, which in turn can predict a variety of pathological symptoms and behaviors (Khalsa & Lapidus, 2016).

Supporting the relevance of interoceptive appraisal for well-being, dysfunctional interoceptive appraisal habits have been associated with a growing number of mental health disorders, including anxiety (Paulus & Stein, 2006), depression (Barrett, Quigley, & Hamilton, 2016), autism (Silani et al., 2008), and eating disorders (Merwin et al., 2010). It is important to note that these disorders are more often associated with abnormal appraisal habits rather than impaired interoceptive accuracy. As a canonical example, anxiety disorders are associated with superior levels of interoceptive accuracy, but accurate identification of physiological change often gives rise to anxious or catastrophic appraisals (Domschke et al., 2010). In panic disorders, small but real changes in interoceptive arousal are often catastrophized, an appraisal that physiological changes reflect an underlying pathological and life-threatening process (Kearney et al., 1997). While interoceptive accuracy seems important for provoking appropriate and adaptive regulatory responses, appraisal tendencies may be the most effective point by which to predict mental health and approach treatment.

To support this claim, evidence from the clinical literature emphasizes that it is not interoceptive accuracy per se but rather the appraisal of interoceptive signals that is most relevant to feelings of wellness or illness (Paulus & Stein, 2010). Studies on the misattribution of arousal suggest that the appraised causes of a detected physiological change can moderate the effects of such change on mood. For example, attributing heightened physiological arousal to a pill reduces the experience of anxiety stemming from such arousal (Zanna & Cooper, 1974). Similarly, anxiety related to public speaking is reduced when one attributes arousal to a source unrelated to the speech act (Olson, 1988). Therefore, the measurement of interoceptive appraisal habits may be a vital step in efforts to characterize whether interoception serves to support or undermine mental health, and the modification of interoceptive appraisal habits may serve as an important treatment target in the presence of affective distress.

To clarify the roles of interoceptive representation and appraisal in determining mental health, this chapter will proceed by presenting an emerging neurobiological model for interoceptive processing, and explaining how this model can be used to characterize aberrant interoceptive processing in various mental disorders. To correct such processing abnormalities, we discuss the theoretical rationale for contemplative interventions such as mindfulness training, and we review our group's neuroscience research on how attention training can improve the fidelity and plasticity of neural interoceptive representations. Finally, we propose a novel behavioral task for assessment of interoceptive function through characterization of appraisal habits following controlled changes in physiological arousal. By experimentally manipulating interoceptive awareness independently from objectively defined arousal, it may be possible directly to assess the influence of interoceptive appraisal habits on affect, cognition, and behavior.

12.2 An emerging neurobiological model

Emerging research supports both the existence of a dedicated neural network for interoceptive representation and the distinction between such representation and its contextualized appraisal. Small diameter (Aδ and C) afferents have long been known to carry information about pain and temperature through the lamina I spinothalamocortical pathway, though it is now apparent that these fibers contain homeostatic information from all tissues of the body (Craig, 2002; Strigo & Craig, 2016). These afferents travel through the ventromedial thalamic nucleus and eventually project to the mid/posterior dorsal insula, which acts as a primary interoceptive cortex (Craig, 2002). This area is organized as a topographical map and appears to be the primary region of viscerosensory fields for body sensation (Brooks et al., 2005). Positron emission tomography (PET) and functional magnetic resonance imaging (fMRI) studies have related that activation in the mid/posterior insula reveals graduated activity to sensual touch, temperature, itch, and pain (Craig, 2002). Using fMRI, our research group has also found graduated activity in right posterior insula to changes in respiration rate (Farb, Segal, & Anderson, 2013a). Attention directed towards respiration was associated with enhanced activation in this primary interoceptive cortex. This is similar to the effect of selective attention on signal gain amplification observed in external senses such as vision (Hillyard, Vogel, & Luck, 1998).

While the posterior insula seems to operate as a primary interoception representation cortex, the appraisal of these representations seems dependent on the propagation of posterior insula representations towards the anterior insula and adjacent prefrontal cortex. Topographically organized interoceptive information from the posterior insula appears to be re-represented in the right anterior insula as an image of the interoceptive state of the body (Craig, 2002, 2009). The right anterior insula is thought to act as an area of integration between interoceptive signals from the body and contextual information from the external environment (Craig, 2009). Imaging studies have commonly implicated right anterior insula activity in tasks that involve interoceptive awareness (Crichley et al., 2004; Pollatos, et al., 2007) as well as during induction of high-arousal affective states (Jabbi, Bastiaansen, & Keysers, 2008; Gu et al., 2013). Given its anatomical role in connecting primary interoceptive cortex in the posterior insula to higher cognitive processes supported by the prefrontal cortex, anterior insula processing is a likely candidate region involved in translating interoceptive sensory signals into appraisals of well-being.

12.3 **Interoceptive appraisal in mental disorders**

In keeping with a theory of interoceptive appraisal constituting the sense of well-being, it is unsurprising that altered activation in the anterior insula is commonly associated with mental health disorders. With regards to depression and anxiety, Paulus and Stein (2010) argue that belief states and top-down processes play a large role in these disorders as well as influence how interoceptive signals are appraised. For instance, it appears that individuals suffering from anxiety disorders tend to overrepresent interoceptive signals and to appraise them as more threatening (Paulus & Stein, 2006). This leads to a state of enhanced sensitivity to aversive interoceptive signals. Accordingly, studies have found that individuals suffering from general anxiety disorder (GAD) were able to detect interoceptive signals associated with autonomic arousal better than controls despite no differences in external measures of physiological arousal (Andor, Gerlach, & Rist, 2008). With regard to brain activation, fMRI studies have found that anxiety-prone individuals show heightened activity in the bilateral insula as well amygdala when shown emotional faces (Stein, et al., 2007), and individuals with phobias tend to show increased activation in the right insula when viewing fearful faces (Wright et al., 2003). Research on anxiety disorders emphasizes the importance of proper appraisal of the interoceptive signal and shows that increased sensitivity to aversive interoceptive signals can be detrimental to mental health. From a neurobiological standpoint, amplification of afferent interoceptive signals in the anterior insula may serve as a biological correlate of the catastrophizing appraisals associated with anxiety disorders.

Major depressive disorder (MDD) may serve as a useful example for why suppression of nominal levels of interoceptive activation is also maladaptive. Although studies have found that individuals suffering from MDD show increased activation in right anterior insula in anticipation to painful stimuli (Strigo et al., 2008), our research has found that depression symptom burden is associated with suppression rather than activation of right insula activity during sadness provocation (Farb et al., 2010). This finding is convergent with clinical reports that people suffering from MDD tend to use maladaptive emotion regulation strategies defined by avoidance and dissociation from body sensations (Naragon-Gainey, McMahon, & Chacko, 2017). A consequence of such suppression is that appraisals of low mood and lethargy are unchallenged by natural variation in physiological arousal. Once again, accuracy in detecting interoceptive signals seems less relevant for mental health than appraisal tendency—both the exaggeration of interoceptive signal importance and the dissociation from such signals seem to support psychopathology, in the form of anxiety and depressive disorders respectively.

In summary, suboptimal integration of interoceptive signals in mental disorders may involve deficits in the detection of these signals, followed by maladaptive appraisal of interoceptive states (Paulus & Stein, 2010). Disorders characterized by feelings of disconnection and isolation seem to involve deficits in actively attending to and appraising interoceptive signals, including both depression (Farb et al., 2010) and autism (Quattrocki & Friston, 2014). Conversely, anxiety disorders are associated with a heightened awareness towards, and a tendency to appraise negatively initial detection of physiological change without attending to the full range of interoceptive information (Paulus & Stein, 2010). Restructuring interoceptive appraisal habits may therefore be beneficial in alleviating symptoms associated with these mental disorders. One approach to restructuring interoceptive appraisal tendencies may lie in contemplative practices that modulate interoceptive attention and appraisal habits, such as mindfulness meditation and other mind–body interventions.

12.4 **Interoception in contemplative interventions**

The past decades have featured an increasing assimilation of contemplative intervention techniques originating from Eastern spiritual traditions into Western clinical practices and broader culture (Farb, 2014). Although there are many variations of meditation and movement-based exercises that are classified as contemplative interventions, they commonly, though not exclusively, feature exploration of one's relationship to physical sensation, and this is a particular focus of mindfulness-based training techniques (Farb et al., 2015). As such, promoting awareness of appraisal habits, and in particular interoceptive appraisals, is a core aspect of these techniques.

Contemplative interventions often progress from focal attention on somatic and interoceptive targets towards an "open monitoring" or diffuse approach to awareness in which mental content is observed as it arises in the present moment (Raffone & Srinivasan, 2010). As Bishop (2004) explains, in order to cultivate this open-monitoring style of attention, contemplative practices often begin by shifting attention towards the interoceptive target of respiration. Interoceptive attention is coupled with instructions on how to structure appraisal of interoceptive signals, such as responding to novel signals with an attitude of acceptance and curiosity (Bishop, 2004). Two popular contemplative interventions used in clinical research are Mindfulness Based Stress Reduction (MBSR) and Mindfulness Based Cognitive Therapy (MBCT), which are both eight-week long programs in a group setting and involve a range of exercises. As their names suggest, both approaches emphasize awareness of interoceptive signals and related appraisal tendencies as an overarching orientation. Critically, both interventions emphasize the suspension of interoceptive appraisal habits as a means by which to improve interoceptive awareness and response (Bishop, 2004).

Clinical research has found both MBSR and MBCT to be moderately effective treatments across a range of disorders, such as chronic pain, depression, and anxiety (Goyal et al., 2014). These interventions have also been shown to be effective in increasing overall measures of subjective well-being (Carmody & Baer, 2008), although the process of developing new interoceptive habits may itself be stressful (Farias et al., 2016). Central to these interventions' theorized efficacy is the intention to restructure one's relationship with experience, and particularly interoceptive experience, to reduce habitual exaggeration or suppression in interoceptive appraisal (Kabat-Zinn, 2009; Segal, Williams, & Teasdale, 2012). This intention is consistent with the finding that maladaptive and inaccurate appraisals tend to be associated with a range of anxiety and affective disorders. MBIs thus offer a unique method of re-attending to primary sensation in an effort to renegotiate chronic interoceptive appraisal tendencies. By reducing habits that pathologically catastrophize or dissociate from interoceptive experience, it may be possible to develop resilience against the translation of interoceptive change into maladaptive feeling states. While definitive validation of these interventions' mechanisms of action are still pursued in the research literature, evidence to date is consistent with the stated intention of these programs to introduce flexibility into the appraisal of interoceptive signals, and by extension, the ability to respond more flexibly and adaptively to life stressors that cue interoceptive signalling.

12.5 The role of attention and precision in interoceptive networks

Emerging neuroscience research supports the notion that interoceptive attention can be transformative when coupled with appropriate appraisal instructions. While feeling states such as hunger, itch, or pain arise in a bottom-up manner signalling homeostatic imbalance or potential tissue damage (Craig, 2003), attention can also influence which interoceptive signals cross the threshold into conscious awareness. First, interoceptive attention promotes precision in the representation of the attended interoceptive signal in interoceptive networks: our research group has shown that interoceptive attention to respiration increases the correlation between variation in respiration rate and variation in posterior insula activation (Farb et al., 2013a).

A second major finding is that contemplative training of interoceptive attention introduces both state-like and trait-like neuroplasticity to interoceptive networks that may be indicative of altered interoceptive appraisal tendencies. Interoceptive training via MBSR was associated both with an increased capacity to engage interoceptive regions such as the right insula and somatosensory association cortex during self-referential thought (Farb et al., 2007), and reduced insula suppression following sadness provocation (Farb et al., 2010). Furthermore, compared to a waitlisted control group, individuals who underwent eight weeks of MBSR training tended to have stronger activation in the right insula as well as decreased activity in dorsomedial prefrontal cortex during attention towards respiration (Farbet al., 2013b). In both the 2007 and 2013 MBSR training studies, connectivity between the insula and prefrontal cortex shifted, with increased connectivity to dorsal regions of the prefrontal cortex associated with executive control, and reduced connectivity to the ventral prefrontal cortex in regions associated with evaluative appraisal. These findings are consistent with an account of shifting interoceptive attention away from habitual appraisal into a state of sensory exploration, which may then potentiate novel or more flexible appraisals of a wide range of interoceptive signals.

Other studies have found that attention training that focuses on interoceptive awareness can lead to changes in the brain. For example, long-term meditators have shown reduced atrophy in right anterior insula compared to age-matched controls (Lazar et al., 2005), suggesting less pruning or fixedness in interoceptive integration supported by the right anterior insula. These findings suggest that MBIs engage interoceptive networks in the brain and reduce appraisal-laden interoceptive integration with prefrontal structures supporting conscious awareness. The ability to continually integrate interoceptive signals in the face of a negative mood stressor in the 2010 study, the reduction of ventral prefrontal connectivity with the posterior insula following training, and the general findings of clinical benefits of MBSR interventions in our research together support a theory of therapeutic efficacy in mindfulness interventions as stemming from a restructuring of interoceptive appraisal habits.

12.6 **A respiration-based task for characterizing interoceptive appraisal habits**

12.6.1 **Rationale**

A significant challenge for interoceptive accounts of well-being is the possibility that abnormal interoception is merely a symptom rather than cause of mental health disorders.

This confusion arises because changes in physiological arousal are often confounded with measurement of interoceptive appraisal. For example, in the anxiety literature, established tasks for provoking interoceptive appraisal also require provocation of physiological arousal, such as being required to run on a treadmill. It is therefore unknown to what degree anxiety stems directly from physiological change as opposed to the appraised meaning of the physiological change. Similarly, in therapy, it is difficult to demonstrate to a patient that seemingly threatening physiological change is innocuous because the patient is generally aware of efforts to induce physiological arousal, thus it is difficult for the patient to have an experience of physiological arousal that is separated from fear or threat appraisal. The critical demonstration that appraisal rather than physiology is determinant of mental health requires that we are able to manipulate physiological arousal independently of appraisal, and ideally to do this repeatedly to characterize an individual's appraisal habits and their influence on subjective well-being reliably.

Here, we present preliminary data on a respiration-focused interoceptive task that allows for independent manipulation of physiological arousal from detectability of physiological change. We suggest that, at a given level of physiological change, contrasting trials with and without accurate change detection allows for the examination of interoceptive appraisal habits, which only occur with awareness, that is, accurate detection of physiological change. The intention in this chapter is only to provide the rationale and "proof of concept" for this task rather than to validate the task's experimental and clinical relevance for interoception research fully, which we hope to provide in future scholarship.

12.6.2 Design

Leveraging the controllability of respiration, the novel task requires that participants entrain their respiration frequency to match an external visual stimulus, such as a circle on a computer screen that "pulses"—expanding and contracting in size over time. Participants are instructed to inhale when the circle expands, and exhale when the circle contracts. On a given trial, participants breathe along with the circle for ~60 seconds, which allows for around 12 to 18 pulses, depending on breathing rate.

The task allows for manipulation of both physiological change and the probability of physiological change detection. Correspondingly, the two independent variables (IV) are (a) total change in respiration frequency and (b) rate of respiration frequency change. For the first IV, we incorporated six levels of total respiration rate change to manipulate physiological change. Three levels of respiration rate change (ΔRR) were employed for both increasing and decreasing respiration rate, at 35%, 50%, and 85% change from baseline respiration rates. For the second IV, we incorporated two rates of respiration frequency change, "quick" and "gradual," to manipulate the probability of physiological change detection. "Quick" trials were designed to enhance the detectability of change, and they involve changing the pulse frequency abruptly between two consecutive pulses in the middle of the trial pulse sequence; "gradual" trials were designed to mask change, and involve changing the pulse frequency very slightly between each pulse. Thus, two trials in which respiration slows by 50% can be manipulated with respect to detectability in "quick" trials by increasing pulse length 1.5 times between two pulses in the middle of the trial, or in "gradual" trials by increasing pulse length with every pulse across the trial by 1.5^{-N} times, where N is the number of pulses in the trial. To summarize, physiological change is manipulated by the extent to which pulse rate changes over a trial, whereas detectability of change is manipulated by how abruptly the pulse change occurs. Unlike most interoceptive tasks that measure individual differences between participants, this task would manipulate physiological change and detectability within-participant and within the same experimental session.

The primary dependent variable in the task is awareness of physiological change. Each trial is followed by a three-alternative forced choice paradigm that asks the participant whether respiration rate changed ("faster," "slower," or "no change"). As discussed in the following, other dependent variables can be appended to measure the effects of physiological change and awareness on various facets of cognition, affect and behavior. Awareness of a given level of physiological change may moderate performance on other measures, and this moderation effect can serve as an individual difference measure of appraisal tendency.

12.6.3 Pilot data

Pilot data from our lab ($N = 16$; 10 women; mean age 20 ± 1.4 yr) confirms the feasibility of this paradigm and the dual manipulation of physiology and detection probability. In this version of the task, trial length was 8 pulses, which were 30 to 70 seconds in length depending on the level of rate change. A respiration belt (Bioharness 3; Zephyr Technology, Annapolis, MD) was used to assess baseline respiration rate and to verify participants correctly entrained their breaths to match the circle stimulus. Raw correlations between circle size and belt size over time were routinely > 0.85, indicating very good entraining of respiration. No participants reported difficulties in understanding task instructions or any feelings of distress or light-headedness from the respiratory rate manipulation.

Even in this modest sample, strong significant effects of both manipulations were observed using the "nlme" package for multilevel modeling (Pinheiro et al., 2016) in the R programming environment (R Core Team, 2014). Prediction of change detection accuracy was modelled progressively compared to the null model, first using the degree of respiratory rate change, then quadratic effects to account for extremity of frequency change regardless of change direction, and finally the effect of gradual versus quick change type conditions (Table 12.1).

All model steps were significant, and so t-scores reported here reflect the final model values. The analysis suggested that detection accuracy was significantly better for rate increases than decreases, $t(146) = 4.23$, $p < 0.001$, and better for more extreme rate changes in either direction, $t(146) = 2.41$, $p = 0.017$. Change type was also a significant predictor of accuracy, $t(14) = 5.08$, $p < 0.001$, with quick rate changes detected more accurately than gradual changes.

Finally, change type interacted with degree of change. There was a trend for the effects of change type to increase with greater extremity of frequency change ($\Delta Rate^2$ *Type),

Table 12.1 Effects of respiratory rate change and change type (quick or gradual) on change detection.

Model	Df	Log Likelihood	Likelihood Ratio	P-Value
Accuracy ~ 1 (Intercept Only)	5	−174.4		
Accuracy ~ ΔRate	6	−170.3	8.2	0.004
Accuracy ~ ΔRate + $\Delta Rate^2$	7	−157.7	25.3	<0.001
Accuracy ~ ΔRate + $\Delta Rate^2$ + Type	8	−149.2	16.9	<0.001
Accuracy ~ (ΔRate + $\Delta Rate^2$) * Type	10	−143.7	11.1	0.004

$t(146) = 1.86$, $p = 0.06$; this trend was driven by a significant interaction between change type and the linear effect of frequency change (ΔRate *Type), $t(146) = -2.77$, $p < 0.01$, that shows greater effects of change type for respiratory slowing than respiratory acceleration (Figure 12.1).

As Figure 12.1 shows, the relationship between total change in respiration rate (ΔRR) and awareness of change (accuracy on forced choice reports of change detection) can be modelled by a similar parabolic function for both gradual-change and quick-change conditions. As expected, more extreme shifts in respiration rate tend to be associated with greater detection of change. However, critical to these findings is the main effect of change type (gradual or quick) in which the ability to manipulate change detectability, and

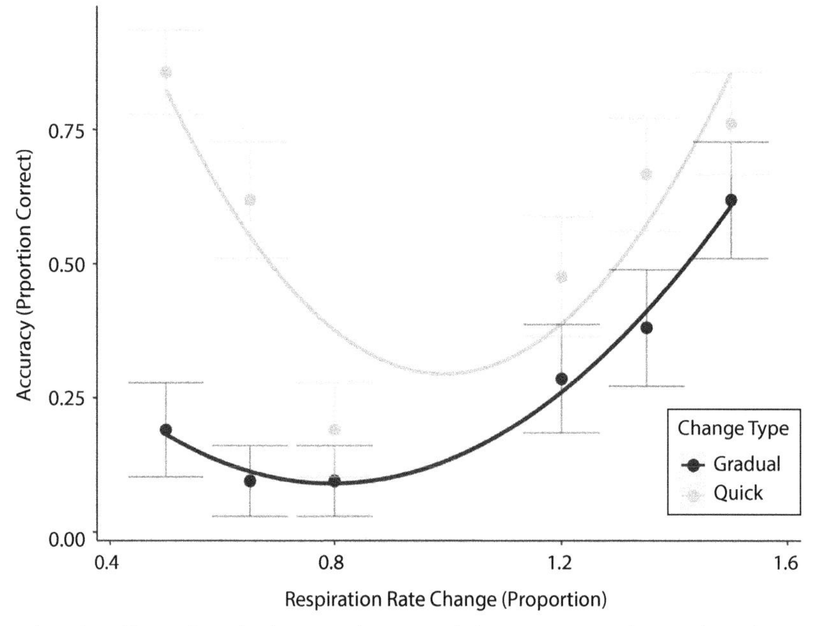

Figure 12.1 The effects of respiration rate change and change type on change detection accuracy.

thereby participant awareness, was demonstrated across various levels of ΔRR. In other words, across all trials participants were less aware of change when it occurred gradually as opposed to quickly. Figure 12.1 also shows that this difference is more pronounced in the trials in which respiration rate was increased compared to decreased.

The ability to examine the effects of interoceptive awareness using a within-participant design affords potential for better understanding of how physiological change and awareness combine to impact cognition across a variety of contexts. The pilot data results support the promise of this paradigm while identifying some areas for improvement. Future piloting will aim to create a more consistent effect of change type in both directions, as the greater accuracy for acceleration than deceleration was unexpected. One solution may be to make trials slightly longer (perhaps ~90 seconds in duration) to allow for more subtle shifts in respiratory rate in the gradual change condition.

12.6.4 Applications

It is important to note that this task is not intended as a measure of interoceptive accuracy but rather a means by which to measure awareness (via the three-alternative forced choice question) and consequences of awareness following experimentally induced changes in respiration rate. As such, it is irrelevant whether or not participants become aware of a change due to visual observation of the circle, or through the physical sense of changing respiration rate. The critical features of the task are instead that: (a) it introduces objectively verifiable changes in physiological states through the manipulation of the respiration rate, and (b) it assesses the presence or absence of awareness of physiological change. The task allows for manipulation of respiration rate independently from the probability of detecting this change. The appraisal consequences of interoceptive awareness of a given level of physiological change could then be measured through measures appended to the task.

There may be several important applications of this experimental design to the assessment of appraisal tendency. There are numerous decisions which may be moderated by awareness of physiological change, with the most obvious being self-appraisal of mood states. Such appraisal can be operationalized simply by asking participants to rate their current subjective mood after each trial. Mood ratings allow for an investigation of the interaction between changes in physiological arousal, manipulated through alterations in the entrained respiration rate, and the awareness of this change, manipulated by the detectability of the respiration change, on subjective appraisals of mood and well-being. Using this task, it may be possible to establish individual differences interoceptive appraisal tendencies, with some participants feeling more anxious following awareness of respiratory acceleration, and some participants feeling more dejected following awareness of respiratory deceleration. Other participants may feel excited or calm following awareness of the same changes. Thus, independent from measurement of interoceptive accuracy, appraisal tendency can become the focus of empirical investigation. Because participants will be generally unaware of the low-detectability change trials, this control condition will allow us to observe the direct effect of physiological change without awareness, isolating the effect of awareness of such changes on subsequent mood ratings and other measures of affect, cognition, and behavior.

As alluded to earlier, our ongoing investigations with this task examine how awareness of respiration change impacts appraisals of mood and subjective well-being. However, the paradigm can also be applied to other forms of decision-making, such as effects on social judgments. There is a substantial literature on the misattribution of arousal in making attractiveness ratings (Payne & Lundberg, 2014). Specifically, trials could be followed by asking participants to rate faces of potential romantic partners or make aesthetic judgment about abstract art. Indeed, anywhere that physiological change has an effect on cognition or behavior, such as choices about food consumption, activity planning, self-assessment of motivation or discomfort, etc., this paradigm may have direct applications. The change in appraisal tendency over time would also be a useful application of this task, with natural extensions in testing the basic tenets of mind–body training techniques such as mindfulness or yoga.

12.7 **Conclusion**

Interoception has long been held to be a central component in our subjective appraisals of well-being. Interoceptive knowledge has been argued to serve as the building blocks of emotional experience (James, 1884, 1890; Lange, 1885), and interoception is thought to be a critical faculty for the ongoing sense of well-being or illness in the body (Farb et al., 2015; Tsakiris & Critchley, 2016; see Chapter 17 in this volume). One of the most intriguing aspects of interoceptive processing is that it often acts at the boundaries of awareness, with more pressing interoceptive signals crossing the threshold for conscious appraisal, whereas other signals may be represented with little to no access to awareness and interpretation.

The rise of mind–body therapies, and their growing evidence base for the treatment of affective disorders, has brought the importance of interoceptive awareness into the spotlight. The ability to adaptively attend and respond to interoceptive signals, and particularly the ability to shift appraisal tendencies away from rigid or dysfunctional patterns of reactivity, is a theoretical cornerstone of many of these interventions and warrants further scientific investigation. By generating more comprehensive, multifaceted assessments of interoceptive awareness, and in particular including assessment of appraisal tendencies in such assessments, it may be possible to translate rich contemplative and clinical accounts of interoception's role into contemporary scientific discourse. In doing so, we may be able to establish the role of interoceptive appraisal in healthy and pathological states with greater care, as well as the mechanisms for restructuring interoceptive access and appraisal to promote greater well-being. It is suggested that innovation is needed to move past unidimensional assessment of interoception through self-report or heart rate monitoring alone, to develop more comprehensive assessment of interoceptive access in relation to mental health. Through novel paradigms such as the one described here, it may be possible to extend substantial progress in characterizing interoceptive accuracy to also experimentally manipulate the roles of awareness and appraisal in responding to interoceptive signals. Together, such efforts will inform our understanding of what it means to engage constructively with the sense of the embodied self.

References

Ainley, V. and **Tsakiris, M.** (2013). Body conscious? Interoceptive awareness, measured by heartbeat perception, is negatively correlated with self-objectification. *PloS One*, *8*(2), e55568.

Andor, T., Gerlach, A. L., and **Rist, F.** (2008). Superior perception of phasic physiological arousal and the detrimental consequences of the conviction to be aroused on worrying and metacognitions in GAD. *Journal of Abnormal Psychology*, *117*(1), 193–205.

Barrett, L. F., Quigley, K. S., and **Hamilton, P.** (2016). An active inference theory of allostasis and interoception in depression. *Philosophical Transactions of the Royal Society B 371*(1708).

Barrett, L. F., Quigley, K. S., Bliss-Moreau, E., and **Aronson, K. R.** (2004). Interoceptive sensitivity and self-reports of emotional experience. *Journal of Personality and Social Psychology*, *87*, 684–97.

Bishop, S. R. (2004). Mindfulness: A proposed operational definition. *Clinical Psychology: Science and Practice*, *11*(3), 230–41.

Brooks, J. C. W., Zambreanu, L., Godinez, A., Craig, A. D., and **Tracey, I.** (2005). Somatotopic organisation of the human insula to painful heat studied with high resolution functional imaging. *Neuroimage*, *27*, 201–9.

Carmody, J. and **Baer, R. A.** (2008). Relationships between mindfulness practice and levels of mindfulness, medical and psychological symptoms and well-being in a mindfulness-based stress reduction program. *Journal of Behavioral Medicine*, *31*(1), 23–33.

Craig, A. D. (2002). How do you feel? Interoception: The sense of the physiological condition of the body. *Nature Reviews Neuroscience*, *3*(8), 655–66.

Craig, A. D. (2003): Interoception: The sense of the physiological condition of the body. *Current Opinions Neurobiology*, *13*, 500–5.

Craig, A. D. (2009). How do you feel—now? The anterior insula and human awareness. *Nature Reviews Neuroscience*, *10*, 59–70.

Critchley, H. D., Wiens, S., Rotshtein, P., Öhman, A., and **Dolan, R. J.** (2004). Neural systems supporting interoceptive awareness. *Nature Neuroscience*, *7*, 189–95.

Critchley, H. D. and **Garfinkel, S. N.** (2017). Interoception and emotion. *Current Opinion in Psychology*, *17*, 7–14.

Damasio, A. and **Carvalho, G. B.** (2013). The nature of feelings: Evolutionary and neurobiological origins. *Nature Reviews Neuroscience*, *14*, 143–52.

Davenport, P. W. and **Kifle, Y.** (2001). Inspiratory resistive load detection in children with life-threatening asthma. *Pediatric Pulmonology*, *32*(1), 44–8.

Domschke, K., Stevens, S., Pfleiderer, B., and **Gerlach, A. L.** (2010). Interoceptive sensitivity in anxiety and anxiety disorders: An overview and integration of neurobiological findings. *Clinical Psychology Review*, *30*, 1–11.

Dunn, B. D., Evans, D., Makarova, D., White, J., and **Clark, L.** (2012). Gut feelings and the reaction to perceived inequity: The interplay between bodily responses, regulation, and perception shapes the rejection of unfair offers on the ultimatum game. *Cognitive, Affective, & Behavioral Neuroscience*, *12*(3), 419–29.

Farb, N. A. S., Segal, Z. V., Mayberg, H., Bean, J., Mckeon, D., Fatima, Z., et al. (2007). Attending to the present: Mindfulness meditation reveals distinct neural modes of self-reference. *Social Cognitive and Affective Neuroscience*, *2*(4), 313–22.

Farb, N. A., Anderson, A. K., Mayberg, H., Bean, J., McKeon, D., and **Segal, Z. V.** (2010). Minding one's emotions: Mindfulness training alters the neural expression of sadness. *Emotion*, *10*(1), 25–33.

Farb, N. A., **Segal, Z. V.**, and **Anderson, A. K.** (2013a). Attentional modulation of primary interoceptive and exteroceptive cortices. *Cerebral Cortex*, *23*(1), 114–26.

Farb, N. A., **Segal, Z. V.**, and **Anderson, A. K.** (2013b). Mindfulness meditation training alters cortical representations of interoceptive attention. *Social Cognitive and Affective Neuroscience*, *8*(1), 15–26.

Farb, N. A. S. (2014). From retreat center to clinic to boardroom? Perils and promises of the modern mindfulness movement. *Religions*, *5*, 1062–86.

Farb, N. A. S., **Daubenmier, J.**, **Price, C. J.**, **Gard, T.**, **Kerr, C.**, **Dunn, B. D.**, et al. (2015). Interoception, contemplative practice, and health. *Frontiers in Psychology*, *7*(1898), 1–26.

Farias, M., **Wikholm, C.**, and **Delmonte, R.** (2016). What is mindfulness-based therapy good for? *Lancet Psychiatry*, *3*(11), 1012–13.

Garfinkel, S. N., **Seth, A. K.**, **Barrett, A. B.**, **Suzuki, K.**, and **Critchley, H. D.** (2015). Knowing your own heart: Distinguishing interoceptive accuracy from interoceptive awareness. *Biological Psychology*, *104*, 65–74.

Goyal, M., **Singh, S.**, **Sibinga, E. M.**, **Gould, N. F.**, **Rowland-Seymour, A.**, **Sharma, R.**, et al. (2014). Meditation programs for psychological stress and well-being: A systematic review and meta-analysis. *JAMA Internal Medicine*, *174*(3), 357–68.

Gu, X., **Hof, P. R.**, **Friston, K. J.**, and **Fan, J.** (2013), Anterior insular cortex and emotional awareness. *Journal of Comparative Neurology*, *521*, 3371–88.

Hackley, S. A. and **Valle-Inclán, F.** (1999). Accessory stimulus effects on response selection: Does arousal speed decision making? *Journal of Cognitive Neuroscience*, *11*(3), 321–9.

Harver, A., **Katkin, E. S.**, and **Bloch, E.** (1993). Signal-detection outcomes on heartbeat and respiratory resistance detection tasks in male and female subjects. *Psychophysiology*, *30*, 223–30.

Herbert, B. M., **Pollatos, O.**, and **Schandry, R.** (2007). Interoceptive sensitivity and emotion processing: An EEG study. *International Journal of Psychophysiology*, *65*, 214–27.

Hillyard, S. A., **Vogel, E. K.**, and **Luck, S. J.** (1998). Sensory gain control (amplification) as a mechanism of selective attention: Electrophysiological and neuroimaging evidence. *Philosophical Transactions of the Royal Society B*, *353*(1373), 1257–70.

Jabbi, M., **Bastiaansen, J.**, and **Keysers, C.** (2008). A common anterior insula representation of disgust observation, experience and imagination shows divergent functional connectivity pathways. *PloS One*, *3*(8), e2939.

James, W. (1884). What is emotion? *Mind*, *9*, 188–205.

James, W. (1890). *Principles of Psychology*. New York, NY: Holt.

Kabat-Zinn, J. (2009). *Full Catastrophe Living: Using the Wisdom of your Body and Mind to Face Stress, Pain, and Illness*. New York, NY: Ballantine Bantam Dell.

Katkin, E., **Wiens, S.**, and **Öhman, A.** (2001). Nonconscious Fear Conditioning, Visceral Perception, and the Development of Gut Feelings. *Psychological Science*, *12*(5), 366–70.

Kearney, C. A., **Albano, A. M.**, **Eisen, A. R.**, **Allan, W. D.**, and **Barlow, D. H.** (1997). The phenomenology of panic disorder in youngsters: An empirical study of a clinical sample. *Journal of Anxiety Disorders*, *11*(1), 49–62.

Khalsa, S. S. and **Lapidus, R. C.** (2016). Can interoception improve the pragmatic search for biomarkers in psychiatry? *Frontiers in Psychiatry*, *7*(121), 1–19.

Lange, C. G. (1885). The mechanism of the emotions. *The Classical Psychologists*. Boston, MA: Houghton Mifflin, pp. 672–84.

Lazar, S. W., **Kerr, C. E.**, **Wasserman, R. H.**, **Gray, J. R.**, **Greve, D. N.**, **Treadway, M. T.**, et al. (2005). Meditation experience is associated with increased cortical thickness. *Neuroreport*, *16*(17), 1893–7.

Merwin, R. M., **Zucker, N. L.**, **Lacy, J. L.**, and **Elliott, C. A.** (2010). Interoceptive awareness in eating disorders: Distinguishing lack of clarity from non-acceptance of internal experience. *Cognition and Emotion*, *24*(5), 892–902.

Naragon-Gainey, K., McMahon, T. P., and **Chacko, T. P.** (2017). The structure of common emotion regulation strategies: A meta-analytic examination. *Psychological Bulletin, 143*(4), 384–427.

Olson, J. M. (1988). Misattribution, preparatory information, and speech anxiety. *Journal of Personality and Social Psychology, 54*(5), 758.

Paulus, M. P. and **Stein, M. B.** (2006). An insular view of anxiety. *Biological Psychiatry, 60*(4), 383–7.

Paulus, M. P. and **Stein, M. B.** (2010). Interoception in anxiety and depression. *Brain Structure and Function, 214*(5-6), 451–63.

Payne, K. and **Lundberg, K.** (2014). The affect misattribution procedure: Ten years of evidence on reliability, validity, and mechanisms. *Social and Personality Psychology Compass, 8*(12), 672–86.

Pinheiro, J., Bates, D., DebRoy, S., Sarkar, D., and **R Core Team** (2016). nlme: Linear and Nonlinear Mixed Effects Models. R package version 3.1-131.1. <http://CRAN.R-project.org/package=nlme>

Pollatos, O., Schandry, R., Auer, D. P., and **Kaufmann, C.** (2007). Brain structures mediating cardiovascular arousal and interoceptive awareness. *Brain Research, 1141*, 178–87.

Quattrocki, E. and **Friston, K.** (2014). Autism, oxytocin and interoception. *Neuroscience & Biobehavioral Reviews, 47*, 410–30.

R Core Team (2014). *R: A language and environment for statistical computing*. Vienna: R Foundation for Statistical Computing. <http://www.R-project.org/>

Raffone, A. and **Srinivasan, N.** (2010). The exploration of meditation in the neuroscience of attention and consciousness. *Cognitive Processing, 11*(1), 1–7.

Rouder, J. N. and **Morey, R. D.** (2009). The nature of psychological thresholds. *Psychological Review, 116*(3), 655–60.

Schachter, S. and **Singer, J.** (1962). Cognitive, social, and physiological determinants of emotional state. *Psychological Review, 69*(5), 379.

Segal, Z. V., Williams, J. M. G., and **Teasdale, J. D.** (2012). *Mindfulness-based Cognitive Therapy for Depression*. New York, NY: Guilford Press.

Seth, A. K. and **Friston, K. J.** (2016). Active interoceptive inference and the emotional brain. *Philosophical Transactions of the Royal Society B, 371*(1708).

Silani, G., Bird, G., Brindley, R., Singer, T., Frith, C., and **Frith, U.** (2008). Levels of emotional awareness and autism: An fMRI study. *Social Neuroscience, 3*(2), 97–112.

Stein, M. B., Simmons, A. N., Feinstein, J. S., and **Paulus, M. P.** (2007). Increased amygdala and insula activation during emotion processing in anxiety-prone subjects. *American Journal of Psychiatry, 164*(2), 318–27.

Strigo, I. A. and **Craig, A. D.** (2016). Interoception, homeostatic emotions and sympathovagal balance. *Philosophical Transactions of the Royal Society Bs, 371*(1708).

Strigo, I. A., Simmons, A. N., Matthews, S. C., Arthur, D., and **Paulus, M. P.** (2008). Association of major depressive disorder with altered functional brain response during anticipation and processing of heat pain. *Archives of General Psychiatry, 65*(11), 1275–84.

Tsakiris, M. and **Critchley, H.** (2016). Interoception beyond homeostasis: Affect, cognition and mental health. *Philosophical Transactions of the Royal Society B, 371*(1708).

White, G. L., Fishbein, S., and **Rutsein, J.** (1981). Passionate love and the misattribution of arousal. *Journal of Personality and Social Psychology, 41*(1), 56.

Wright, C. I., Martis, B., McMullin, K., Shin, L. M., and **Rauch, S. L.** (2003). Amygdala and insular responses to emotionally valenced human faces in small animal specific phobia. *Biological Psychiatry, 54*(10), 1067–76.

Zanna, M. P. and **Cooper, J.** (1974). Dissonance and the pill: An attribution approach to studying the arousal properties of dissonance. *Journal of Personality and Social Psychology, 29*(5), 703–9.

PART IV

Toward a philosophy of interoception

Subjectivity and experience

Chapter 13

From physiology to experience: Enriching existing conceptions of "arousal" in affective science

Giovanna Colombetti and Neil Harrison

13.1 Introduction

"Arousal" is a key notion in the interdisciplinary field of "affective science", which includes primarily the psychology and neuroscience of emotion, but also philosophical and computational approaches to emotion (Davidson, Scherer, & Goldsmith, 2003; Scarantino, forthcoming). Roughly and preliminarily, we can say that "arousal" refers to how more or less "excited" or "activated" one is during an emotion; for example, someone who is very scared is often said to be highly aroused, whereas sadness and contentment are often regarded as involving low degrees of arousal. Several affective scientists regard arousal not just as an important dimension of emotion, but even as a necessary one: part of what it is to be in an emotional state is to be more or less aroused (e.g. Russell, 2003). Importantly for the topic of this volume, arousal is often regarded as interlinked with interoception.

What is it to be aroused during an emotion, exactly? As it turns out, no short definition can capture the various meanings that the term "arousal" has in affective science; moreover, these different meanings are often not clearly discriminated (Colombetti & Kuppens, forthcoming). One goal of this chapter is to bring some clarity by distinguishing the two main meanings of this term; that is, what we call *physiological* and *experienced* arousal.[1] Another goal is to clarify the relationship between these two meanings of arousal, and interoception, understood broadly as "sensitivity to stimuli arising inside the organism"—where "sensitivity" does not necessarily entail conscious perception. In particular, we argue that it is restrictive and inaccurate to reduce physiological arousal to a single dimension of sympathetic activation, or even to just autonomic activation[2] (psychological

[1] In this chapter we limit our analysis to arousal as a component or dimension of emotion and other affective states, such as moods.

[2] "Autonomic activation" commonly refers to activation of the autonomic nervous system (ANS). The ANS is a division of the peripheral nervous system, and is itself divided into the sympathetic and the parasympathetic nervous system. The other two divisions of the peripheral nervous system are the somatic nervous system, which controls the voluntary muscles and more generally the musculoskeletal system, and the enteric nervous system, which both alone and together with the ANS controls activity within the gastrointestinal tract. Until recently the enteric nervous system was regarded as a part of the ANS; it is now recognized as a mainly independent system.

studies that include "physiological measurements," for example, often measure only a few dimensions of autonomic activation, such as skin conductance responses, heart rate, and blood pressure; see Fox, 2008, pp. 32–4). As for experienced arousal, we argue, relatedly, that it is restrictive and inaccurate to reduce it to the conscious perception of organismic changes signalled just via visceral afferents (the afferent partner of the autonomic nervous system). Experienced arousal, we suggest, additionally includes the perception of circulating substances mediated via humoral interoceptive pathways, as well as various somatic sensations and what we call "background bodily feelings."

13.2 **Two main meanings of "arousal"**

In contemporary affective science, "arousal" has two main meanings. First, it refers to what we term *experienced arousal*, the lived, first-personal, or subjective experience of being (more or less) aroused during an emotion. Second, it refers to what we term *physiological arousal*, the third-personal or objective biological processes that occur in the organism during an emotion. These two meanings of arousal are clearly different but they are sometimes conflated, and it is often assumed that experienced arousal provides veridical information about physiological arousal. For example, Scherer and Wallbott (1994) addressed the question of whether at least some emotions exhibit the same patterns of "physiological symptoms" (their term) across cultures. To do this, they used questionnaires that asked participants how they felt their body when experiencing various emotions, but did not actually record any physiological measurements. Likewise, Grewe, Nagel, Kopiez, and Altenmuller (2007) studied "physiological responses" to music with questionnaires asking participants to "report their perceived bodily reactions" (p. 779). They actually also measured physiological responses to music in the form of skin conductance and facial muscle activity. Throughout the paper, however, they conflate "physiological changes" with "reported (or experienced) physiological changes." More recently, Nummenmaa, Glerean, Hari, and Hietanen (2014) identified different "bodily sensations maps" for 13 different emotions. Although they make it clear that this study was about experienced arousal, they assume throughout their paper that bodily sensations "represent" (their term) physiological processes.

How experienced arousal relates to physiological arousal, however, needs to be assessed empirically. Suppose you are feeling very agitated (experienced arousal) as part of being worried about an imminent job interview. Your feeling of agitation may include specific sensations such as feeling your heart pounding heavily in your chest, and your mouth and throat being dry. Now, it is natural and not implausible in this case to think that your heart is in fact beating differently from when you are calmer, and that your mouth and throat are in fact drier (physiological arousal). Whether this is really the case, however, needs to be confirmed by conducting actual measurements on the state of your heart, mouth, and throat. One cannot simply infer the physiological condition of any specific body part from how the person feels, for a variety of reasons. One is that the person's reports of her bodily feelings may be influenced by "social schemata" (Rimé, Philippot, & Cisamolo, 1990), that is, learnt templates of how one is expected to feel in specific situations. Another reason is that there are individual differences in how accurately people can perceive their actual bodily changes (usually measured with heartbeat detection tasks)—a capacity termed "interoceptive accuracy" (Garfinkel et al., 2015). Furthermore, the same person can be more or less accurate depending on the task performed, context, stress, etc. (Schulz et al., 2013). Finally, even though some of us can, at times, accurately feel what is going on in some parts of our body, there is much going on in our body that is inaccessible consciously (Critchley & Harrison, 2013). For example, we cannot feel our pupils dilating or our blood pressure rising. Thus, how bodily aroused a person feels (experienced arousal) provides at best only a partial look into her physiological arousal. At worst, it provides an inaccurate or distorted view of the latter.

The upshot is that we need to distinguish clearly between the subjective experience, or feeling, of being aroused, excited, or activated (all terms found in the literature and used as synonyms), and what is actually going on in the organism during an emotional episode. Having clarified this, let us now examine both phenomena more closely.

13.3 **Physiological arousal**

That our organism often undergoes physiological changes during emotional episodes is something we can easily witness, and often do: we see our hands shaking when we are nervous, and a mirror can show our skin getting red when we are embarrassed. This is such a commonplace observation that it is not surprising to find it in ancient philosophical texts. At the beginning of *De Anima*, for example, Aristotle noted that in "anger, mildness, fear, pity, hope and even joy and love and hating . . . the body is affected in some way" (1986, p. 128). The Stoics and Galen also recognized the contribution of the body to our emotional states (Gill, 2010).

There is thus a sense in which we have always known that our body gets more or less "excited" during different emotions. It is worth noting, though, that contemporary empirical studies of emotion typically measure physiological arousal by measuring something very specific, that is, changes in the organism ascribed (sometimes incorrectly) to activation of the *sympathetic* division of the ANS, such as increases in heart rate and skin conductance, alterations in skin temperature, and pupillary dilation (Berntson & Cacioppo, 2009).[3] Walter Cannon famously associated the sympathetic nervous system with the "fight or flight response," and the narrow identification of physiological arousal with sympathetic activation can be traced back to the work on fear and rage he conducted in the 1910s and 1920s (Cannon, 1929). Cannon also conceptualized sympathetic activation as mutually exclusive with, and antagonistic to, activation of the parasympathetic system, whose contribution to emotion he generally disregarded. Finally, Cannon is also

[3] Acute increases in heart rate and pupil size are actually initiated by a withdrawal in parasympathetic tone (Robinson et al., 1966; Barbur, 2004).

responsible for characterizing sympathetic activation as generally uniform and undifferentiated. Though these ideas were challenged by Cannon's contemporaries (see Dror, 2014), they influenced scientific conceptions of arousal throughout the twentieth century, and still do so. Most famously, Schachter and Singer (1962, pp. 381–2) maintained that the same state of (sympathetic) physiological arousal (induced using an adrenaline injection) "could be labelled 'joy' or 'fury' or 'jealousy' or any of a great diversity of emotional labels depending on the cognitive aspects of the situation." These authors also suggested (despite previous studies to the contrary, e.g. Ax, 1953; Wolf & Wolff, 1947), that "emotional states may . . . be generally characterized by a high level of sympathetic activation with few if any physiological distinguishers among the many emotional states" (Schachter & Singer, 1962, pp. 397).

Our view is that this conception of arousal during emotion is superseded and too narrow, and needs to be abandoned, for the following four reasons.

1. The term "autonomic nervous system" (ANS) and its division into sympathetic and para- (meaning "by the side of," "alongside") sympathetic components was introduced by Langley (1900) on the basis of predominantly neuroanatomical, rather than functional, considerations. To talk of global sympathetic and parasympathetic functions (e.g. fight and flight versus rest and digest) has the potential to generate misunderstandings and to create an overly simplistic impression of the functional architecture of the ANS (for more details, see Harrison, Kreibig, & Critchley, 2013). For example, empirical data acquired over the last half-century show that pre- and postganglionic neurons of both the sympathetic and parasympathetic nervous system link together in multiple *functionally distinct pathways* that facilitate the generation of a huge variety of highly differentiated and specific responses (Jänig, 2006). This has undermined previous false assumptions that sympathetic preganglionic neurons diverge widely and synapse with postganglionic neurons with multiple diverse functions, dispelling the belief that the sympathetic nervous system operates in a monolithic all-or-nothing fashion. This research also demonstrates that the ANS can support emotion-specific physiological patterning.
2. A consideration that invites broadening the traditional conception of physiological arousal is that autonomic activation is also influenced by afferent (from periphery to brain) neural and humoral feedback pathways (for details see Critchley & Harrison, 2013). Visceral afferent fibers innervate almost all tissues of the body and fall into two broad groups: first, those that carry motivational information such as hunger, satiety, thirst, nausea, and respiratory sensations, and travel mainly along cranial (e.g. vagus and glossopharyngeal) nerves to terminate within the nucleus of the solitary tract; second, spinal visceral afferents that project to the dorsal horns of the spinal cord and, via spinal laminar 1, into the spinothalamic tract. These fibers tend to have a more prominent role in signalling tissue damage. Humoral feedback is largely processed through the circumventricular organs (regions of the brain that lack a normal blood-brain barrier), though some (e.g. core temperature, glucose, and insulin) can also

be sensed directly within brain regions such as the hypothalamus. Additionally, inflammatory mediators can modulate brain function through microglial transduction pathways, resulting in a wave of microglial activation that propagates across the brain (Rivest, 2009; Saper, Romanovsky, & Scammell, 2012). Efferent activation is continuously modulated by this afferent, "interoceptive" feedback, so that it is misleading to restrict autonomic arousal occurring during emotion only to the outcome of neural efferent processes without including the continuous regulatory afferent feedback that co-occurs with those processes.

3. A further and partly related challenge to narrow conceptions of physiological arousal comes from psychoneuroendocrinology and psychoneuroimmunology. Developments in these fields have shown that the central and peripheral nervous system bi-directionally interact with both endocrine and immune processes, and that these interactions influence, and are influenced by, our emotional states. We know for example that the stress response includes the release of hormones from the brain into the adrenal glands and the bloodstream, which in turn influence hypothalamic-pituitary activity in the brain (Charmandari, Tsigos, & Chrousos, 2005; Spiga et al., 2015). We also know that during illness, the immune system produces pro-inflammatory proteins (cytokines) that influence brain activity (Harrison, 2017) and that appear to play a contributory role in at least some patients with depression (Dantzer et al., 2008); in turn, the brain responds by sending signals to inhibit this inflammatory process (Tracey, 2002). Given this bi-directional interactivity, in our view it is arbitrary to identify arousal with activation of any one system alone (the ANS, the endocrine system, etc.), or of any subset of it. Bi-directional interactivity also implies that it would still be arbitrary to regard the ANS (or any other system alone) as the "most relevant" or "most basic" arousal system, with the other systems making only a "peripheral contribution" to arousal. The existence of reciprocal influences entails that the systems involved are coupled, such that without additional criteria or reasons, no system alone can be picked out as the one having the causally most relevant role. In the presence of this complexity, we think it more plausible to regard the combined activity of all systems involved as constituting physiological arousal.

The reason why endocrine and immune changes are generally not included in definitions of physiological arousal may have to do with the widespread assumption, in affective science, that emotions are short-lived episodes that involve brief but intense changes in the body. Changes in the endocrine and immune systems are typically regarded to unfold on a longer time frame, and thus arguably do not qualify as candidates for arousal. Indeed, sometimes arousal in emotion is explicitly characterized as "phasic" (temporary, short-lived; see e.g. Fowles, 2009, p. 50), which excludes longer-lasting physiological processes (see also Bradley & Lang, 2007, p. 601). However, it is not obvious that emotions are always short lived: whereas sometimes we are upset, annoyed, or scared for a few seconds or minutes, we are also often upset, annoyed, or scared (as well as jealous, envious, angry, happy, and so on) for hours or even longer. Arousal, in the latter cases, may well involve physiological processes that unfold and change over hours or even days. Moreover, it is not just emotions, defined as short-lived affective episodes, that involve a certain level of arousal; moods, often characterized as lasting longer than emotions, also do (see Thayer, 1996). Perhaps, one might suggest, the main difference between emotions and moods is precisely that, in the former, physiological arousal corresponds to brief patterns of activation of the ANS, whereas in the latter it also involves longer-lasting endocrine and immune changes.[4] This is in part, of course, an empirical question, yet, importantly, emotions typically occur in the context of a mood that makes some emotions more likely than others (e.g. one is more likely to get angry at someone when in an irritable mood); the physiological profile of a certain mood is thus likely to affect one of these emotions so that short-lived activation of the ANS would occur in a specific endocrine and immune context, which should then be regarded as part and parcel of the physiological arousal profile of the emotions in question.

4. Yet another challenge to narrow conceptions of physiological arousal comes from research on the bacteria that live in our organism. They are found in almost all parts of the body, with the highest concentration in the guts. The human guts contain nearly 10^{14}–10^{15} bacteria, which is 10–100 times the number of eukaryotic cells of the human organism (10^{13}). The many different functions of these bacteria have only recently begun to be revealed. Importantly, we now know that they influence, and are influenced by, the central nervous system, along the so-called microbiota-gut–brain axis. Particularly relevant for present purposes is recent evidence indicating that stress-related mood disorders, such as anxiety and depression, alter the composition of gut bacteria, and that, in turn, the composition of gut bacteria influences those states (for reviews, see Cryan & Dinan, 2012; Foster & McVey Neufeld, 2013; Mayer et al., 2014). In a landmark study on mice, Sudo, Chida, Aiba, and colleagues (2004) showed that gut microbiota influence the development of the hypothalamic-pituitary-adrenal system, responsible for the endocrine response to stress. Since then, further evidence has been gathered indicating that, in humans too, microbiota influence brain processes and behaviors relevant to anxiety-related stress disorders, and even individuals' susceptibility to depression (see reviews listed earlier for references). This influence appears to occur via neural, hormonal, and immune routes: many of the effects of gut microbiota on brain and behavior are dependent on activation of visceral afferents travelling in the vagus nerve; gut microbiota also generate neurotransmitters and neuromodulators known to influence mood, such as GABA, serotonin, noradrenaline, dopamine, and acetylcholine; and gut microbiota can also influence circulating levels of pro-inflammatory cytokines produced by innate immune cells which, as we saw, affect brain function. Less is known about the relation between microbiota and

[4] Thanks again to an anonymous reviewer for raising this possibility.

short-lived emotions, but given the influence of moods on the latter, microbiota are likely to influence them as well.

Conceptually, this body of work raises the question of where the natural boundaries of physiological arousal lie: what is the physical entity that gets aroused? The more conservative answer is that physiological arousal recruits subsystems and processes of the organism "traditionally conceived" (i.e. formed by cells with the same DNA), and that gut microbiota are different living forms (cells with different DNA) that causally influence those subsystems and processes. In other words, bacteria are not part of the organism, and thus not of physiological arousal either; rather, they constitute an external context that modulates, and is modulated by, the organism "proper." A less intuitive, yet arguably more coherent, answer is that gut microbiota can be constitutive parts of the physiological arousal that characterizes affective processes. The reasoning is the same we applied earlier to the recognition of the existence of reciprocal influences between the sympathetic and parasympathetic system, and more generally between the central nervous system (CNS), ANS, endocrine, and immune systems: given the complex mutual relations interconnecting all these systems and the gut microbiota, it is arguably conceptually problematic and even arbitrary to maintain that only processes of the organism traditionally conceived can constitute physiological arousal, and that microbial processes are mere external factors or extrinsic (non-constitutive) causes. Rather, it seems more coherent to regard microbiotic processes as constitutive of physiological arousal.

In sum, together these four sets of considerations indicate that it is misleading to regard physiological arousal during an emotion as a temporary upsurge from a baseline state of "non-aroused physiology" of the organism traditionally conceived. Our physiology (i.e. the totality of the processes that contribute to sustaining our living condition) is continuously changing and shifting, with the CNS influencing, and being influenced by, a multitude of processes taking place at many different timescales in the (various divisions of) the peripheral nervous system, the endocrine and immune systems, and even beyond them.

13.4 **Experienced arousal**

Let us now take a closer look at the notion of experienced, or subjective, arousal. Again, we can begin by noting that there is nothing surprising or controversial in claiming that during some emotions we feel more agitated or excited than during others. Indeed, that emotions can vary in how upset or excited one feels was noted long before the birth of modern psychology. Just to mention a few examples, the Stoics distinguished the "passions" from the "good emotions," where the former are intense and overwhelming, and the latter are calm and under control (Graver, 2007). Later, and possibly under the influence of the Stoics, in his *Treatise of Human Nature* (2003 [1739–40]) David Hume distinguished the violent passions from the calm ones. The calm passions include the moral sentiments and the aesthetic sense, which cause "no disorder in the soul" (*Treatise*,

2.3.3.8) and are known more by their effects than by any immediate feeling; the violent passions (love, hate, grief, joy, pride, humility), on the other hand, are characterized by the felt quality of "turbulence."[5]

As for contemporary affective science, Jim Russell, for example, characterizes arousal as "one's sense of mobilization and energy" (Russell, 2003, p. 148). Similarly, Fox (2008, p. 120) writes that "*arousal* or *activation* are often interpreted as the amount of energy we feel we have available." A recent neuroscientific paper defines arousal as "the degree of activation experienced during an instance of emotion, ranging from calm to excited" (Kragel & LaBar, 2016, p. 445).

Whereas it is relatively uncontroversial to say that we feel more or less activated during an emotion, it is surprisingly hard to specify *what it is* to feel more or less activated, energized, mobilized, and/or under the control of a "turbulent passion." A common view (consistent with the popular identification, discussed in the section 13.3, of "physiological arousal" with autonomic or even sympathetic activation) is to characterize experienced arousal as the conscious perception of bodily changes induced by the ANS.[6] According to this view, to feel aroused during an episode of fear, for example, is to feel one's own heart beating fast, or one's own skin sweating profusely or changing temperature (famously, this view was originally proposed by James, 1884; it is still influential today. See e.g. references at the beginning of section 13.2).

Intuitively, it indeed seems to be the case that these sensations contribute to feeling aroused during an emotion, and also that they contribute to the felt *intensity* of arousal: the more (less, respectively) one feels certain parts of one's body, the more (less) aroused one feels. By analogy, at first glance at least, this appears to be what happens when one feels sexually aroused, which partly involves feeling changes in erogenous areas of the body controlled by the ANS: the "more" one feels those areas, the more sexually aroused one feels.[7] Similarly, it would seem, in the case of arousal during an emotion. Moreover, the more aroused one feels, the less in control one feels; the traditionally recognized overwhelming character of a passion, in other words, appears to owe much to the uncontrollable nature of visceral sensations of autonomic origin. Finally, in addition to contributing to the intensity of experienced arousal, these sensations also appear to contribute to the intensity of an emotional experience. Back in 1964, Schachter had already proposed that experienced arousal contributes to felt emotional intensity. Relatedly, Wiens, Mezzacappa, and Katkin (2000) showed that subjects who are better

[5] See Dixon (2003) for a historical overview of other philosophical accounts that distinguished the 'unruly passions' from the calmer 'affects' or 'affections'.

[6] In the rest of the chapter we call these, for lack of a better term, visceral sensations "of autonomic origin" or "due to the ANS," to distinguish them from other visceral sensations due to the interoception of substances circulating in the blood stream (as described in section 13.3).

[7] But note that feelings of sexual arousal are likely mediated by a combination of visceral and somatic afferents.

at perceiving their physiological arousal and report more subjective arousal also experience emotions more intensely.

In our view, this is a plausible but still *partial* account of what it is to feel aroused during an emotion. Similar to the case of physiological arousal discussed in the section 13.3, to regard experienced arousal as constituted only by sensations of bodily changes induced by the ANS is too narrow, and does not account for other ways in which we can feel aroused during an emotion; in particular: (a) some visceral sensations are due to the interoception of substances circulating in the bloodstream; (b) non-visceral somatic sensations also contribute to feeling aroused; and (c) experienced arousal also appears to involve conscious experiences that are not feelings *of* bodily changes. We already discussed the first point briefly in section 13.3.2. Here we consider the other two points in turn.

1. William James (1884) already noted that emotional experience also involves the perception of bodily changes mediated by the somatic nervous system (the division of the peripheral nervous system that controls the musculoskeletal system; see footnote 2). We can call them "somatic sensations." Important somatic sensations that contribute to feeling aroused come from facial expressions (smiling, frowning, pouting, grinning, and so on) and from bodily posture, and also include felt urges to act in specific ways. For example, feeling angry and anxious often involves the conscious perception of one's tense facial muscles (such as tense jaws and/or forehead) and other bodily muscles (especially in the upper back, neck, and shoulders); feeling sad often involves feeling one's drooping jaws and eye corners, slouched posture, and so on.

In addition, feeling aroused during an emotion often involves the experience of wanting to move one way or the other (felt urges to act). This experience partly constitutes the motivational aspect of emotion. For example, during an aggressive face-to-face confrontation, we may experience wanting to shout at, or even physically attack, the person we are angry at. Most of the time in this kind of scenario we repress our outward behavior because of social rules, yet even if we do not assail the opponent, the urge to do so is there and is felt in one's own body tensing up, preparing to attack, and restraining itself. Note that, especially in the moment, we may not be able to clearly discriminate these felt urges to act from other types of sensations (e.g. the angry person may also feel her heart pounding hard). Similar considerations readily apply to experiences of fear, great joy, contempt, pride, jealousy, and many others. In affective science, the term that best captures this aspect of emotion experience is *action readiness awareness* (Frijda, 1986, pp. 231–40). "Action readiness," as the word indicates, refers to a state of being ready to act in a certain way. The awareness of this state is a bodily feeling, in the sense that it involves the conscious perception of one's own body, constituted by proprioceptive sensations of position, and state of tension or calmness. As in the case of visceral sensations of autonomic origin, felt urges to act appear to contribute significantly to experienced arousal during an emotion, and also to the intensity of the emotion: for example, the more I want to shout at someone, the more aroused, agitated, or upset I feel as part of my experience of anger, and arguably also the "more angry" or "more intensely angry" I feel.

2. The other reason why experienced arousal during emotion cannot be reduced to perception of bodily changes due to the ANS is that it arguably includes also conscious states that are not feelings of bodily changes. This possibility splits into two: (a) experienced arousal includes non-bodily experiences; that is, experiences with no "bodily phenomenology"; (b) experienced emotional arousal involves bodily feelings that are not feelings *of* the body but feelings of the world shaped *through* bodily self-awareness; here, experienced emotional arousal does include bodily phenomenology, but this remains "in the background," as we explain in the following.

According to (a), it is possible to be highly aroused during an emotion without feeling one's own body. Mostly philosophers supporting a cognitivist view of emotions tend to make this claim. For example, Claire Armon-Jones (1986, p. 51) writes: "whether or not I feel any twinges or palpitations, if my thoughts are totally consumed by a 'strong desire for an object which I do not possess and which belongs to another', then I can be said to feel 'extremely envious'." According to this view, one can be very worried that his child might have a life-threatening condition, for example, without experiencing any bodily sensation (neither visceral nor somatic). What constitutes feeling worried, here, is likely to be the conscious thoughts that one's child may suffer and die young, say, with the frequency and disruptive character of these thoughts determining the level of experienced arousal. Uriah Kriegel's (2015) recent account of emotional phenomenology also supports this possibility. In his view, emotional experience is reducible to a combination of cognitive, conative, and algedonic (pain–pleasure) phenomenology, none of which, he argues, necessarily involves bodily feelings. He briefly suggests that conative phenomenology contributes to felt emotional intensity (2015, p. 135), however not in virtue of any bodily sensation.

Our view is that possibility (a) is implausible. Although it is the case that "cognitive phenomenology" (thoughts, predictions, memories) can constitute much of our experience of being aroused during an emotion, it is not clear to us that it is deprived of any bodily phenomenology. We think that cognitivist accounts of this sort overlook possibility (b), that is, the existence of bodily feelings that are not feelings *of* the body but experiences of the body *through* which certain aspects of the world (one's current situation, imagined future events, etc.) are experienced as emotionally salient (see also Colombetti, 2014, Chapter 5); because these bodily experiences are often subtle and inconspicuous, they can be mistaken for "purely mental" (Kriegel, 2015, p. 89). To illustrate this second possibility, consider again Armon-Jones's example of her experience of an alleged "non-bodily" envy. As she describes this case, she says that her thoughts "are totally consumed by a 'strong desire for an object which I do not possess and which belongs to another,' " and that these thoughts exhaust her experience of envy. However, it does not seem to be phenomenologically accurate to say that one can be "totally consumed" by a "strong desire" (note the intensity of the described experience) for an object without *any* bodily phenomenology. Even if we grant that the desired object is quite abstract (e.g. respect and admiration, rather than a new modern kitchen) and that being "totally consumed" by a desire for it consists in cognitive rumination, it seems inaccurate to maintain that bodily feelings are entirely absent from this experience. In particular, we suggest that the experience of envy, for example, is shaped by inconspicuous *background* bodily feelings that "color" what the person attends to in her thoughts and ruminations (much like looking through a colored pair of lenses makes the world show up as colored, while the lenses themselves are not noted, and are rather that *through* which the world appears tinted). These background bodily feelings may not be noted by the envious person but they nevertheless contribute to feelings of tension and unpleasantness that, arguably, partly constitute the experience of envy described by Armon-Jones. In addition, emotional experiences typically take place in the context of more general mood experiences—such as feeling up or down, sluggish or energized, tense or calm (Thayer, 1996). These feelings, we propose, are bodily feelings that constitute a "background bodily phenomenology" against which the occurrent emotional experiences can stand out (in the foreground).[8] So, even if one granted that, sometimes at least, emotional experiences include primarily "purely mental" cognitive or conative phenomenology, it would still be the case that bodily feelings constituting background moods shape and structure what is in the foreground. Taken together, these considerations complement, at the experiential level, the point we made in section 13.3 about the existence of several bi-directional pathways between brain and body, such that it does not seem possible to "silence" all sources of feedback from the body.

13.5 **Conclusion**

In sum, then, in this chapter we have argued that the notion of arousal used in affective science needs to be characterized broadly, both at the physiological and experiential level, and cannot be reduced to narrow conceptions of interoception limited to the perception (conscious and not) of ANS activation. At the physiological level, we need to move beyond Cannon's (1929) and Schachter and Singer's (1962) conceptualization of arousal as a uniform pattern of sympathetic activation. The sympathetic and parasympathetic systems are complexly interrelated and work together to generate specific patterns of autonomic arousal; additionally, autonomic activity includes not just neural efferent processes but is also influenced by afferent neural and humoral feedback. Third, autonomic activation does not happen in isolation from other bodily processes, rather it is complexly interrelated via bi-directional pathways with the CNS and the endocrine and immune system. Fourth, we suggested that the notion of physiological arousal may be extended even beyond processes taking place within the organism traditionally conceived, so as to include (at least) those gut bacteria known to influence and be influenced by neural, endocrine, and immune processes relevant to emotions and moods.

At the experiential level, we have argued that arousal cannot be reduced to visceral sensations of autonomic origin but instead additionally includes perception of circulating substances mediated via humoral interoceptive pathways as well as specific somatic

[8] See also Damasio (1999) for the related notion of 'background feeling', and Colombetti (2014, Chapter 5) for a discussion of this and other notions of background bodily experiences.

sensations: feedback from facial muscles and bodily posture and felt urges to act (perception of muscle tension in preparation for action). We also proposed to regard "background bodily feelings" as constituting the experience of being aroused during emotion, where these are feelings in which bodily self-awareness is present but is not conspicuous, and is best characterized as shaping the person's experience from, or through, the background.

References

Aristotle. (1986). *De anima (On the soul).* (trans. H. Lawson-Tancred). London: Penguin.

Armon-Jones, C. (1986). The thesis of constructionism. In: R. Harré (ed.), *The Social Construction of Emotions*. Oxford: Blackwell, pp. 32–56.

Ax, A. F. (1953). The physiological differentiation between fear and anger in humans. *Psychosomatic Medicine, 15*(5), 433–42.

Barbur, J. L. (2004). Learning from the pupil: Studies of basic mechanisms and clinical applications. In: L. M. Chalupa and J. S. Werner (eds), *The Visual Neurosciences*, Vol. **1**. Cambridge, MA: MIT Press, pp. 641–56.

Berntson, G. G. and **Cacioppo, J. T.** (2009). Autonomic nervous system. In: D. Sander and K. R. Scherer (eds), *Oxford Companion to Emotion and the Affective Sciences*. Oxford: Oxford University Press, pp. 65–7.

Bradley, M. M. and **Lang, P. J.** (2007). Emotion and motivation. In: J. Cacioppo, L. G. Tassinary, and G. G. Berntson (eds), *Handbook of Psychophysiology*, 3rd edn. New York, NY: Cambridge University Press, pp. 581–607.

Cannon, W. B. (1929). *Bodily Changes in Pain, Hunger, Fear and Rage*, 2nd edn. Boston, MA: Charles Branford.

Charmandari, E., Tsigos, C., and **Chrousos, G.** (2005). Endocrinology of the stress response. *Annual Review of Physiology, 67*(1), 259–84.

Colombetti, G. (2014). *The Feeling Body: Affective Science Meets the Enactive Mind*. Cambridge, MA: MIT Press.

Colombetti, G. and **Kuppens, P.** (forthcoming). Valence, arousal and their relation: Conceptual clarifications and empirical issues. In: A. Scarantino (ed.), *The Routledge Handbook of Emotion Theory*. Oxford: Routledge.

Critchley, H. D. and **Harrison, N. A.** (2013). Visceral influences on brain and behavior. *Neuron, 77*(4), 624–38.

Cryan, J. F. and **Dinan, T. G.** (2012). Mind-altering microorganisms: The impact of the gut microbiota on brain and behaviour. *Nature Reviews Neuroscience, 13*(10), 701–12.

Damasio, A. R. (1999). *The Feeling of What Happens: Body, Emotion and the Making of Consciousness*. London: Vintage.

Dantzer, R., O'Connor, J. C., Freund, G. G., Johnson, R. W., and **Kelley, K. W.** (2008). From inflammation to sickness and depression: When the immune system subjugates the brain. *Nature Reviews Neuroscience, 9*(1), 46–56.

Davidson, R. J., Scherer, K. R., and Goldsmith, H. H. (eds), (2003). *Handbook of Affective Sciences*. Oxford: Oxford University Press.

Dixon, T. (2003). *From Passions to Emotions: The Creation of a Secular Psychological Category*. Cambridge: Cambridge University Press.

Dror, O. E. (2014). The Cannon–Bard thalamic theory of emotions: A brief genealogy and reappraisal. *Emotion Review, 6*(1), 13–20.

Foster, J. A. and **McVey Neufeld, K.-A.** (2013). Gut–brain axis: How the microbiome influences anxiety and depression. *Trends in Neurosciences, 36*(5), 305–12.

Fowles, D. C. (2009). Arousal. In: D. Sander and K. R. Scherer (eds), *Oxford Companion to Emotion and the Affective Sciences*. Oxford: Oxford University Press, p. 50.

Fox, E. (2008). *Emotion Science: Cognitive and Neuroscientific Approaches to Understanding Human Emotions*. Basingstoke: Palgrave Macmillan.

Frijda, N. H. (1986). *The Emotions*. Cambridge: Cambridge University Press.

Garfinkel, S. N., Seth, A. K., Barrett, A. B., Suzuki, K., and **Critchley, H. D.** (2015). Knowing your own heart: Distinguishing interoceptive accuracy from interoceptive awareness. *Biological Psychology, 104*, 65–74.

Gill, C. (2010). *Naturalistic Psychology in Galen and Stoicism*. New York, NY: Oxford University Press.

Graver, M. R. (2007). *Stoicism and Emotion*. Chicago, IL: University Of Chicago Press.

Grewe, O., Nagel, F., and **Kopiez, R.,** and **Altenmuller, E.** (2007). Emotions over time: Synchronicity and development of subjective, physiological, and facial affective reactions to music. *Emotion, 7*, 774–88.

Harrison, N. A. (2017). Brain structures implicated in inflammation-associated depression. *Current Topics in Behavioral Neuroscience, 31*, 221–48.

Harrison, N. A., Kreibig, S. D., and **Critchley, H. D.** (2013). A two-way road: Efferent and afferent pathways of autonomic activity in emotion. In: J. Armony and P. Vuilleumier (eds), *Cambridge Handbook of Human Affective Neuroscience*. Cambridge: Cambridge University Press, pp. 82–106.

Hume, D. (1739–40 [2003]). *A Treatise of Human Nature*. London: Everyman.

James, W. (1884). What is an emotion? *Mind, 9*, 188–205.

Jänig, W. (2006). *The Integrative Action of the Autonomic Nervous System: Neurobiology of Homeostasis*. Cambridge: Cambridge University Press.

Kragel, P. A. and **LaBar, K. S.** (2016). Decoding the nature of emotion in the brain. *Trends in Cognitive Sciences, 20*(6), 444–55.

Kriegel, U. (2015). *The Varieties of Consciousness*. Oxford: Oxford University Press.

Langley, J. N. (1900). The sympathetic and other related systems of nerves. In: E. A. Sharpey-Schäfer (ed.), *Textbook of Physiology*. London: Young J. Pentland, pp. 616–96.

Mayer, E. A., Knight, R., Mazmanian, S. K., Cryan, J. F., and **Tillisch, K.** (2014). Gut microbes and the brain: Paradigm shift in neuroscience. *Journal of Neuroscience, 34*(46), 15490–6.

Nummenmaa, L., Glerean, E., Hari, R., and **Hietanen, J. K.** (2014). Bodily maps of emotions. *Proceedings of the National Academy of Sciences, 111*(2), 646–51.

Rimé, B., Philippot, P., and **Cisamolo, D.** (1990). Social schemata of peripheral changes in emotion. *Journal of Personality and Social Psychology, 59*(1), 38–49.

Rivest, S. (2009). Regulation of innate immune responses in the brain. *Nature Reviews Immunology, 9*(6), 429–39.

Robinson, B. F., Epstein, S. E., Beiser, G. D., and **Braunwald, E.** (1966). Control of heart rate by the autonomic nervous system: Studies in man on the interrelation between baroreceptor mechanisms and exercise. *Circulation Research, 19*(2), 400–11.

Russell, J. A. (2003). Core affect and the psychological construction of emotion. *Psychological Review, 110*(1), 145–72.

Saper, C. B., Romanovsky, A. A., and **Scammell, T. E.** (2012). Neural circuitry engaged by prostaglandins during the sickness syndrome. *Nature Neuroscience, 15*(8), 1088–95.

Scarantino, A. (ed.), (forthcoming). *The Routledge Handbook of Emotion Theory*. Oxford: Routledge.

Schachter, S. (1964). The interaction of cognitive and physiological determinants of emotional state. In: L. Berkowitz (ed.), *Advances in Experimental Social Psychology*. New York, NY: Academic Press, pp. 49–80.

Schachter, S. and **Singer, J.** (1962). Cognitive, social, and physiological determinants of emotional state. *Psychological Review, 69*(5), 379–99.

Scherer, K. R. and **Wallbott, H. G.** (1994). Evidence for universality and cultural variation of differential emotion response patterning. *Journal of Personality and Social Psychology*, *66*, 310–28.

Schulz, A., **Lass-Hennemann, J.**, **Sütterlin, S.**, **Schächinger, H.**, and **Vögele, C.** (2013). Cold pressor stress induces opposite effects on cardioceptive accuracy dependent on assessment paradigm. *Biological Psychology*, *93*(1), 167–74.

Spiga, F., **Walker, J. J.**, **Gupta, R.**, **Terry, J. R.**, and **Lightman, S. L.** (2015). 60 Years of neuroendocrinology. Glucocorticoid dynamics: Insights from mathematical, experimental and clinical studies. *Journal of Endocrinology*, *226*(2), T55–T66.

Sudo, N., **Chida, Y.**, **Aiba, Y.**, **Sonoda, J.**, **Oyama, N.**, **Yu, X.-N.**, et al. (2004). Postnatal microbial colonization programs the hypothalamic–pituitary–adrenal system for stress response in mice. *Journal of Physiology*, *558*(1), 263–75.

Thayer, R. E. (1996). *The Origin of Everyday Moods: Managing Energy, Tension, and Stress*. Oxford: Oxford University Press.

Tracey, K. J. (2002). The inflammatory reflex. *Nature*, *420*(6917), 853–9.

Wiens, S., **Mezzacappa, E. S.**, and **Katkin, E. S.** (2000). Heartbeat detection and the experience of emotions. *Cognition & Emotion*, *14*(3), 417–27.

Wolf, S. and **Wolff, H. G.** (1947). *Human Gastric Function*. New York, NY: Oxford University Press.

Chapter 14

Was Descartes right after all? An affective background for bodily awareness

Frédérique de Vignemont

14.1 Introduction

These last 20 years have seen an explosion of experimental work on interoception. Recent accounts of interoception have highlighted its role for self-awareness, positing it at the core of what is sometimes called the "sentient self" (Craig, 2010), the "proto-self" (Damasio, 1999), the "embodied self" (Seth, 2013), or the "material me" (Tsakiris, 2017). What gives such a privileged status to interoception compared to other sources of information about the body, and is it actually warranted?

In this chapter, I shall leave aside the empirical investigation of interoception and more simply return to Descartes's *Meditations on First Philosophy*.[1] Although he is mainly known for his dualism and sometimes even perceived as an enemy of interoception (e.g. Damasio, 1994), one should not forget that he also strongly emphasizes the unity between the body and the self:

> Nature likewise teaches me by these sensations of pain, hunger, thirst, etc., that I am not only lodged in my body as a pilot in a vessel, but that I am besides so intimately conjoined, and as it were intermixed with it, that my mind and body compose a certain unity. For if this were not the case, I should not feel pain when my body is hurt, seeing I am merely a thinking thing, but should perceive the wound by the understanding alone, just as a pilot perceives by sight when any part of his vessel is damaged; and when my body has need of food or drink, I should have a clear knowledge of this, and not be made aware of it by the confused sensations of hunger and thirst: for, in truth, all these sensations of hunger, thirst, pain, etc., are nothing more than certain confused modes of thinking, arising from the union and apparent fusion of mind and body. (Descartes, 2016 [1641] *Meditation VI*, p. 56)

What is interesting is that Descartes uses the examples of pain, thirst, and hunger to show that we have a unique relationship with our body. Descartes might thus have been the first advocate of the significance of interoception for bodily awareness. In this chapter I shall first explore the many ways one might understand the notion of interoception. I shall then assess its contribution for the awareness of one's body as one's own.

[1] See also *The Passions of the Soul* (1649).

14.2 The manifold of interoception

The first question one may ask is whether the notion of interoception corresponds to a *natural kind* since it might sometimes seem that it results more from an artificial taxonomy than from the structure of the natural world. However, there is no easy answer insofar as many disagree on the ontological status and the exact criterion for natural kinds. Leaving aside these delicate issues, one may still question the homogeneity of the notion of interoception. What should be included or not is indeed not always clear. Consider the following three definitional attempts:

- *The sole-object definition*: Interoception consists of information that is exclusively about one's body.
- *The insider definition*: Interoception consists of information about what is internal to the body and not about what is at its surface.
- *The regulator definition*: Interoception consists of information that plays a role in internal regulation and monitoring.

Each definition is problematic. Consider for instance proprioception, which informs the organism about joint angle, muscle stretch, and tendon tension. It meets both the sole-object and the insider criteria and yet it is usually distinguished from interoception. The regulator definition does not fare better. On this interpretation, an efferent copy sent when moving should qualify as interoceptive and yet nobody includes it in interoception. On the other hand, pain and affective touch are sometimes—but not always—conceived of as being part of interoception and yet they are felt to be located on the surface of the skin. One could go on like that without finding a single unifying criterion that is not too broad. The best strategy may then be to return to Sherrington's (1906) original definition since he was the first to coin the term (for review see Ceunen, Vlaeyen, & Van Diest, 2016):

- *The visceral definition*: Interoception consists of information coming from internal organs.

Sherrington's definition includes neither nociception nor thermal perception nor affective touch. It is thus narrower than most definitions but one may still question its unity because each internal organ is different and sends different types of signals. One may then talk of the "modalities" of interoception in the same way that we talk of the modalities of exteroception, such as sight and audition (e.g. Crucianelli et al., in press; Garfinkel et al., 2016; Herbert et al., 2012). A further source of complexity is that we need to distinguish between three levels at which one can analyse interoception:

- *Physiological level*: interoceptive signals originating from internal organs.
- *Phenomenological level*: interoceptive sensations (e.g. feeling one's bladder or stomach full) and interoceptive feelings (e.g. feeling hungry or thirsty).
- *Introspective level*: interoceptive accuracy (as measured by heartbeat counting, for instance), interoceptive sensibility (as measured by the confidence in one's interoceptive

accuracy), and interoceptive awareness (as measured by the relationship between accuracy and sensibility) (Garfinkel et al., 2015).

Most current literature focuses either on the physiological level itself (e.g. Babo-Rebelo et al., 2016; Critchley & Harrison, 2013) or on the introspective level (e.g. Seth, 2013; Tsakiris, 2017), but it largely neglects the phenomenological one. However, it is important to note that the way it is operationalized, interoceptive awareness involves more than being conscious of interoceptive signals. Consider interoceptive accuracy: it requires a reflective act of attention that turns to one's bodily signals in order to perform a cognitive task (e.g. counting one's heartbeat). The "interoceptive score" is then computed either directly on the basis of the reliability of the judgment or more indirectly by comparing the reliability of the judgment with the confidence that one has in it. It is thus disconnected from the function of interoception to maintain optimal homeostasis: interoceptive accuracy by itself has no positive or negative valence and it plays no motivational role. One may then legitimately wonder to what extent it can actually be taken as a proxy to interoception as such. It rather seems to be a proxy for interoceptive *top-down attention*: the capacity to voluntarily switch the focus of attention from the external world (on which it usually is) to the internal world, and to access and process the information that is then available. Interoceptive awareness further involves *metacognitive processes*. These are interesting capacities and many studies have shown that the capacity to pay attention inward *modulates* the reliability of bodily judgments and the sensitivity to bodily illusions, such as the Rubber Hand Illusion (for review see Tsakiris, 2017), but we are a long way from the primitive self-regulatory function of interoception.

Many might easily grant that interoceptive awareness is far from perfect but still argue that it remains the best proxy available. After all, we can spontaneously feel our heart beating too fast or feel our bladder full. Interoceptive awareness is simply a way to voluntarily pay attention to these interoceptive sensations. However, I do not think that these kinds of sensations, even when experienced spontaneously, are the right starting point to investigate the significance of interoception for self-awareness. Indeed, I want to propose that they are *indirect* or impure, so to speak: they inform us about the state of our internal organs but they do not result from interoceptive signals only. Consider the example of the full bladder, which is sometimes experimentally used as a measure for interoception. What we actually experience is a sensation of pressure, as if something were pushing the surface of our body from the inside, as well as the sensation of our skin stretching. The sensation is then not only interoceptive but also tactile.[2] Something along the same lines could be said about the heartbeat sensation, which also involves tactile sensations of the blood in our veins and arteries tapping too fast on the surface. It might also involve internal auditory sensations of the heart pumping and the blood rushing. These non-interoceptive signals contribute to the way we are aware of the internal state of our body and play a crucial role for homeostasis. However, because they involve other modalities

[2] See de Vignemont and Massin (2015) for a definition of touch in terms of pressure.

(touch, audition), there is too many potential confound and one cannot control what comes from interoception per se. I shall thus leave aside these interoceptive sensations from now on. Instead, I will focus on what I call *interoceptive feelings*.

It was Armstrong (1962) who first distinguishes between bodily feelings and sensations. His criterion could be phrased as follows: sensations, such as touch and pain, are local whereas feelings, such as thirst, hunger, fatigue, sleepiness, dizziness, and shortness of breath, are global. For instance, you can contrast the sensation of the pinprick at the tip of your index finger with the diffuse feeling of fatigue in your whole body. Or consider the case of thirst: it reveals the general state of the entirety of your body missing water. More generally, interoceptive feelings inform us about the welfare of the organism as a whole.[3] Their spatial principle of organization is thus holistic.

Despite these apparent differences, one may question the validity of the distinction between interoceptive sensations and interoceptive feelings. In other words, are interoceptive feelings really global? Although it is true that they do not activate specific areas of Penfield's Homunculus in the primary somatosensory cortex, Craig (2010) argues that there are interoceptive maps which are organized somatotopically. The difficulty here is that in his definition of interoception he includes pain, thermal perception, and affective touch which are clearly localized on the surface of the body. My claim is restricted to thirst, hunger, fatigue, and so forth. Is there a somatotopic representation of these feelings? One way to test their spatial organization is to investigate the consequences of local anaesthesia. It is true that one can feel a sensation of dryness in the throat when one feels thirsty but does this entail that you cannot feel thirsty during a local anaesthesia of the throat? I doubt it. Alternatively, one may try to perform some classic tasks in psychophysics such as judgments of spatial distance: you can judge whether two tactile stimuli are farther apart than two other tactile stimuli but can you do it for interoceptive feelings? Again, this seems unlikely.[4] Hence, the spatiality of interoceptive feelings is limited. Their role is not to attract attention to a specific part of the body but rather to adjust one's behavior to reinstate the internal equilibrium that has been disturbed.[5] Hence, we generally do not

[3] Interoceptive feelings are tightly connected to emotions. According to the James–Lange theory, they actually constitute emotions. However, they should not be confused because emotions are not only about the body, they are also about the object or the event in the world that is taken as the source of the emotion (e.g. I am afraid of *the dog*). One may then suggest that interoceptive feelings are similar or even identical to moods. Moods indeed lack intentional objects. For instance, when I feel anxious, I may not feel anxious about anything particular, my feeling seems to be primarily bodily, something like a negative form of arousal. Nonetheless, moods and bodily feelings do not play the same motivational role. In brief, I should stop eating if I feel full but there is no salient action that I should perform if I feel anxious and the behavior that I might adopt is directed toward the external world (e.g. paying more attention to potential threats in the environment) and not toward my body.

[4] Even for painful sensations, which are localized, subjects have difficulties judging their distance (Mancini et al., 2015).

[5] Still it should be noted that in some occasions their affective valence can be positive and they can feel pleasant (e.g. feeling full).

need voluntarily to pay attention to interoceptive feelings. We spontaneously experience them when needed (they can even invade our whole mental life).

As mentioned earlier, interoceptive feelings are rarely investigated in the recent literature on interoception. It is easy to see why: they are indeed difficult to operationalize in experimental context. Roughly speaking, one does not want to starve one's subjects not one time but 60 times to have reliable data. Furthermore, one would have to be able to dissociate cases with and without interoceptive feelings but they are pervasive in our life and almost never fully impaired, leading, for instance, to the complete absence of thirst (i.e. hypodipsia). Even in pain asymbolia, patients who seem to no longer care about their body still drink and eat normally (Bain, 2014). Nonetheless, interoceptive feelings might be disturbed in some disorders like depersonalization (Billon, 2017), anorexia nervosa (Holsen & Goldstein, 2015 see Chapter 9 in the present volume), and addiction (Naqvi et. al., 2014) but the difficulty is that many other factors intervene to explain these disorders, which makes difficult any conclusion about the specific role of interoception. My approach here will thus be mainly based on conceptual analysis. I shall first describe what it takes to be aware of one's body as being one's own and then determine what role, if any, interoceptive feelings play.

14.3 The bodyguard hypothesis of bodily ownership

Consider the following basic example: I touch the table with my hand. My tactile sensation includes sensations of resistance, texture, and temperature, as well as the sensation of the location at which I feel the pressure to occur, namely the hand. I am also aware that the hand on which I feel touch is mine. This type of self-awareness is known as the sense of bodily ownership, for want of a better name. It might seem indeed that I do not "own" my body; I only own my laptop, my flat, and my books, while I have a more privileged relation with my body than with any other objects, one might even say a relation of identity. The fact is that numerous other languages—although not English—use different suffixes to indicate the possession of alienable (e.g. my flat) and inalienable entities (e.g. my hand) (Kemmerer, 2014). The relation that we have with our body, however, cannot be characterized only by the fact that it is inalienable. Indeed, I can also qualify my relation to my son in the same way. We thus need to go beyond this in our description and ask what it actually means to experience one's body as one's own.

Let me start with a first approximation by drawing a parallel with *nationalistic feelings*. Consider what was called the Russian "Patriotic War" of 1812. In the nineteenth century, people who lived in the Russian Empire were characterized by the heterogeneity of their cultures and religions and the enormous distances that separated them. It was only at the time when Napoleon invaded Russia and burnt Moscow down that the Russians felt that they belonged to the one country. More generally, it has been noted in social psychology that feeling one's country as one's own involves not just being aware of its borders, nor being aware that one can vote; it also involves being aware that what happens to the country matters, and this feeling is especially salient when the country is under threat. One can then experience a feeling of national unity against the common enemy. To some extent this characterization applies to the sense of bodily ownership (de Vignemont, 2018). To fix the boundaries of the body that one feels as one's own, I propose that it is not sufficient to fix where the body stops and the rest of the world starts; one must also fix what matters for self-preservation. It is not sufficient to be aware of the boundaries of the body, one must also be aware of the valence of these boundaries: one must be aware that these boundaries are the ones to care about and to protect if one wants to survive and that it is important to keep track of them.

My claim is relatively simple and uncontroversial: one's own body matters for survival and needs to be defended. Because of the significance of the body for the organism's survival, I propose that a specific representation to fix the body that must be protected, which I call a *protective body map*, evolved to increase the organism's chance of survival. Consequently, one does not protect one's biological body, one protects the body that one takes oneself to have. The protective body map represents the body that has a special value for the organism's evolutionary needs. I further propose that the protective body map grounds the sense of bodily ownership.

> *The bodyguard hypothesis:* One experiences as one's own any body parts that are incorporated in the protective body map.

The protective body map informs the brain about the potential relevance of the location of the sensation for the organism's needs. Hence, if a spider crawls on my hand, I feel its contact as being located within the frame of the body to protect. Thanks to their protective reference frame, bodily experiences involve the awareness of the body as having a special import for the self. They are thus endowed with a specific affective coloring that goes beyond their sensory phenomenology. This affective quality constitutes the phenomenology of bodily ownership: feeling your body as your own consists in feeling that it has a special significance for you.

Evidence in favor of the bodyguard hypothesis can be found in borderline cases of ownership. Physiological response to threat (measured by skin conductance response, or SCR) has become the main implicit measure of the Rubber Hand Illusion (RHI), which is conceived of as the main experimental paradigm to test the sense of bodily ownership. It has been repeatedly shown that participants react when the rubber hand is threatened, but only when they report it as their own after synchronous stroking, and the strength of their reaction is correlated with their ownership rating in questionnaires (e.g. Ehrsson et al., 2007). Conversely, patients with somatoparaphrenia who no longer experience their limb as their own show a lack of increase of SCR when their "alien" hand is threatened (Romano et al., 2014). This finding is consistent with their broad pattern of attitudes. Many somatoparaphrenic patients try to get rid of their "alien" limb by pulling it out of their bed, giving it to the doctor, putting it in the garbage, and so forth.

Further evidence in favor of the bodyguard hypothesis can be found in congenital pain insensitivity. Patients with congenital pain insensitivity are characterized by dramatic impairment of pain sensations since birth, caused by a hereditary neuropathy or channelopathy. They show a complete lack of discomfort, grimacing, or withdrawal reaction to prolonged pinpricks, strong pressure, soft tissue pinching, and noxious thermal stimuli. Interestingly, they can describe that their body feels like an external object, a kind of tool (Danziger, 2010). An 18-year-old boy with congenital pain insensitivity reported: "A body is like a car, it can be dented but it pops out again and can be fixed like a car. Someone can get in and use it but the body isn't you, you just inhabit it" Frances & Gale, 1975, pp. 116–17).

Descartes was right: without pain, one is only as a pilot in a vessel.[6] This does not mean that it is only when the body is in danger that we feel our body as our own. I defend a weaker conception, according to which there is a stage in development in which it is important, possibly even necessary, to experience pain (or other affectively loaded bodily sensations) in order to give affective significance to the boundaries of the body, a significance that is at the origin of the sense of bodily ownership. In short, past experiences that the boundaries of the body could be at risk make these boundaries the boundaries of the body that we experience as our own now. Hence, it appears that without pain expertise and without pain expectation, bodily boundaries are just spatial boundaries, and this is not sufficient for the sense of bodily ownership (de Vignemont, 2017).

One may object at this point that one does not always protect the body that one experiences as one's own, and that one protects many things—including many bodies—besides one's own body without having a sense of ownership of them. However, this is not an objection against the bodyguard hypothesis. First, one should not neglect that protective behaviors can be analysed at many different levels, and only the lowest one is relevant here. Consider the pleasure that some people experience in extreme sports, for instance. Even if the mountain biker is ready to risk his life by going downhill on a very steep and dangerous slope, he also pays extreme attention to its immediate environment and he is ready to react in case of obstacles. More generally, the affective conception that I defend does not assume that the protective body map is the only factor that decides which body is to be protected, even at the most primitive level. Like any other behavior, protective behaviors can result from complex decision-making processes, involving a variety of beliefs, desires, emotions, moral considerations, and so forth.

To recapitulate, it is a fact of the matter that there is a specific body that one should protect to survive and reproduce and it is the function of the protective body map to covariate reliably with it. The protective body map is normally recruited as a spatial frame of reference for bodily experiences, ascribing an affective value to the body that one experiences.

[6] Interestingly, patients with congenital pain insensitivity often engage in self-mutilation, including burns and auto-amputations of fingertips and tongues (Danziger & Willer, 2009; Nagasako, Oaklander, & Dworkin, 2003). Similar self-inflicted injuries can also be found in animals raised in isolation preserved from pain (Melzack & Scott, 1957; Lichstein & Sackett, 1971). Injuring one' s body may be a way to test whose body it is. Feeling something can then strengthen a fading feeling of confidence in the sense of bodily ownership, whereas feeling nothing can confirm that this body has nothing to do with oneself, or it might be that one simply feels no sense of ownership whatsoever. If so, one is not voluntarily injuring oneself, rather one is injuring *a body*, which happens to be one's own.

One is then aware of one's body as one's own and one is motivated to protect it. The feeling of bodily ownership should thus be conceived of in affective terms. For all that, does the bodyguard hypothesis qualify as an *interoceptive* theory of ownership?

14.4. Disembodied interoception

We have just seen that pain plays a key role for the sense of bodily ownership. It may then seem that interoceptive feelings should play the same role: they are affective-loaded experiences, which are essential for self-preservation. However, as I shall now argue, their significance is of a different kind.

Imagine a creature that only receives interoceptive signals and that only experiences interoceptive feelings. It receives information about its body, and its body only. It thus has self-specific information, but does it have a sense of bodily ownership? Not necessarily, I argue. There is indeed a difference between self-specificity and self-reference. Self-specific information corresponds to information exclusively about the body that happens to be one's own; self-reference corresponds to the awareness of the body *qua* one's own. Self-specific information is thus necessary for the sense of ownership but it is not sufficient. In other words, it does not suffice to be aware exclusively of one's body for one to be aware of it *as one's own*. The sense of ownership cannot be reduced to a privileged informational link to one's body. It also involves being able to discriminate one's body from what is not one's body. The problem is that on the basis of interoception only, one is locked in one's body: the body is only an inside. Since our creature receives no information about the outside world, and thus about other bodies, it does not have to discriminate its body from what is not its body. It is so fixated on its own body that it can dispense with representing whose body is hungry or thirsty. Following a principle of cognitive parsimony, we may then conclude that if there is no need to individuate the body that it feels as being its own, then the creature simply does not do it. To show that interoception is not sufficient for the sense of bodily ownership is clearly illustrated by the many cases in which patients—with spinal cord injuries, peripheral deafferentation, right parietal lesion, or congenital pain insensitivity—report a sense of disownership toward their body despite still receiving interoceptive signals and experiencing interoceptive feelings.

The fact is that one usually says "I am thirsty," "I am out of breath," or "I am full" without any explicit reference to the body. There is only a unique occurrence of the first-person pronoun, which refers to the *mental* subject, the subject who experiences the sensation. By contrast, when I say "I feel touch on my hand," the body is an explicit part of the content and there are two occurrences of the first person: there is the "I" that experiences the tactile sensation but there is also "my" hand, which individuates the limb as being part of my body. In interoceptive feelings, there is no such "myness," no specific limb that one experiences as one's own. As O'Shaughnessy (1980) notes, there is no feeling of "immediate presence" when it comes to our kidneys, unlike our legs or our hands. This is so because the function of interoceptive feelings is to inform the individual about the state of the *whole body* for self-regulation. What matters is not the kidney as such but whether the organism gets rid of its toxins. By being so much about what is inside, interoceptive feelings are unable to contrast what is inside from what is outside, and thus to fix the spatial boundaries of the body. If one conceives of the body as being primarily a "*res extensa*" as Descartes puts it—that is, as a material entity extended in space—then interoceptive feelings might almost qualify as being *disembodied*.

14.5 **An affective background**

None of the advocates of interoception for the embodied self actually assumes that interoception on its own could suffice for self-awareness. Instead, the view is that it is in the interaction between interoceptive and exteroceptive information that the sense of self can emerge. They say very little, however, on the nature of these interactions. What is the special contribution provided by interoception and how is interoception integrated with exteroception?

Tsakiris (2017), for instance, suggests that there is both integration and competition between interoception and exteroception. These two types of interaction involve a common denominator that can bring together exteroceptive and interoceptive information, but what can it be? One might reply that interoceptive awareness competes with exteroceptive awareness for the focus of attention. In everyday life when we are not counting our heartbeats, however, is interoception in such a competitive situation? At the physiological level, interoceptive signals are sent whether one pays attention to them or not. Furthermore, attention clearly does not suffice to integrate information together. What else is required?

Consider a classic example of multisensory integration such as the RHI. The visual information about the rubber hand being stroked is integrated with the tactile and proprioceptive information about the subject's hand leading the subject to experience touch on the rubber hand and to mislocate her hand in the direction of the location of the rubber hand. This process of integrative binding involves redundant information (i.e. about the same property of the object) and aims at reliability: it is important to have more than one source of information because informational redundancy increases robustness and compensates for sensory noises. Integrative binding is successful only if the information that is bound is actually about the same object or event. It thus involves *selecting* the relevant information to bind in order to avoid bringing together features or experiences that have nothing to do with each other, as in the RHI. There are then two main criteria used to guide the selection: one binds together the sensory states that carry information about the same location and/or about the same object. For instance, it has been shown that there are spatial constraints for the RHI: the rubber hand needs to be located in the peripersonal space of the subject's hand for visual information to be integrated with tactile and proprioception information (Lloyd, 2007). Furthermore, the RHI does not work if one visually presents a rectangular piece of wood while one strokes the subject's hand (Tsakiris et al., 2010).

What about the interaction between interoception and the other senses? Tsakiris (2017, p. 350) seems to suggest similar processes:

> The exteroceptive evidence suggests that what I am looking at (i.e., the rubber hand) is my hand. However if this is my hand, then there are interoceptive prediction errors that need to be explained away between how my true hand feels (i.e., the interoceptive prediction) and the fact that I cannot feel the rubber hand interoceptively.

However, do we really have interoceptive feelings of our hands? If we use Sherrington's visceral definition, this is not obvious. I do not feel the rubber hand interoceptively, but neither do I feel my own hand interoceptively. What I feel is the stretching of my skin, its temperature, its position, and possibly pressure exerted on it, pain, itches, or tickles, but no visceral sensation. In brief, there are no interoceptive feelings experienced in one's hand or in one's foot. How then could one integrate them with localized visual, tactile, and proprioceptive experiences? In addition, most information carried by interoception is not redundant with information coming from other sensory modalities.[7] In all the integrative models of the bodily self that have been recently proposed, it is paradoxically often forgotten how unique interoception is. In short, interoception cannot be integrated with proprioception and touch in the same way that vision is. What form, then, can its interaction take with the other senses?

Here I suggest that one should consider another type of perceptual binding, not integrative binding, but *additive binding* (de Vignemont, 2014). In additive binding, modality-specific experiences complement each other: the perceptual system collects all the pieces of information that are not redundant in order to have as rich and complete an experience of the perceived object as possible. Now what is bound together can be of different types. One can bring together different properties of the same object or different parts of it. There is a further dimension that might be more relevant here, however, which is the relationship figure/ground. The proposal, which is still very sketchy, is thus the following. At the phenomenological level, interoceptive feelings, which are about the global state of the body, constitute the ground on which local bodily sensations are experienced and they are bound together for a rich awareness of the body. Insofar as interoceptive feelings are affectively loaded, the background that they provide is affective. They thus provide an affective coloring to bodily awareness. We can now try to refine the proposal further and become more precise about the exact affective shade of interoceptive feelings.

Interoceptive feelings aim at protecting the organism. They have what Kathleen Akins (1996) calls a narcissistic function: they aim at securing what is best for the organism. On her view, sensory systems are not just servile detection systems that aim to be as reliable as possible in carrying information about the states with which they co-vary. Narcissistic perception is not about what is perceived but about the impact of what is

[7] The exception is rhythm, which can be internally felt but also seen and heard. One can then envisage interaction with other sensory modalities.

perceived for the subject. This theory of perception can already be found in Descartes's *Sixth Meditation*: "These perceptions of the senses, although given me by nature, merely to signify to my mind what things are beneficial and hurtful to the composite whole of which it is a part."[8] To illustrate her narcissistic hypothesis, Akins considers the case of thermal sensations, which indicate what is safe or dangerous for the body given its thermal needs:

> What the organism is worried about, in the best of narcissistic traditions, is its own comfort. The system is not asking, "What is it like out there?", a question about the objective temperature states of the body's skin. Rather it is doing something—informing the brain about the presence of any relevant thermal events. Relevant, of course, to itself. (Akins, 1996, p. 349)

Narcissistic principles are especially plausible in the case of interoception: what matters is not to track one's heartbeats in order to be able to count them; what matters is to determine whether the rhythm is neither too fast nor too slow. As said earlier, the function of interoception is to regulate the physiological balance of the organism. Therefore, interoception is not about the state of the body *simpliciter*; it is about the state of the body given the organism's needs and interests. One might also say that it is about the state of the body *for the self*. According to Akins, the narcissistic question can indeed be phrased as follows: "But how does this all relate to ME?" (Akins, 1996, p. 345). On her view, this question does not only affect the content of my experiences, filtering only what is relevant to me; it also marks the structure, or the format, of my experiences, like a signature: "by asking the narcissistic question, the *form* of the answer is compromised: it always has a self-entered (sic) glow" (Akins, 1996, p. 345). One may then suggest that by being narcissistic, interoceptive feelings that are at the background of bodily sensations give a "self-centered glow" to bodily awareness.

14.6 **Conclusion**

In this chapter I proposed to return to the original functional meaning of interoception, which is to ensure the physiological stability of the organism as a whole. To do so, one needs to leave aside interoceptive awareness, which is primarily about attention control and reliability, and focus on self-regulatory interoceptive feelings such as thirst and hunger, which are too often neglected in the recent literature. I then argued that interoceptive feelings cannot provide a contrast between inside and outside of the body because they only present the body as being an inside. Consequently, on their own they cannot ground the distinction between self and non-self. What they can do, however, is to provide a narcissistic coloring to our bodily sensations. All sensations are experienced not only on the spatial background of the protective body map but also on the affective background of our interoceptive feelings: this is not any body that we are aware of, this is the body that matters the most for our survival.

[8] For more detail on Descartes's view see Simmons (2008).

References

Akins, K. (1996). Of sensory systems and the "aboutness" of mental states. *Journal of Philosophy*, **93**(7), 337–72.

Armstrong, D. (1962). *Bodily Sensations*. London: Routledge.

Babo-Rebelo, M., Wolpert, N., Adam, C., Hasboun, D., and **Tallon-Baudry, C.** (2016). Is the cardiac monitoring function related to the self in both the default network and right anterior insula? *Philosophical Transactions of the Royal Society of London B, Biological Sciences*, **371**(1708), 20160004.

Bain, D. (2014). Pains that don't hurt. *Australasian Journal of Philosophy*, *92*(2), 305–20.

Billon, A. (2017). Mineness first. In: F. de Vignemont and A. Alsmith (eds), *The Subject's Matter: Self-Consciousness and the Body*. Cambridge, MA: MIT Press, pp. 189–216.

Ceunen, E., Vlaeyen, J. W. S., and **Van Diest, I.** (2016). On the origin of interoception. *Frontiers in Psychology*, *7*, 743.

Critchley, H. D. and **Harrison, N. A.** (2013). Visceral influences on brain and behavior. *Neuron*, *77*(4), 624–38.

Craig, A. D. B. (2010). The sentient self. *Brain Structure and Function*, *214*(5), 563–77.

Crucianelli, L., Krahé, C., Jenkinson, P. M., and **Fotopoulou, A. K.** (in press). Interoceptive ingredients of body ownership: Affective touch and cardiac awareness in the rubber hand illusion. *Cortex*.

Damasio, A. R. (1994). *Descartes' Error: Emotion, Reason and the Human Brain*. New York, NY: Putnam.

Damasio, A. R. (1999). *The Feeling of What Happens*. London: William Heinemann.

Danziger, N. and **Willer, J. C.** (2009). Congenital insensitivity to pain. *Revue Neurologique* (Paris), **165**(2), 129–36.

Danziger, N. (2010). *Vivre sans la douleur*. Paris: Odile Jacob.

Descartes, R. (1649). *The Passions of the Soul*. Indianapolis, IN: Hackett.

Descartes, R., Williams, B., and **Cottingham, J.** (2016 [1641]). *René Descartes: Meditations On First Philosophy: With Selections from the Objections and Replies*. Cambridge: Cambridge University Press.

Ehrsson, H. H., Wiech, K., Weiskopf, N., Dolan, R. J., and **Passingham, R. E.** (2007). Threatening a rubber hand that you feel is yours elicits a cortical anxiety response. *Proceedings of the National Academy of Sciences of the USA*, *104*(23), 9828–33.

Frances, A. and **Gale L.** (1975). The proprioceptive body image in self-object differentiation—a case of congenital indifference to pain and head-banging. *Psychoanalytic Quarterly*, *44*(1), 107–26.

Garfinkel, S. N., Seth, A. K., Barrett, A. B., Suzuki, K., and **Critchley, H. D.** (2015). Knowing your own heart: Distinguishing interoceptive accuracy from interoceptive awareness. *Biological Psychology*, *104*, 65–74.

Garfinkel, S. N., Manassei, M. F., Hamilton-Fletcher, G., In den Bosch, Y., Critchley, H. D., and **Engels, M.** (2016). Interoceptive dimensions across cardiac and respiratory axes. *Philosophical Transactions of the Royal Society of London B*, *371*(1708), 20160014.

Herbert, B. M., Muth, E. R., Pollatos, O., and **Herbert, C.** (2012). Interoception across modalities: On the relationship between cardiac awareness and the sensitivity for gastric functions. *PLoS One*, *7*(5), e36646.

Holsen, L. M. and **Goldstein, J. M.** (2015). Valuation and cognitive circuitry in anorexia nervosa: Disentangling appetite from the effort to obtain a reward. *Biological Psychiatry*, *77*(7), 604–6.

Kemmerer, D. (2014). Body ownership and beyond: Connections between cognitive neuroscience and linguistic typology. *Consciousness and Cognition*, *26*(1), 189–96.

Lichstein L. and **Sackett G. P.** (1971). Reactions by differentially raised rhesus monkeys to noxious stimulation. *Developmental Psychobiology*, *4*(4), 339–52.

Mancini, F., Steinitz, H., Steckelmacher, J., Iannetti, G., and **Haggard, P.** (2015). Poor judgment of distance between nociceptive stimuli. *Cognition*, **143**, 41–7.

O'Shaughnessy, B. (1980). *The Will*, Vol. 1. Cambridge: Cambridge University Press.

Lloyd, D. M. (2007). Spatial limits on referred touch to an alien limb may reflect boundaries of visuo-tactile peripersonal space surrounding the hand. *Brain and Cognition*, *64*(1), 104–9.

Melzack R. and **Scott, T. H.** (1957). The effects of early experience on the response to pain. *Journal of Comparative and Physiological Psychology*, *50*(2), 155–61.

Nagasako, E. M., Oaklander, A. L., and **Dworkin, R. H.** (2003). Congenital insensitivity to pain: An update. *Pain*, *101*(3), 213–19.

Naqvi, N. H., Gaznick, N., Tranel, D., and **Bechara, A.** (2014). The insula: A critical neural substrate for craving and drug seeking under conflict and risk. *Annals of the New York Academy of Sciences*, **1316**, 53–70.

Romano, D., Gandola, M., Bottini, G., and **Maravita, A.** (2014). Arousal responses to noxious stimuli in somatoparaphrenia and anosognosia: Clues to body awareness. *Brain*, **137**(Pt 4): 1213–23.

Seth, A. (2013). Interoceptive inference, emotion, and the embodied self. *Trends in Cognitive Sciences*, *17*(11), 565–73.

Sherrington, C. S. (1906). *The Integrative Action of the Nervous System*. New Haven, CT: Yale University Press.

Simmons, A. (2008). Guarding the body: A Cartesian phenomenology of perception. In: P. Hoffman and G. Yaffe (eds), *Contemporary Perspectives on Early Modern Philosophy: Essays in Honor of Vere Chappell*. Peterborough, Ont: Broadview Press, pp. 81–113.

Tsakiris, M., Carpenter, L., James, D., and **Fotopoulou, A.** (2010). Hands only illusion: Multisensory integration elicits sense of ownership for body parts but not for non-corporeal objects. *Experimental Brain Research*, *204*(3), 343–52.

Tsakiris, M. (2017). The material me. In: F. de Vignemont and A. Alsmith (eds), *The Subject's Matter: Self-Consciousness and the Body*. Cambridge, MA: MIT Press, pp. 33–361.

de Vignemont, F. (2014). Multimodal unity and multimodal binding. In: D. Bennett and C. Hill (eds), *Sensory Integration and the Unity of Consciousness*. Cambridge, MA: MIT Press, pp. 125–50.

de Vignemont, F. and **Massin, O.** (2015). Touch. In: M. Matthen (ed.), *Oxford Handbook of Philosophy of Perception*. Oxford: Oxford University Press, pp. 294–311.

de Vignemont, F. (2017). Pain and touch. *The Monist*, *100*(4), 465–77.

de Vignemont, F. (2018). *Mind the Body*. Oxford: Oxford University Press.

Chapter 15

Allostasis, interoception, and the free energy principle: Feeling our way forward

Andrew W. Corcoran and Jakob Hohwy

15.1 Introduction

The free energy principle (Friston, 2010) invokes variational Bayesian methods to explain how biological systems maximize evidence for their predictive models via the minimization of variational free energy, a tractable information-theoretic quantification of prediction error. This account, which was originally proposed to explain sensory learning, has evolved into a much broader scheme encompassing action and motor control, decision-making, attention, communication, and many other aspects of mental function (for overviews see Clark, 2013, 2016; Hohwy, 2013). Under the free energy principle, minimization of free energy is what any self-organizing system is compelled to do in order to resist dissipation and maximize the evidence for its own existence (i.e. self-evidencing through active inference; Hohwy, 2016).

Recent years have witnessed a growing interest in extending the conceptual apparatus of the free energy principle to the interoceptive domain. A number of investigators have sought to explain the influence of interoceptive modes of prediction error minimization on various cognitive processes and disruptions (for recent reviews see Barrett, 2017; Khalsa et al., in press; Seth & Friston, 2016, Smith et al., 2017). Central to such *interoceptive inference* perspectives is the notion that interoceptive signals encode representations of the internal (physiological) state of the body, thus providing vital information about how well the organism is managing to preserve the biological viability of its internal environment. Traditionally, the latter has been conceived in terms of *homeostasis*, a concept that usually refers (minimally) to the process of maintaining the internal conditions of complex, thermodynamically open, self-organizing biological systems in stable, far-from-equilibrium states (Yates, 1996). From the perspective of the free energy principle, homeostasis translates to the process of restricting the organism to visiting a relatively small number of states that are conducive to its ongoing existence, with interoceptive prediction error playing a particularly important role in signaling deviation from these attractive states (technically, these are known as attracting sets).

Notably, the centrality of homeostasis in some free energy-inspired accounts of interoceptive processing has started to give way to the newer concept of *allostasis*. According to proponents of the latter, homeostasis fails to capture the rich variety of self-regulatory processes that biological systems engage in in order to conserve their own integrity. Allostasis tries to address this shortcoming through various theoretical innovations, chief amongst which is a core emphasis on predictive or anticipatory modes of regulation. This is to say that, rather than merely responding to physiological perturbations in order to ensure the internal conditions of the body remain within homeostatic bounds, allostasis enables the organism to proactively prepare for such disturbances *before* they occur.

While this account carries obvious appeal from the perspective of predictive model-based theories of interoceptive processing, attempts to marry the two have given rise to a number of divergent interpretations of allostatic regulation. As it turns out, the history of allostasis is a history of contested definitions; some 30 years on from its inception, there appears to be no definitive consensus as to its precise meaning. The key aims of this chapter, then, are to establish (a) how allostasis might be best understood as a distinctive concept in the overall scheme of biological regulation, and (b) how this construal might inform (and indeed, be informed by) free energy-inspired theories of interoceptive inference.

15.2 **Discovering "the wisdom of the body": Homeostasis**

A standard account of the history of homeostasis might trace its source to the nineteenth century physiologist Claude Bernard, whose pioneering work on the role of the nervous system in maintaining the relative constancy of internal states (*le milieu intérieur*, i.e. the extracellular fluid environment that envelops the cell) would prove highly influential (Cooper, 2008; Woods & Ramsay, 2007). The key ideas at the core of Bernard's thinking—notions of harmony, equilibrium, and regulation—are, however, much older, dating as far back as the pre-Socratics (see Adolph, 1961, for a historical review). Bernard refined the ancient insight that organisms maintain a healthy constitution by engaging in certain self-regulatory behaviors (e.g. consuming nutrients, excreting waste)—and deviate from well-being whenever subject to certain unfavorable physiological imbalances—by drawing attention to the physiological mechanisms that ensure the continuity of a stable internal environment. Such compensatory adjustments act to cancel out internal disturbances that would otherwise be caused by fluctuations in the external environment. This capacity to meet environmental impingements with countervailing responses thus grants the organism an adaptive coupling with—and a special kind of autonomy from—its environmental niche.

Benefitting from Bernard's keen insights and some 50 years of subsequent experimental research, Walter Cannon (1929, 1939) coined the term "homeostasis" to describe the organism's capacity to maintain a "steady state" or intrinsic uniformity despite ongoing fluctuations in its internal and external processes. Cannon was at pains, however, to stress that his neologism was intended to characterize a complex process in which multiple physiological mechanisms are recruited to ensure the continued stability of the organism's internal milieu, where stability is construed in terms of a more or less variable range of acceptable (i.e. viable) values. This latter point is crucial for distinguishing

Cannon's conception of homeostasis from Bernard's emphasis on the fixed, invariant nature of internal conditions, in as much as homeostatic processes admit a space of permissible states. Also important was Cannon's concern to elucidate the autonomic mechanisms responsible for mediating adaptive physiological responses (e.g. increased respiratory rate) to altered internal conditions (e.g. decreased blood pH, increased carbon dioxide concentration) (Cooper, 2008), a subtle reorientation that would prove highly influential for later work in cybernetics.

The basic concept of homeostasis elaborated by Cannon (and extended by contemporaries such as Curt Richter; see Woods & Ramsay, 2007) would become one of, if not *the* core theoretical principle of modern physiology (Michael & McFarland, 2011; Michael et al., 2009). One essential element of modern conceptions of homeostasis that was, however, still missing from the Cannonian picture was a formal account of negative feedback (Modell et al., 2015). From a control-theoretic perspective, Cannon's careful analysis of particular homeostatic processes can be conceived according to a generic scheme of error detection (i.e. where some regulated variable, for instance blood glucose concentration, is found to deviate from some desirable value or *setpoint*) and correction (i.e. where some effector mechanism is activated in order to restore the regulated variable to the prescribed setpoint). It is important to note here that the notion of a setpoint generally conforms to Cannon's conception of a (broader or narrower) range of acceptable values, rather than any singular, fixed level (Modell et al., 2015). This set of values can thus be construed as a model against which the actual (sensed) state of the regulated variable is compared. The error signal elicited when the current state of the monitored tissue deviates from its setpoint reference represents a threat to organismic viability, and must therefore be corrected via mobilization of the appropriate effector system(s). Recasting homeostasis in this light thus furnishes a powerful conceptual framework in which the processes responsible for maintaining internal stability achieve this goal through the communication of information between peripheral tissues and a central controller (such as the central nervous system).

15.3 Allostasis: The future of homeostatic regulation?

As mentioned in our introduction, several recent theoretical frameworks of interoceptive inference co-opt notions of allostasis in order to situate the autonomic regulation of the internal milieu within the broader scheme of hierarchical predictive processing. Various theorists have argued that the basic concept of homeostasis is somehow insufficient to account for the rich complexity of self-regulatory behavior evinced by humans and other animals, advocating allostasis as a necessary theoretical supplement or corrective. To what extent allostasis extends, encompasses, or eliminates homeostasis is, however, unclear, not least because the characteristic features of allostatic regulation have been espoused in ambiguous or inconsistent terms across the literature (Lowe, Almér, & Dodig-Crnkovic, 2017; Power, 2004; Schulkin, 2004). This section thus aims to canvass some of the most influential accounts of allostasis to have emerged over the past three decades.

15.3.1 Achieving stability through change

The term "allostasis" was originally introduced by Sterling and Eyer (1988) to describe the integrated, hierarchical mechanisms through which the nervous system maintains organismic integrity. In this scheme, the brain is responsible for orchestrating complex, multisystem responses to physiological perturbations, resulting in a cascade of mutually reinforcing effects that are designed to maintain "stability through change" (Sterling & Eyer, 1988, p. 636). Multilevel allostatic regulation is supposedly accomplished through a fine-grained network of feedforward and feedback mechanisms, thus affording a more flexible and coordinated means of physiological control than the rather more primitive negative feedback loops typically attributed to homeostatic regulation. One key advantage of this arrangement is that it enables anticipatory alterations of physiological parameters *prior* to undergoing some perturbation (e.g. increasing blood pressure before standing up from a chair, rather than correcting the hypotension induced by the postural change after the fact). Under this allostatic regime, the body benefits from the brain's capacity to learn from experience by forecasting the organism's physiological needs ahead of time. As such, allostasis represents a rather more sophisticated system of internal regulation, one which minimizes reliance upon the kind of error signaling required to drive homeostatic correction.

Sterling and Eyer argued that the concept of homeostasis is fatally deficient, and ought thus to be "superseded" by their notion of allostasis (1988, p. 646; see also Sterling, 2004, 2012; Sterling & Laughlin, 2015). However, the validity of this assertion has been challenged by critics who argue that it turns on a fundamentally mistaken construal of homeostatic regulation (Carpenter, 2004; Day, 2005). The source of this error is twofold. First, the careful nuance of Cannon's (1929, 1939) definition of homeostasis is ignored in this account, giving rise to the overly simplistic (and arguably misleading) impression that homeostasis is supposed to "clamp each internal parameter at a 'setpoint'" (Sterling, 2004, p. 17), except in response to emergency (i.e. potentially life-threatening) situations. Second, Sterling and Eyer (1988) conflate the physiological variables that are the target of homeostatic regulation with the control mechanisms tasked with the job of maintaining such variables within acceptable bounds. The idea that physiological parameters such as blood pressure should fluctuate significantly throughout the day does not constitute a counterexample to the homeostatic model; rather, these fluctuations are in the service of homeostasis precisely insofar as they ensure that the vital constituents and properties of the fluid matrix (e.g. blood pH, oxygen tension) remain suitable for cell functioning. On this reading then, allostasis appears little more than "an unnecessary re-statement of the concept of homeostasis" (Day, 2005, p. 1196).

15.3.2 Allostatic means for homeostatic ends

Since Sterling and Eyer's (1988) introduction of the concept, less radical versions of allostasis have been developed that seek to complement or extend the scope of homeostatic regulation, rather than reject it wholesale. Early work by McEwen, Schulkin, and colleagues (McEwen & Stellar, 1993; Schulkin, McEwen, & Gold, 1994) embraced allostasis as a promising framework for studying complex relations between stress, behavior, and chronic disease, and set about developing the concept of *allostatic load* to account for the potentially deleterious consequences of resisting stressful stimuli. (Although an important dimension of the allostatic framework developed by McEwen and others, notions relating to allostatic load/overload will not be considered here—but see Peters, McEwen, & Friston, 2017).

As these theories matured, however, a more distinctive articulation of the base concept of allostasis started to emerge. McEwen began to conceive of allostasis as "an essential component of maintaining homeostasis" (1998, p. 37); where the latter is limited to "systems . . . that are truly essential for life" (2000b, p. 173). According to this view, allostasis describes "the process for actively maintaining homeostasis" (McEwen, 2000b, p. 173); or alternatively, "the means by which the body re-establishes homeostasis in the face of a challenge" (McEwen, 2000a, p. 25). In collaboration with Wingfield, McEwen's notion of allostatic regulation was further expanded to include setpoint adjustments in anticipation of cyclical changes across various temporal scales (McEwen & Wingfield, 2003, 2010). This conceptual development highlighted the circadian modulation of homeostatic parameters implicit in Sterling and Eyer's (1988) paradigmatic example of allostatic change (i.e. the diurnal variation of blood pressure upon which phasic modulations are superposed), while also extending the scope of allostatic processes to incorporate broader aspects of animal well-being, reproduction, and ontogenetic adaptation (e.g. seasonal variations in physiology and behavior in preparation for hibernation or migration).

McEwen concedes that his construal of allostasis might seem almost identical to broader conceptions of homeostasis, such as the view promulgated by Cannon (McEwen, 2000b, 2004; McEwen & Wingfield, 2003). He insists, however, that the notion of the "steady state" at the core of Cannonian homeostasis is inherently vague, insofar as it fails to delineate vital (homeostatic) systems from those mechanisms which work to maintain their stability. It is not entirely clear though why such a distinction ought to be desired, or indeed, if it is even coherent in the context of McEwen's broader framework. Dallman (2003) argued that so-called allostatic systems do not manifest qualitatively distinct properties as compared to their homeostatic counterparts, on the basis that such systems are responsible for a great deal of essential physiological and behavioral functions. Indeed, it seems strange to claim that allostatic mechanisms are not equally essential to survival if such adaptive systems play a crucial role in enabling the organism to flee (or better yet, entirely avoid) a deadly predator, for example.

Although arguments of this sort might be blunted by a more charitable interpretation of the key idea underlying McEwen's proposed distinction (namely, that allostatic systems accommodate large fluctuations precisely so that those physiological parameters which cannot tolerate such lability are not pushed beyond their narrow limits; e.g. McEwen, 1998), it seems plausible that significant enough deviations in allostatic systems should likewise prove fatal. Furthermore, cross-species analysis suggests that setpoint flexibility does not constitute a reliable indicator of the relative importance of a given physiological parameter (see Boulos & Rosenwasser, 2004). Nevertheless, McEwen and Wingfield's (2003) thematization of the multiple layers of predictive regulation that unfold across the life cycle strikes us a valuable addition to the allostasis framework, one which we take to be a genuine departure from traditional notions of homeostasis.

15.3.3 Two modes of sustained viability

Another account of allostatic regulation that seeks to integrate (rather than replace) conventional notions of homeostatic control was put forth by Schulkin and colleagues (Power & Schulkin, 2012; Rosen & Schulkin, 2004; Schulkin, 2003a, 2003b). Schulkin (2003a, 2003b) credits Cannon's conception of homeostasis with greater scope and sophistication than Sterling and Eyer (1988), while maintaining that some kind of supplementary concept is necessary in order to capture the full gamut of regulatory strategies exhibited by complex organisms (Power & Schulkin, 2012; Schulkin, 2003b). Schulkin expounds a version of allostasis in which brain-driven regulatory mechanisms effect fluctuating physiological and psychological states in the absence of any clear setpoint boundary. In particular, anticipatory (feedforward) hormonal processes are posited to play a crucial role in the emergence of many appetitive, self-protective, and socially orientated motivational drives (Schulkin, 2003b, 2011), as well as explaining the affective valence of emotional experiences that accompany such states (Rosen & Schulkin, 2004). Schulkin and colleagues (Power & Schulkin, 2012; Rosen & Schulkin, 2004; Schulkin, 2003b, 2004) thus advocate a broad conception of biological regulation, one in which homeostasis and allostasis constitute equally important (yet functionally opponent) mechanisms for maintaining the biological viability of the internal milieu.

In some sense, we might regard Schulkin's framework as a kind of synthesis of prior allostatic concepts. It clearly inherits from Sterling and Eyer's (1988) original conception of allostasis, retaining as it does an explicit emphasis on the role of anticipatory physiological changes in efficient adaptation to environmental diversity. It also takes up McEwen and Wingfield's (2003) temporal expansion of the concept to account for longer-term adaptive changes in response to various ecological and life cycle contexts (Schulkin, 2003b, 2004). However, by balancing the homeostatic imperative to conserve stability with the allostatic impulse towards dynamic state transition, Schulkin and colleagues thematize the deeper continuity uniting these apparently contradictory concepts. At the heart of these regulatory principles is not so much the immediate influence they exert over target physiological parameters (i.e. internal constancy versus variability) but rather the overarching goal that these mechanisms dually subserve: namely, the ongoing survival and reproductive success (i.e. evolutionary fitness) of the organism (Power & Schulkin, 2012; Schulkin, 2004; see also Power, 2004).

This is not to say that the regulatory frameworks described by Sterling, McEwen, and others do not also ground the emergence of allostatic mechanisms in the selective advantages they confer. The point here, rather, is that sustained biological viability (rather than some other criterion such as internal stability) seems to us the most plausible target towards which physiological and behavioral regulatory mechanisms are striving. By these lights, there is no inherent contradiction between homeostatic and allostatic principles; they are merely different routes to the same end.

15.4 Allostasis and interoceptive inference

The imperative to maintain biological viability over time is at the very core of the free energy principle (Friston, 2010). Briefly, this principle begins with the observation that living entities must "maintain their sensory states within physiological bounds," and that they do so by engaging in actions which maintain the integrity of their structural and dynamical organization (Friston, 2013, pp. 1–2). This restates the cybernetic insight that biological organisms resist the tendency towards disorder wrought by variable external conditions (Ashby, 1947, 1962). The central element of the principle is that such self-preserving adaptation is achieved via environmental exchanges enabled by the minimization of free energy (or, under simplifying assumptions, the long-term average of prediction error; Friston, 2010). Under most accounts invoking the free energy principle, the process of maintaining the biological agent's internal milieu within the limited subset of states conducive to its ongoing existence is that of homeostasis (where homeostasis is understood more precisely in terms of minimizing the free energy of internal state trajectories in order to avoid surprise, i.e. minimize prediction error; Friston, 2010).

The concept of allostasis started to infiltrate this picture in conjunction with remarks on the necessity of maintaining homeostasis for survival (e.g. Friston, 2012; Friston et al., 2014; Moran et al., 2014). Such comments typically invoked allostasis in the same breath as homeostasis, without offering any indication as to how the two terms might refer to differentiated aspects of biological regulation. To our knowledge, the first attempt at characterizing a substantive notion of allostasis as an independent mode of physiological regulation within the context of free energy minimization was made by Gu and FitzGerald (2014). In the short period that has elapsed since, a number of investigators have imported allostasis into their own free energy-inspired accounts of interoceptive inference. Much like the original development of allostasis in the biomedical and ethological literatures however, the precise nature of allostatic control in these schemes has been elaborated in various ways. The time is ripe then to take stock of this nascent body of research, both to establish its continuities with—and departures from—pre-existing notions of allostasis, and to assess which interpretation(s) of the concept seem most promising from the free energy perspective.

For convenience, we divide these recent allostatic treatments of interoceptive inference into three broad classes: *behavioral, teleological*, and *diachronic* (see Figure 15.1). This division is not meant to be taken as absolute; indeed, these accounts share many similarities by dint of their common theoretical origins.

15.4.1 Behavioral allostasis

In their commentary on Seth's (2013) theory of interoceptive inference, Gu and FitzGerald argue that the scope of predictive interoceptive processing should be extended beyond

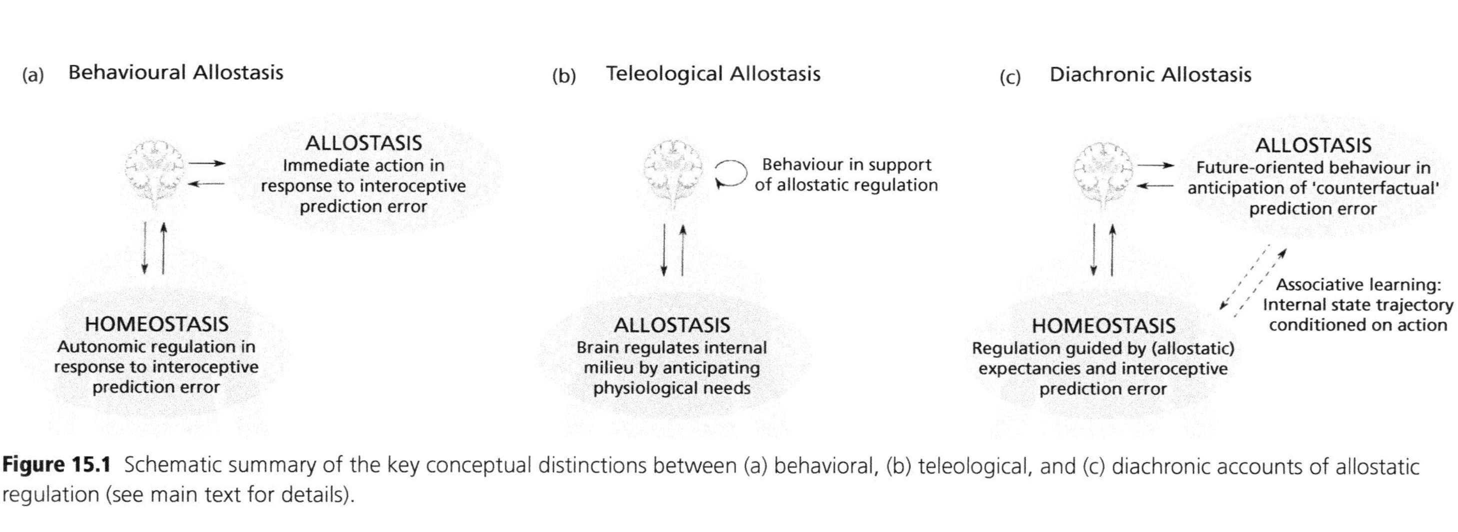

Figure 15.1 Schematic summary of the key conceptual distinctions between (a) behavioral, (b) teleological, and (c) diachronic accounts of allostatic regulation (see main text for details).

"homeostatic control of the internal milieu" to incorporate "allostatic actions on the external world" (2014, p. 269). At first, their position sounds isomorphic to that espoused by McEwen, insofar as allostasis is defined as "the process of achieving homeostasis" (Gu & FitzGerald, 2014, p. 269). It becomes quickly apparent, however, that Gu and FitzGerald (2014) conceive of homeostasis and allostasis in rather different terms. Here, homeostasis consists of autonomic reflexes that resist substantial fluctuations in the physiological conditions of the body (e.g. metabolizing stored fat in response to declining blood glucose levels), while allostasis corresponds to the behavioral actions that the agent undertakes in order to ameliorate some internal perturbation (e.g. consuming food in response to glucose decline). Gu and FitzGerald (2014) thus advocate a framework in which homeostatic (brain–internal world) and allostatic (brain–external world) loops offer alternative pathways to the same ultimate goal; namely, that of keeping the organism within the subset of biophysical states most conducive to its survival (in other words, minimizing the surprise or free energy indexed by interoceptive prediction error).

Gu and FitzGerald's (2014) behavior-orientated characterization of allostasis is adopted and further elaborated by Seth (2015). Thematizing the continuity between Ross Ashby's pioneering work in cybernetics (Ashby, 1956, 1960) and the free energy principle, Seth (2015) seeks to map homeostasis and allostasis onto the "ultrastable" scheme exemplified by Ashby's (1960) *homeostat*. Briefly, this device consists of four modular subsystems which dynamically interact to influence one another's essential variables. If these interactions fail to preserve essential variables within an acceptable range, a regulatory switch intervenes to randomly reconfigure the system's behavior. If the homeostat's new organization fails to stabilize essential variables within range, it will continue to transition through its repertoire of possible configurations until stability is restored, or until the system disintegrates (see Cariani, 2009, for a more detailed explication of the homeostat's functional architecture). Seth compares homeostasis to the first-order feedback loop constituted by the dynamic interplay of each module's inputs and outputs, and allostasis to the second-order reorganization of these interactions (although allostatic behavior constitutes a purposeful, rather than random, attempt to transform system dynamics). On this account, then, allostatic behavior functions to alter the organism's relation to its environment when homeostatic compensation fails to maintain physiological parameters within viable bounds.

Implementing these ideas within the context of free energy minimization, Seth (2015) argues that interoceptive prediction error can be minimized in one of three ways: (a) by adjusting model predictions in order to better approximate the incoming sensory signal (equivalently, updating one's emotional state; i.e. perceptual inference); (b) by enlisting autonomic reflexes to alter internal conditions such that they correspond with the predicted internal state (i.e. active inference or first-order (homeostatic) control); or (c) by engaging in goal-directed behavior to act on the environment in such a way that brings about the predicted internal state (i.e. second-order (allostatic) control). Here, then, allostasis is not only distinguished from the physiological mechanisms responsible for regulating the internal milieu, but also construed as an alternative mode of achieving organismic viability.

An interesting aspect of Seth's (2015) analysis is the claim that perception simply "falls out" of the fundamental necessity to achieve homeostatic control. It is not entirely clear whether Seth subscribes to a kind of anti-realism which denies the veridicality of perceptual experience, or whether he wants to say that our rich perceptual experiences of the world are merely an accidental consequence of (or a useful tool for) the homeostatic imperative. In any case, Seth interprets the free energy principle in a way that assigns primacy to interoception (over exteroceptive perception), insofar as interoceptive inference is regarded as playing an instrumental role in steering the agent towards its homeostatic states. We shall encounter a similar view in section 15.4.2, hence we postpone further consideration of its implications until later. Let us first review the allostatic picture presented here.

Perhaps the most striking feature of these initial attempts to assimilate allostatic principles within a broader predictive processing framework is the surprisingly *reactive* way in which allostasis is depicted. Rather than presenting a paradigmatic example of *anticipatory* behavior in the service of some homeostatic goal (e.g. consuming food *prior* to the decline of blood glucose concentration), Gu and FitzGerald (2014) portray allostatic actions as a kind of external-world equivalent to the corrective autonomic responses orchestrated by homeostatic control mechanisms. Seth (2015) likewise articulates what seems to be a distinctly reactive form of allostatic regulation. Indeed, the ultrastable system to which Seth draws conceptual allusion is entirely dependent on negative feedback responses to the perturbation of essential variables. Although the second-order feedback loop is functionally analogous to McEwen's conception of allostasis as the means by which homeostatic variables are stabilized, this arrangement lacks the capacity to anticipate and offset such deviations before they occur (a vital feature of all allostatic frameworks reviewed in section 15.3). Consequently, the notion of allostasis invoked by these "behavioral" accounts does not obviously pick out any process that is distinctively predictive in nature.

Arguably, these fundamentally reactive models of allostasis derive from a partitioning of biological regulation along the lines of internal/autonomic (i.e. homeostatic) and external/goal-directed (i.e. allostatic) responses. Such a distinction is to our knowledge unprecedented in the allostasis literature, inasmuch as allostatic mechanisms have always been conceived as a suite of actions traversing the physiological—behavioral continuum. Here, notably, allostasis seems instead to refer exclusively to the behavioral strategies an agent can engage in response to mounting interoceptive prediction error, rather than a process that participates in the proactive avoidance of such surprising states. It is however unclear to us what substantive insights can be gleaned from this sort of picture. Indeed, it is so obvious that organisms must interact with their environment in order to satisfy their basic homeostatic needs (e.g. seeking out and drinking fluids to quench thirst) that such behavioral repertoires are a well-established feature of homeostatic theory (see e.g. Richter, 1942–43). Simply reassigning such activities under the rubric of allostasis is thus likely to revive the kind of criticism engendered by earlier renditions of the theory (e.g. that allostasis is essentially redundant insofar as it "represent[s] nothing that has not always been part of the ordinary conceptual basis of homeostatic control," Carpenter, 2004, p. 180).

On balance then, these interpretations risk diluting the concept of allostasis to the point where it constitutes little more than a particular mode of homeostasis, a behavioral rearguard for occasions when autonomic mechanisms prove insufficient. As such, these inherently reactive accounts do not seem to carry us far beyond the insights availed by traditional homeostatic principles.

15.4.2 Teleological allostasis

The Embodied Predictive Interoception Coding model (EPIC; Barrett & Simmons, 2015) offers another free-energy inspired account grounding interoceptive experience in the physiological status of homeostatic variables. Initially, the authors of this model also defined allostasis in instrumental terms, describing it as the "process of activating physiological systems (such as hormonal, autonomic, or immune systems) with the aim of returning the body to homeostasis" (Barrett & Simmons, 2015, p. 422; Chanes & Barrett, 2016, p. 97). However, allostasis assumes a more pivotal role in subsequent work by Barrett and colleagues (Barrett, 2017; Barrett et al., 2016; Kleckner et al., 2017); the focus shifting from a reactive-mechanistic interpretation (i.e. where allostatic processes are recruited in response to homeostatic perturbation, similar to McEwen's (1998, 2004) definition), to a broader perspective emphasizing its fundamentally predictive nature (i.e. where bodily conditions are efficiently regulated through the coordinated allocation of energy resources in anticipation of upcoming demands, similar to Sterling's (2004, 2012; Sterling & Eyer, 1988) position). In this view, allostasis (and its interoceptive consequents) is assigned primary importance in the brain's computational economy such that the predictive models posited to underpin cognitive representation are entirely subservient to the efficient satisfaction of the body's physiological requirements (Barrett, 2017; Barrett et al., 2016).

Barrett and colleagues' more recent characterizations of allostasis as the primary design feature driving brain evolution involves a number of important theoretical commitments. First, this expanded version of allostasis apparently subsumes the homeostatic functions that allostatic processes had previously been supposed to support. In eliminating all talk of homeostasis in favor of a more comprehensively encompassing model of predictive regulation, Barrett and colleagues (Barrett, 2017; Barrett et al., 2016; Kleckner et al., 2017) align themselves with Sterling's (2004, 2012; Sterling & Laughlin, 2015) more radical allostatic agenda. It is not immediately clear that this sort of move is necessary for Barrett and colleagues' more recent formulations to cohere, especially since their explicit concern with metabolic exchange and energy regulation would seem to sit just as comfortably within McEwen and Wingfield's (2003) framework.

The second notable claim deriving from this framework is that the brain's computational architecture has evolved in order to optimize allostatic regulation, rather than for purposes such as veridical perception or reasoned action (Barrett, 2017; Barrett et al.,

2016; Kleckner et al., 2017). This is to say that the brain's internal model (or "embodied simulation") of the body and the ecological niche it inhabits is fundamentally attuned to its physiological needs, such that only those features (i.e. statistical regularities) of the body–niche dyad relevant to allostatic regulation are represented (Barrett, 2017). Furthermore, Barrett and colleagues (Barrett, 2017; Barrett et al., 2016) propose that interoceptive representations emerge as a consequence of allostatic processing, and that such affective sensations form a fundamental and pervasive feature of conscious awareness. By implication, other sensory domains (and presumably, volitional motor activity) figure as secondary or derivative phenomena, the metabolic costs of which are tolerated only insofar as they furnish additional support to the brain's primary allostatic–interoceptive axis (Barrett, 2017).

This picture is reminiscent of Seth's (2015) argument for the primacy of interoceptive inference and physiological regulation. It is not entirely clear whether Barrett and colleagues consider higher-level cognitive functions to be useful adjuncts for maintaining allostasis, or whether they simply emerge as a byproduct of the brain's allostatic machinery. It is clear, however, that Barrett (2017) considers perceptual experience to be fundamentally driven by allostatic and interoceptive processing, such that one's subjective grasp of reality is modelled according to one's physiological needs. The upshot of this hypothesis is a constructivist account in which allostasis functions as the author and arbiter of phenomenological experience, both insofar as the imperative to optimize allostasis has carved out an evolutionary trajectory that has endowed the creature with a particular cognitive architecture and set of sensory capacities, and insofar as the experiential possibilities afforded by these devices are constrained and modulated in ways designed to realize this imperative in a given context.

The brain's evolution into a highly efficient allostatic machine, rather than (say) a rational decision-maker or accurate perceiver of the world, does not necessarily preclude the possibility that it should realize these additional properties also. Indeed, Seth, Barrett, and their colleagues may well agree that providing a creature with the capacity to accurately model the hidden causes of its external perturbations would, over the long-run, improve its capacity to maintain the viability of its internal milieu, as well as engage in other intrinsically rewarding (and evolutionarily relevant) projects such as reproductive activity. As Barrett (2017) points out, however, creatures need only be informed about hidden causes that are (potentially) relevant to their ongoing allostatic needs and priorities (for instance, evolution has endowed humans with a sensorium that is indifferent to infrared light stimulation). In this sense, then, these authors are correct to say that human perception does not afford a "true" picture of the world, at least insofar as the latter is construed as some complete account of the totality of measurable phenomena. Indeed, it is hard to imagine how the kind of experience that would obtain in the event that we really could perceive "everything" could be of much use, as dense with (predominantly irrelevant) information as it would be. There seems to be good *prima facie* reason then to think that (exteroceptive) sensation has evolved precisely to the extent that it is *useful*, and adaptive self-regulatory activity (maximizing the likelihood of well-being and successful reproduction) would seem a reasonable object *for which* it ought to be useful.

These considerations notwithstanding, we note a general doubt about the plausibility of any thoroughgoing distinction between interoception and exteroception (independent of the specific role accorded to allostasis). Although it is true that the free energy principle allows for the possibility of inherited model parameters, and hence the newborn may come into the world equipped with certain expectations about the kinds of states its various sensory receptors ought to entertain, it is unclear why information conveyed via interoceptive afferents should be recognized by the brain as somehow different in kind to that received via exteroceptive (or proprioceptive) channels. From a brain-centric perspective, the external world to be modelled is that which lies beyond its neural projections, irrespective of whether this environment happens to be within or without the boundary formed by the body (Friston, 2010). In this respect, then, there is no meaningful distinction (for the brain) between the internal and external milieu; rather, there is only a Markov blanket (see Hohwy, 2017) separating a nervous system on the one side, and a hidden world of glucose molecules, blood vessels, muscles, fires, kittens, and so on, on the other. Collapsing this distinction leaves no principled rationale for privileging interoception over alternative forms sensory input; all channels furnish the brain with equally vital information about the state of play beyond the Markov blanket, from which its models profit.

A further, rather abstract concern about the teleological perspective presented here relates subtly to the conceptual role of the free energy principle. A key justification for the subordination of perceptual experience to homeostatic or allostatic regulation is made by way of appeal to the free energy principle's central concern with the persistent integrity of self-organized systems in the face of uncertain environmental conditions. Although we opened this section with a somewhat similar comment on the vital import of sustained biological viability in Friston's (2010) account, we urge caution in equating this with any so-called "fundamental imperative towards homeostasis" (Seth, 2015, p. 3). Rather, it would be more precise to say that the free energy principle captures something essential about the sorts of properties a biological system must possess in order to live (e.g. Friston & Stephan, 2007). It might be better then to say something like the following: any biological entity that consists of some form of sensorimotor interface through which it can enter into a dynamic exchange of energy and information with its environment, and which comprises an internal organization that enables it to minimize the free energy that bounds the surprise on its sensory states, is likely to endure; and in so doing, any such entity will thus *appear* to conform to the assumed imperative for the conservation of its biophysical integrity via self-regulatory processes. In other words, if a free energy-minimizing system exists, then it must indeed do so in virtue of possessing the right kind of internal configuration, and having entered into the right kind of circular-causal relationship with its environment, to be able to model the causes of its sensory states and engage in (what will look like) adaptive, self-regulatory activity (cf. Allen & Friston, 2018). As such, the apparent imperative towards self-regulatory behavior (be it homeostatic, allostatic, or whatever) seems to fall out of the ongoing minimization of free energy in much the same way as the apparent teleological force driving evolutionary "design" emerges as a consequence of the intricate, non-teleological dynamics driving natural selection.

15.4.3 Diachronic allostasis

We turn finally to two remaining inferential formulations of allostasis, which we refer to as "diachronic" on account of the important implications they have for regulatory activity over various timescales.

Pezzulo, Rigoli, and Friston (2015) set out to explain how prospective and goal-directed (i.e. allostatic) forms of control might have evolved from more primitive mechanisms subserving homeostatic regulation. Here, homeostasis is construed along control-theoretic/cybernetic lines of negative feedback and setpoint control, where autonomic and behavioral reflexes are enlisted to correct deviations in physiological variables (see also Pezzulo, 2013; Seth, 2013). By contrast, allostasis refers to the flexible, context-specific engagement of complex, adaptive behavioral repertoires for the purposes of achieving some future outcome. Like the accounts surveyed in section 15.4.1, then, homeostasis and allostasis are equated with "direct" and "indirect" modes of eliminating interoceptive prediction error, respectively. Note however that the distinction here is more nuanced, insofar as homeostatic responses extend to the innate behavioral sets (e.g. approach/avoidance behavior) that equip animals to survive in the absence of associative learning.

If complex behavioral policies are to offer an effective means of controlling the physiological conditions of the body, it is essential that they deliver the right kinds of state transitions at the right time. This requirement is inherently challenging, however, since the consequences of a particular policy are necessarily realized some time after those conditions that triggered its initiation. Such delays are nontrivial in the context of homeostatic control, where a process causing physiological conditions to deteriorate may precipitate catastrophic damage if not promptly addressed. Pezzulo, Rigoli, and Friston's (2015) solution to this problem leverages the free energy minimizing agent's ability to acquire sophisticated internal models of the hidden environmental causes of its sensory states. Specifically, they argue that such generative interoceptive models enable such agents to predict the temporal evolution of interoceptive state trajectories (i.e. how interoceptive signals are likely to change over time), and encode how these trajectories correlate with sensorimotor events in the external world (cf. Friston et al., 2017). In virtue of the higher-level integration of sensory information converging from interoceptive, exteroceptive, and proprioceptive streams, the agent is thus able to acquire a rich understanding of how behavioral activities come to influence interoceptive states across various contexts. By linking interoceptive prediction errors and their suppression through active inference (i.e. engagement of allostatic behavior) via such associative learning processes, Pezzulo and colleagues (2015) provide a compelling explanation of (a) how the allostatic anticipation of future homeostatic needs might systematically arise, and (b) why allostatic behavioral policies should be endorsed despite potentially lengthy delays in their homeostatic payoff.

On this construal, allostatic processing turns out to be fundamentally *counterfactual* in nature. Higher (or deeper) hierarchical representations map the relation between increasingly distal outcome states and the behavioral policies that would lead towards their accomplishment. This account thus renders a smooth continuum of adaptive action selection, ranging from the primitive drives that work, for instance, to sate appetite via exploitation of the immediate environment, to the complex deliberative activities serving various motivations extending well beyond the basic requirements of the internal milieu (see also Pezzulo, 2017). Indeed, Pezzulo and colleagues (2015) observe that the capacity to learn the counterfactual relations that enable the agent to engage in prospective planning, and to choose amongst various available policies, confers an unparalleled degree of autonomy from the exigencies of the homeostatic imperative. Thus, in much the same way as Bernard and Cannon recognized how the capacity to maintain the stability of the internal milieu granted complex biological systems a remarkable degree of autonomy from the caprices of their external environments, allostasis under this scheme extends such freedom even further. Capable of holding the immediate demands of homeostasis in abeyance to some supraordinate desired (i.e. unsurprising and attracting) state, the autonomous horizon of the allostatic organism expands beyond the conditions of the present into a predictable (albeit uncertain) future.

Finally, Stephan, Manjaly, Mathis, and colleagues (2016) propose a formalized Bayesian implementation of hierarchical allostatic control that likewise operates across various temporal grains. Allostasis is defined here as the mode of active inference which performs "anticipatory homeostatic control" (Stephan et al., 2016, p. 5). This is achieved via the modulation of prior beliefs concerning the expected state trajectory of a given homeostatic setpoint. Expectancies about setpoint values are construed in terms of a probability distribution, such that beliefs propagated from higher-level circuits influence both the mean value of the controlled variable, and its associated variability (or precision). In other words, the traditional notion of a homeostatic negative feedback loop is situated at the lowest level of the processing hierarchy, with its target setpoint (i.e. the expected physiological state) conditioned by top-down information received from higher (allostatic) circuits. These higher (or deeper) hierarchical levels are posited to model increasingly broader, domain-general representations of the present state of the body and its environment, as well as predictions about changes in those states. Consequently, this account of allostatic regulation incorporates an important temporal dimension, where higher-level generative models are able to inform and update lower-level homeostatic control mechanisms in accordance with predictions about upcoming state transitions.

Stephan and colleagues (2016) set out their model of allostatically regulated homeostatic reflexes in accordance with the basic computational architecture assumed by the free energy principle. Homeostatic control thus depends on both the perception of salient features within the internal and external milieu (comprising both physical and social dynamics), and selection of appropriate actions designed to prevent dangerous (i.e. surprising) deviations of physiological parameters. Inference is divided into interoceptive and exteroceptive sensory processing. Prediction concerns how internal and external states will evolve over time, as well as the degree to which possible actions will maintain internal states within the bounds of a given homeostatic setpoint over time. In other words, allostatic prior beliefs set expectations about the space of bodily states that the organism ought to inhabit (i.e. that delimited set of attracting states which engender low entropy), which homeostatic systems subsequently attempt to realize. Importantly, this generic active inference scheme is extended beyond the context of low-level homeostatic reflexes to encompass the higher-level implementation of flexible behavioral policies designed to avoid homeostatic surprise (in a similar vein to Pezzulo et al., 2015).

Stephan and colleagues (2016) present the first mathematically concrete account of allostatic control within the context of free energy minimization. Although more work needs to be done to flesh out this formal scheme with respect to the complex dynamics involved in the integrated regulation of complex physiological systems, it provides a plausible theoretical framework for explaining a number of core allostatic phenomena. The notion of a Bayesian reflex arc whose setpoint is adaptively defined and constrained by higher-order (allostatic) dynamics provides an elegant explanation of setpoint variability; one that seems equally capable of incorporating other (i.e. non-allostatic) accounts of flexible setpoint control (e.g. Cabanac, 2006). Embedding this arc within a hierarchical architecture also provides a principled mechanistic explanation of how certain higher-order parameters might be prioritized at the expense of less-urgent homeostatic needs, and how maladaptive psychological states might be entrained by persistent interoceptive prediction error. This perspective thus offers a deeply unifying picture of homeostatic and allostatic control as a dynamic coupling or closed loop, with lower-level homeostatic inferences and higher-level allostatic predictions reciprocally informing and modulating one another as the joint conditions of the agent–niche dyad evolve.

Aside from some minor technicalities concerning the precise definitional boundaries of homeostatic and allostatic control, we consider the diachronic theories reviewed in this section to be broadly compatible and complementary. We prefer Stephan and colleagues' (2016) Bayesian reflex formulation insofar as it expands the scope of allostatic control to the modulation of internal conditions (rather than limiting it to the domain of external, goal-directed behavior). This perspective is more consistent with the historical development of the allostatic framework (as examined in section 15.3), all prominent versions of which assume allostasis to consist of a repertoire of mechanisms that include the capacity to influence internal conditions directly by harnessing physiological effectors. Happily, the Bayesian reflex account invokes a principled distinction between homeostatic and allostatic control which succeeds in preserving the key functional characteristics of both modes of regulation (i.e. it neither collapses one concept into the other, nor relies on arbitrary or vague criteria for distinguishing their respective remits), while still allowing for the kind of higher-level, temporally-extended allostatic behavior articulated by Pezzulo and colleagues (2015). Furthermore, we find Stephan and colleagues' (2016) framework a potentially more useful starting point for future inquiry into the general nature of biological regulation, insofar as it affords the basic computational elements for scaffolding the emergence of less flexible, non-counterfactual forms of allostatic regulation (e.g.

circadian, circannual, and ontogenetic). By integrating the complementary perspectives provided by both diachronic theories, we arrive at a nuanced and fecund account of self-regulation that accommodates multiple scales of biological and cognitive complexity.

15.5 The future of the history of allostasis

Our review of the origins of allostasis, and analysis of its recent uptake in theories of interoceptive inference, might give the impression that the concept is as protean as the phenomena which inspired its coinage. This may be a consequence of zealous category splitting on our part, motivated by our intent to differentiate meaningful distinctions amongst a cluster of intersecting (and not entirely consistent) theoretical perspectives. However, the various interpretations and treatments allostasis has received over the years have tended to congeal around a more or less stable core of organizing principles (e.g. Schulkin, 2004). Mature versions of Sterling's (2004, 2012) and McEwen's (e.g. 2004, 2007) frameworks have understandably evolved into more expansive and nuanced iterations of their progenitors, benefitting from empirical advances and critical discussion. These influential accounts have thus reached a point of quasi-consensus, in as much as they lack the diversity of a genuine pluralism, but fail to converge fully on a coherent, unified account of what allostasis is or does. This leaves us in the somewhat precarious position of possessing a theoretical construct that appears well established and valid, but comprises a heterogeneous and not entirely coherent set of commitments. Part of the motivation of this chapter was therefore to highlight this situation, given that free energy theorists have started helping themselves to aspects of the allostasis construct without necessarily being explicit about which particular interpretation(s) of it they wish to endorse.

A useful illustration might be drawn from our distinction between what we dubbed the teleological and the diachronic interpretations of allostasis. Indeed, those familiar with the former might protest that it too invokes a hierarchical architecture which, much like the diachronic accounts, also admits of higher generative models encoding predictions extending across increasingly extended temporal windows. As such, it might seem somewhat disingenuous to exclude this model from our favored diachronic category. Our point, however, is that these frameworks are founded on rather different understandings of allostasis, giving rise to subtle but deep conceptual disagreements. The teleological perspective considers exteroception as secondary to interoception, which in turn emerges as a consequence of allostasis. The diachronic perspectives, on the other hand, seem to hold each domain of sensory information in equal standing; interoception, exteroception, and proprioception are blended together at a suitably high level of hierarchical modelling and without any indication that any stream is more fundamental than the others.

We urge care about which aspects of allostatic theory are imported into predictive model-based accounts of interoception. Indeed, it is notable that none of the interoceptive inference theories reviewed in this chapter acknowledge the accusations of redundancy, inconsistency, and ambiguity that have been levelled against the allostasis literature, even after some of these authors had substantially revised their own application of the concept.

Ignoring such issues not only belies the contested nature of allostatic control, it has the potential to propagate further confusion as disparate elements of the construct are selectively sampled and fused together.

If the future of allostasis is to disclose meaningful theoretical insights concerning the predictive processes that support biological regulation and interoceptive inference, then the next phase of its conceptual development requires us to work out a clear and precise understanding of its core principles and entailments. We have tried to clarify some of the confusion that has plagued the allostasis literature since its inception, and argued in favor of an inclusive view that reconciles homeostasis and allostasis as complementary strategies for sustaining biological viability. We have also attempted to shed light on some of the idiosyncratic ways in which allostasis has been deployed in recent characterizations of interoceptive inference, and suggest that future progress in this line of research will be hindered if these conceptual inconsistencies are not subject to critical scrutiny.

Acknowledgments

We thank the anonymous reviewer for their suggested improvements to an earlier version of this chapter. AWC is supported by an Australian Government Research Training Program (RTP) scholarship. JH is supported by The Australian Research Council DP160102770 and by the Research School Bochum and the Center for Mind, Brain and Cognitive Evolution, Ruhr-University Bochum. Author ORCIDs are as follows: AWC is 0000-0002-0449-4883; JH is 0000-0003-3906-3060.

References

Adolph, E. F. (1961). Early concepts of physiological regulations. *Physiological Reviews, 41*(4), 737–70.

Allen, M. and **Friston, K. J.** (2018). From cognitivism to autopoiesis: Towards a computational framework for the embodied mind. *Synthese, 195*(6), 2459–82.

Ashby, W. R. (1947). The nervous system as physical machine: With special reference to the origin of adaptive behavior. *Mind, 56*(221), 44–59.

Ashby, W. R. (1956). *An Introduction to Cybernetics*. London: Chapman & Hall Ltd.

Ashby, W. R. (1960). *Design for a Brain: The Origin of Adaptive Behaviour*, 2nd edn. London: Chapman & Hall Ltd.

Ashby, W. R. (1962). Principles of the self-organizing system. In: H. Von Foerster and G. W. Zopf Jr. (eds), *Principles of Self-Organization: Transactions of the University of Illinois Symposium*. London: Pergamon Press, pp. 255–78.

Barrett, L. F. and **Simmons, W. K.** (2015). Interoceptive predictions in the brain. *Nature Reviews Neuroscience, 16*(7), 419–29.

Barrett, L. F., **Quigley, K. S.**, and **Hamilton, P.** (2016). An active inference theory of allostasis and interoception in depression. *Philosophical Transactions of the Royal Society B, 371*(20160011), 1–17.

Barrett, L. F. (2017). The theory of constructed emotion: An active inference account of interoception and categorization. *Social Cognitive & Affective Neuroscience, 12*(1), 1–23.

Boulos, Z. and **Rosenwasser, A. M.** (2004). A chronobiological perspective on allostasis and its application to shift work. In: J. Schulkin (ed.), *Allostasis, Homeostasis, and the Costs of Physiological Adaptation*. Cambridge: Cambridge University Press, pp. 228–301.

Cabanac, M. (2006). Adjustable set point: To honor Harold T. Hammel. *Journal of Applied Physiology, 100*(4), 1338–46.

Cannon, W. B. (1929). Organization for physiological homeostasis. *Physiological Reviews, 9*(3), 399–431.

Cannon, W. B. (1939). *The Wisdom of the Body*. New York, NY: W. W. Norton & Company, Inc.

Cariani, P. A. (2009). The homeostat as embodiment of adaptive control. *International Journal of General Systems, 38*(2), 139–54.

Carpenter, R. H. S. (2004). Homeostasis: A plea for a unified approach. *Advances in Physiology Education, 28*, 180–7.

Chanes, L. and **Barrett, L. F.** (2016). Redefining the role of limbic areas in cortical processing. *Trends in Cognitive Sciences, 20*(2), 96–106.

Clark, A. (2013). Whatever next? Predictive brains, situated agents, and the future of cognitive science. *Behavioral Brain Sciences, 36*(3), 181–253.

Clark, A. (2016). *Surfing Uncertainty: Prediction, Action, and the Embodied Mind*. Oxford: Oxford University Press.

Cooper, S. J. (2008). From Claude Bernard to Walter Cannon. Emergence of the concept of homeostasis. *Appetite, 51*(3), 419–27.

Dallman, M. F. (2003). Stress by any other name? *Hormones & Behavior, 43*(1), 18–20.

Day, T. A. (2005). Defining stress as a prelude to mapping its neurocircuitry: No help from allostasis. *Progress in Neuro-Psychopharmacology & Biological Psychiatry, 29*(8), 1195–200.

Friston, K. J. and **Stephan, K. E.** (2007). Free-energy and the brain. *Synthese, 159*(3), 417–58.

Friston, K. J. (2010). The free-energy principle: A unified brain theory? *Nature Reviews Neuroscience, 11*(2), 127–38.

Friston, K. J. (2012). Embodied inference and spatial cognition. *Cognitive Processing, 13*(Suppl. 1) S171–77.

Friston, K. J. (2013). Life as we know it. *Journal of the Royal Society Interface, 10*(86), 20130475.

Friston, K. J., Rosch, R., Parr, T., Price, C., and **Bowman, H.** (2017). Deep temporal models and active inference. *Neuroscience & Biobehavioral Reviews, 77*, 388–402.

Friston, K. J., Schwartenbeck, P., FitzGerald, T., Moutoussis, M., Behrens, T., and **Dolan, R. J.** (2014). The anatomy of choice: Dopamine and decision-making. *Philosophical Transactions of the Royal Society B, 369*(20130481), 1–12.

Gu, X. and **FitzGerald, T. H. B.** (2014). Interoceptive inference: Homeostasis and decision-making. *Trends in Cognitive Sciences, 18*(6), 269–70.

Hohwy, J. (2013). *The Predictive Mind*. Oxford: Oxford University Press.

Hohwy, J. (2016). The self-evidencing brain. *Noûs, 50*(2), 259–85.

Hohwy, J. (2017). How to entrain your evil demon. In: T. Metzinger and W. Wiese (eds), *Philosophy and Predictive Processing*. Frankfurt am Main: MIND Group, pp. 1–15.

Khalsa, S. S., Adolphs, R., Cameron, O. G., Critchley, H. D., Davenport, J. S., Feinstein, J. S., et al. (in press). Interoception and mental health: A roadmap. *Biological Psychiatry: Cognitive Neuroscience & Neuroimaging*.

Kleckner, I. R., Zhang, J., Touroutoglou, A., Chanes, L., Xia, C., Simmons, W. K., et al. (2017). Evidence for a large-scale brain system supporting allostasis and interoception in humans. *Nature Human Behaviour, 1*(0069), 1–14.

Lowe, R., Almér, A., and **Dodig-Crnkovic, G.** (2017). Predictive regulation in affective and adaptive behaviour: An allostatic-cybernetics perspective. In: J. Vallverdú, M. Mazzara, M. Talanov, S. Distefano, and R. Lowe (eds), *Advanced Research on Biologically Inspired Cognitive Architectures*. Hershey, PA: IGI Global, pp. 148–77.

McEwen, B. S. and **Stellar, E.** (1993). Stress and the individual: Mechanisms leading to disease. *Archives of Internal Medicine, 153*(18), 2093–101.

McEwen, B. S. (1998). Stress, adaptation, and disease: Allostasis and allostatic load. *Annals of the New York Academy of Sciences, 840*, 33–44.

McEwen, B. S. (2000a). Protective and damaging effects of stress mediators: Central role of the brain. In: E. A. Mayer and C. B. Saper (eds), *Progress in Brain Research*, Vol. **122**. Amsterdam: Elsevier Science, pp. 25–34.

McEwen, B. S. (2000b). The neurobiology of stress: From serendipity to clinical relevance. *Brain Research, 886*(1–2), 172–89.

McEwen, B. S. and **Wingfield, J. C.** (2003). The concept of allostasis in biology and biomedicine. *Hormones & Behavior, 43*(1), 2–15.

McEwen, B. S. (2004). Protective and damaging effects of mediators of stress: Allostasis and allostatic load. In: J. Schulkin (ed.), *Allostasis, Homeostasis, and the Costs of Physiological Adaptation.* Cambridge, MA: MIT Press, pp. 65–98.

McEwen, B. S. (2007). Physiology and neurobiology of stress and adaptation: Central role of the brain. *Physiological Reviews, 87*(3), 873–904.

McEwen, B. S. and **Wingfield, J. C.** (2010). What is in a name? Integrating homeostasis, allostasis and stress. *Hormones & Behavior, 57*(2), 105–11.

Michael, J., **Modell, H.**, **McFarland, J.**, and **Cliff, W.** (2009). The "core principles" of physiology: What should students understand? *Advances in Physiology Education, 33*(1), 10–16.

Michael, J. and **McFarland, J.** (2011). The core principles ("big ideas") of physiology: Results of faculty surveys. *Advances in Physiology Education, 35*(4), 336–341.

Modell, H., **Cliff, W.**, **Michael, J.**, **McFarland, J.**, **Wenderoth, M. P.**, and **Wright, A.** (2015). A physiologist's view of homeostasis. *Advances in Physiology Education, 39*(4), 259–66.

Moran, R. J., **Symmonds, M.**, **Dolan, R. J.**, and **Friston, K. J.** (2014). The brain ages optimally to model its environment: Evidence from sensory learning over the adult lifespan. *PLoS Computational Biology, 10*(1), e1003422.

Peters, A., **McEwen, B. S.**, and **Friston, K. J.** (2017). Uncertainty and stress: Why it causes diseases and how it is mastered by the brain. *Progress in Neurobiology*, **156**, 164–88.

Pezzulo, G. (2013). Why do you fear the bogeyman? An embodied predictive coding model of perceptual inference. *Cognitive, Affective, & Behavioral Neuroscience, 14*(3), 902–11.

Pezzulo, G., **Rigoli, F.**, and **Friston, K. J.** (2015). Active inference, homeostatic regulation and adaptive behavioural control. *Progress in Neurobiology, 134*, 17–35.

Pezzulo, G. (2017). Tracing the roots of cognition in predictive processing. In: T. Metzinger and W. Wiese (eds), *Philosophy and Predictive Processing.* Frankfurt am Main: MIND Group, pp. 1–20.

Power, M. L. (2004). Commentary: Viability as opposed to stability: An evolutionary perspective on physiological regulation. In: J. Schulkin (ed.), *Allostasis, Homeostasis, and the Costs of Physiological Adaptation.* Cambridge: Cambridge University Press, pp. 343–64.

Power, M. L. and **Schulkin, J.** (2012). Maternal obesity, metabolic disease, and allostatic load. *Physiology & Behavior, 106*(1), 22–8.

Richter, C. P. (1942–43). Total self-regulatory functions in animals and human beings. *Harvey Lecture Series, 38*, 63–103.

Rosen, J. B. and **Schulkin, J.** (2004). Adaptive fear, allostasis, and the pathology of anxiety and depression. In: J. Schulkin (ed.), *Allostasis, Homeostasis, and the Costs of Physiological Adaptation.* Cambridge: Cambridge University Press, pp. 164–227.

Schulkin, J., **McEwen, B. S.**, and **Gold, P. W.** (1994). Allostasis, amygdala, and anticipatory angst. *Neuroscience & Biobehavioral Reviews, 18*(3), 385–96.

Schulkin, J. (2003a). Allostasis: A neural behavioral perspective. *Hormones & Behavior*, *43*(1), 21–7.

Schulkin, J. (2003b). *Rethinking Homeostasis: Allostatic Regulation in Physiology and Pathophysiology*. Cambridge, MA: MIT Press.

Schulkin, J. (2004). Introduction. In: J. Schulkin (ed.), *Allostasis, Homeostasis, and the Costs of Physiological Adaptation*. Cambridge: Cambridge University Press, pp. 1–16.

Schulkin, J. (2011). Social allostasis: Anticipatory regulation of the internal milieu. *Frontiers in Evolutionary Neuroscience*, *2*(111), 1–15.

Seth, A. K. (2013). Interoceptive inference, emotion, and the embodied self. *Trends in Cognitive Sciences*, *17*(11), 565–73.

Seth, A. K. (2015). The cybernetic Bayesian brain: From interoceptive inference to sensorimotor contingencies. In: T. Metzinger and J. M. Windt (eds), *Open Mind*. Frankfurt am Main: MIND Group, pp. 1–24.

Seth, A. K. and **Friston, K. J.** (2016). Active interoceptive inference and the emotional brain. *Philosophical Transactions of the Royal Society B*, *371*(1708), 1–10.

Smith, R., **Thayer, J. F.**, **Khalsa, S. S.**, and **Lane, R. D.** (2017). The hierarchical basis of neurovisceral integration. *Neuroscience & Biobehavioral Reviews*, 75, 274–96.

Stephan, K. E., **Manjaly, Z. M.**, **Mathys, C. D.**, **Weber, L. A. E.**, **Paliwal, S.**, **Gard, T.**, et al. (2016). Allostatic self-efficacy: A metacognitive theory of dyshomeostasis-induced fatigue and depression. *Frontiers in Human Neuroscience*, *10*(550), 1–27.

Sterling, P. and **Eyer, J.** (1988). Allostasis: A new paradigm to explain arousal pathology. In: S. Fisher and J. Reason (eds), *Handbook of Life Stress, Cognition and Health*. John Wiley & Sons Ltd, pp. 629–49.

Sterling, P. (2004). Principles of allostasis: Optimal design, predictive regulation, pathophysiology and rational therapeutics. In: J. Schulkin (ed.), *Allostasis, Homeostasis, and the Costs of Physiological Adaptation* . Cambridge: Cambridge University Press, pp. 17–64.

Sterling, P. (2012). Allostasis: A model of predictive regulation. *Physiology & Behavior*, *106*(1), 5–15.

Sterling, P. and **Laughlin, S.** (2015). *Principles of Neural Design*. Cambridge, MA: MIT Press.

Woods, S. C. and **Ramsay, D. S.** (2007). Homeostasis: Beyond Curt Richter. *Appetite*, *49*(2), 388–98.

Yates, F. E. (1996). Homeostasis. In: J. E. Birren (ed.), *Encyclopedia of Gerontology: Age, Aging, and the Aged*, Vol. 1. San Diego, CA: Academic Press, pp. 679–86).

Chapter 16

Subjectivity as a sentient perspective and the role of interoception

Helena De Preester

The essence of subjectivity is affectivity.
(Henry, 1973, p. 476)

16.1 Introduction

Subjects and objects are radically different beings, distinguished by a basic feature that all subjects have in common and that all objects seem to lack. Objects seem to rest in themselves, unaware of, not sensitive to, and unconcerned about what is happening to them or in the environment. A subject, by contrast, is a sentient perspective that breaches the self-enclosed state of objects and opens up a world.[1]

This chapter argues that the most basic form of subjectivity is different from and more fundamental than having a self. It also posits a hypothesis about the origin of subjectivity in terms of interoception. Both topics have been on the agenda of philosophers, psychologists, and neuroscientists before, but now a consensus concerning the homeostatic-interoceptive origin of subjectivity is growing in these domains of research. This chapter critically explores that growing consensus. In particular, it argues that the idea that the brain *topographically represents* bodily states is unfit for thinking about the coming about of subjectivity. The reason is that representation implies objectification—and thus the irreparable disappearance—of subjectivity. We therefore present an approach that preserves the importance of interoceptive processes for the coming about of subjectivity, but gives due attention to its inherent characteristics.

In the first part, four inherent characteristics of subjectivity are discussed from a philosophical point of view. First, the most basic form of subjectivity consists in being a sentient perspective. Second, subjectivity necessarily implies self-awareness but not necessarily the existence of a self. Third, in contrast to a self, subjectivity in its most basic form lacks

[1] There are different possible ways of characterizing objects in opposition to subjects. One may argue that objects cannot be self-enclosed because they lack a proper self-identity. In that case, objects are considered as mere nexuses in a causal network. If we oppose objects and subjects in that way, subjects would differ from objects in the sense that the network matters to them; this means, it matters to them from their perspective. Objects, by contrast, would not take a stance toward the network. What is important in either characterization, however, is that subjectivity and having a world are co-originary.

spatial extension. Finally, it is marked by self-affectivity. The second part explores whether an approach to subjectivity in which interoception maintains its crucial role is possible without relying on topographic representations of the in-depth body, and giving due attention to the inherent characteristics of subjectivity.

16.2 Four inherent characteristics of subjectivity

16.2.1 Subjectivity as a sentient perspective

Subjectivity is a sentient form of being a perspective. Sentience, or awareness, refers to the capacity to feel or to be affected—internally by one's own body or externally by the environment. We use the terms "sentience" and "awareness" interchangeably, and we prefer to avoid the term "consciousness" for the basic form of subjectivity discussed here. A graded approach to subjectivity allows the conceptual and terminological distinction between a basic form of subjectivity in terms of a sentient perspective, characterized by the four inherent characteristics discussed in this chapter, and the full-fledged and articulate form we often associate with human consciousness. Whereas the existence of a sentient perspective may be a necessary condition for consciousness, we do not claim that its four characteristics fully capture it or are sufficient for it.

Subjectivity is difficult to grasp without changing the way it manifests itself to us when it is not observed but lived through while it is unfolding in time. Subjectivity is not only impossible to grasp from a third-person approach but even a first-person thematic or reflective access to it is hard as well. As the point of view that makes things visible, a perspective is itself not visible as a thing. "Perspective," from the Latin *perspicere* or "looking through," is etymologically indeed related to the idea of transparency or invisibility. Therefore, when subjectivity is observed or made thematic, it is not grasped the way in which it pre-reflectively unfolds (Legrand, 2007). The shift from lived-through subjectivity to the objectification of it in an act of reflection turns a perspective into something it is not, losing sight of its inherent characteristics. Objectification, however, does not mean that subjectivity is turned into an object in the way that stones and tables are objects. It means that we approach the subjective perspective *from another point of view*, stepping out of the former and losing its lived-through, unmediated presence.

16.2.2 Subjectivity, self-awareness, and self

The lived-through presence of subjectivity is not wholly inaccessible from a first-person perspective, however. In a non-thematical or non-reflective way, subjectivity is aware of itself as sentient. In other words, to be sentient or to feel would imply to be aware of this feeling. For the sake of conceptual clarity, we use "self-awareness" in the sense of being aware of feeling, not in the sense of an articulate form of reflective self-consciousness. Moreover, on the basic level of subjectivity, there is no divide between awareness and its so-called object (the "self" of self-awareness). Self-awareness is built into subjectivity itself. A subjective perspective is like a beam of light in which a world appears, but this beam of light does not need to shine on itself in order to appear in awareness. Many philosophers have tried to point out exactly this, but in the context and terminology of consciousness: consciousness *is* self-consciousness; self-awareness is an intrinsic feature of consciousness (see, e.g. Legrand, 2007; Zahavi, 2005; Shoemaker, 1996; Frankfurt, 1988). Language somehow leads us astray in separating awareness from self-awareness. The conceptual and terminological distinction between sentience and the awareness of being sentient, or between feeling and the feeling that one feels, may be unwarranted.

Many philosophers of consciousness have tried to spell out that strictly speaking, self-consciousness is not consciousness *of* itself, because it does not follow the perception model in which an act of consciousness is directed toward an object (see Frank, 2007). Consciousness does not stand in a subject-object relation to itself but is *non-relational*; consciousness and self-consciousness coincide at the pole of subjectivity. That explains why, in order to explore the phenomenon of subjectivity, we should not shift from lived-through subjectivity to the objectification of it in an act of reflection (see section 16.2.1). Philosophers sometimes use the term "pre-reflective self-consciousness" (Legrand, 2007) in order to refer to self-consciousness in the sense of consciousness of the self as the *subject* (and not the object) of experience. The term "first-person perspective" is also often used in order to emphasize that dimension of consciousness (Zahavi, 2005).

That the full-fledged form of subjectivity called "consciousness" is capable of an articulate, reflective, and relational mode of self-consciousness hinders a good understanding of *basic* self-awareness. The articulate mode of self-consciousness is active when a subject, from a first-person perspective ("I"), turns to itself and takes itself reflectively as the object of thinking or feeling, resulting in a "me" or a self that is the object of a thought, a feeling, etc. When I consider myself clumsy, recognize myself in the mirror, or remember myself as a child, a reflective mode of self-consciousness is active. That mode of consciousness relates to a self—my self—with all the characteristics proper to it: self-identity, individuation, biographic narrative, etc.

Self-awareness, by contrast, does not require the existence of a person, an "I," or a subject (we talk about "subjectivity," not about "subjects") that reflects on itself. Too often, the notion of "self" evokes the idea of a self as in reflective self-consciousness, leaping over the minimal notion of "self" involved in self-awareness. The following descriptions aim to point out such a minimal notion of "self." For example, Zahavi concludes that "there is a minimal sense of self present whenever there is self-awareness. Self-awareness is there . . . whenever there is something it is like for me to have the experience. In other words, pre-reflective self-awareness and a minimal sense of self are integral parts of our experiential life" (Zahavi, 2005, p. 146). "Minimal self" refers to the basic, immediate, or primitive self, devoid of anything that is not essential to a self. It is defined as a bare locus of consciousness, devoid of personality. It is "a consciousness of oneself as an immediate subject of experience, unextended in time" (Gallagher, 2000, p. 15; see also Strawson, 1999).

Whereas these philosophers, in trying to get down to the bedrock of subjectivity, carefully avoid a too inflated notion of self, elements from the complex and sophisticated phenomenon of self-consciousness are too often incorporated. As the second part of this chapter shows, that happens in a number of influential neuroscience approaches to self and subjectivity. A careful consideration of the idea that in its most basic form, subjectivity is a sentient perspective that is *non-relationally* self-aware, may advance neuroscience and neuropsychological approaches of subjectivity. However, most research in cognitive science still focuses on the self as the result of a relation between a subject ("I") and itself ("me"), such as the self as object of perception in self-recognition (Legrand, 2007). It is the self to which acts of consciousness, such as perception, attention, or representation, are directed. Any of these acts objectifies the self, and that is why neuro(psycho)logical research needs a shift away from the self-as-object to the self-as-subject (Legrand, 2007; Christoff et al., 2011). In the vein of William James' (1893) classical distinction between "me" and "I," Christoff, Cosmelli, Legrand, and colleagues (2011) focus on the "I" *as agent* (of perception, action, cognition, and emotion) instead of the "me" as object (of perception, action, cognition, and emotion). This is a step in a much-needed direction in the scientific study of subjectivity.

However, if we want to study the most basic form of subjectivity, the notion of "I" already suggests too much, such as a central, unified, or unifying point of experience, somehow "owning" consciousness (or "owning" a subjective perspective). A subjective perspective, however, does not need an owner in order to exist. Subjectivity as such does not presuppose an ego or an "I" standing above or floating along with the stream of consciousness. In terms of the distinction between egological and non-egological theories of consciousness (see Gurwitsch, 1941), the subjective perspective is ego-less or anonymous.

16.2.3 **Temporal extension of the subjective perspective versus spatial extension of the self**

A third basic characteristic of basic subjectivity is its temporal extension. This may be surprising because it is often stated that a minimal form of consciousness is present in singular and transitory experiences and that it does not enjoy any diachronic persistency or identity in a plurality of experiences (see Damasio, 1999; Gallagher, 2000). In contrast, more sophisticated versions of consciousness and self, such as a narrative or autobiographic self, are considered as extended over periods of time, ranging from seconds to decades.

This marked contrast between minimal and more extended interpretations of the self hides the fact that basic subjectivity too is temporally extended over small stretches of time. These small stretches of time can be identified as instances of the specious present (James, 1893, p. 609). The temporal structure of the most basic layer of subjectivity was also analysed in great detail by the phenomenological philosopher Edmund Husserl (1859–1938). His analysis, which happens in terms of "consciousness," not only explains how we can be conscious of temporal objects (e.g. a piece of music) but also how consciousness is a phenomenon *of* time (and not only *in* time). The question of how the stream of consciousness inevitably is conscious of itself is tackled in a reflection on the temporal nature of consciousness (De Preester, 2007; Kortooms, 2002; Husserl, 1991). Husserl speaks of "inner" consciousness when he emphasizes the self-conscious nature of consciousness. In his account, consciousness is not only responsible for its objects of perception but it also constitutes *itself* as a temporally extended unity[2] (for technical details see De Preester, 2007; Zahavi, 2005; Kortooms, 2002). The crucial idea is that in this operation of auto-constitution, the stream appears to itself (*Selbsterscheinung*, Husserl, 1966, p. 83). Consciousness exists as a stream, and it appears to itself as a stream. Whatever the value of the details of his account, and of his explanation for the self-conscious nature of consciousness, Husserl gives due attention to the temporal nature of the subjective perspective.

Many objects of consciousness (including the self) are experienced as spatially existing, whereas the subjective perspective itself cannot be experienced as extended in space. Since it is the point of origin where experience starts from and which opens up onto a world, it itself cannot appear in a perspective, enjoying spatial extension. Spatial appearance is impossible for the most basic form of subjectivity. The subjective perspective's temporal nature, its irreducibility to objecthood, and its self-awareness (or self-consciousness, in Husserl's account) inherently cohere.

The self, in contrast, in its articulate form of self-consciousness, does not resist spatialization. On the contrary, the self as object of reflection, memory, perception, etc., and spatial extension of the self often go hand in hand. Even the bodily roots of the self in the body image (conceptually or perceptually related to the self) or the body schema (related to the self via movement and proprioception) enjoy spatial extension (De Preester & Knockaert, 2005).

16.2.4 Subjectivity, self-affectivity, and sensibility

We pointed out that the stream of consciousness not only makes a world appear but also appears to itself in a process of auto-constitution (see Husserl's *Selbsterscheinung*). In this section we have a closer look at this self-awareness proper to subjectivity, relying on the work of another phenomenological philosopher, Michel Henry (1922–2002). A notion central to Henry's phenomenology is "self-affectivity." Whereas "affection" implies a difference between an object sensed/affecting and an affected/sensing pole (a subject), self-affection does not imply a relation between two poles. There is no subject–object dichotomy on the level of self-affection (Henry, 1973; Zahavi, 2005).

That means that there is more than one way of appearing or manifestation. To appear is not always to be given as an object (to a subject). The subjective perspective too appears to itself, but not in terms of a splitting between an object and a subject.

[2] The idea of auto-constitution is Husserl's solution for the problem of an infinite regress of layers of consciousness responsible for the unity on higher levels of consciousness. The infinite regress is related to the thought that a succession of phases of consciousness is not yet in itself a consciousness of a succession. The problem has the shape of an infinite regress because we have to presuppose again and again an underlying "absolute" consciousness constituting units of the level above. According to Husserl, consciousness, implying self-consciousness, constitutes *itself* as a temporal unity on the basis of an interweaving of the formal-temporal structure the stream of consciousness (for more details see De Preester, 2007).

Subjectivity presents itself to itself, not as a foreign reality (i.e. as an object) but as the reality it itself is (i.e. as subjectivity). We already indicated this mode of appearing in self-awareness as 'non-relational' (see section 16.2.2). This mode of appearing is possible because of self-affectivity (Henry, 1973, p. 243). As the idea of self-affectivity will play a major part when we discuss the issue of interoception in relation to subjectivity, three features of it are briefly discussed here. Central to Henry's (1963) idea of self-affection is that "the self-manifestation of subjectivity is an *immediate, non-objectifying* and *passive* occurrence" (Zahavi, 2007, p. 137). First, the immediacy of the occurrence means that there is no difference, distance, or mediation between that which affects and that which is affected. In that sense, self-affection is non-relational. Second, the self-manifestation of subjectivity does not objectify the subjective perspective precisely because it is non-relational. Third, the passivity of the occurrence implies that the subjective perspective affects itself and cannot break this bond. It is unfree, delivered to self-experience, and bound to itself (Henry, 1973, p. 468, pp. 470–1). Henry calls this the "helplessness of feeling" (not to be confused with a feeling of helplessness) because in feeling, subjectivity cannot free itself from itself (Henry, 1973, p. 473). Feeling is a gift that cannot be refused (Henry, 1973, p. 457). The "helplessness of feeling" deepens the idea that feeling implies the feeling of this feeling or, in other words, that awareness implies self-awareness.

In line with the idea that subjectivity is self-aware in a non-relational way, Henry states that subjectivity affects itself *without the mediation of a sense* (Henry, 1973, p. 461). Two kinds of feeling are distinguished. On the one hand, there is sensibility, or affection that takes place through the intermediary of a sense. On the other hand, there is feeling of self or auto-affection (Henry, 1973, p. 463). The two should not be confused, and Henry reserves the term "sensibility" for the former kind of feeling, and "affectivity" for the latter. Nonetheless, affectivity is always present in sensibility because what constitutes the feeling aspect of any sensation or perception is not sensation or perception itself, but affectivity. "Affectivity is the condition of sensibility" (Henry, 1973, p. 479, see also p. 481, p. 498, p. 502). In other words, the possibility of being aware of an object depends on being self-aware. Without self-affectivity, perception would lack feeling (the so-called qualia of today's analytic philosophy) or subjectivity. Without it, there may be a machine-like perspective, a registering and interpretation of signals, but such a perspective would lack self-affectivity and thus subjectivity or feeling.

The reverse, however, is not true: affectivity is never sensible! Henry criticizes both common sense and the "positive" sciences that attempt to found affectivity in sensibility or the senses (Henry, 1973, p. 498). According to Henry, it is not possible to found feeling on a part of the sensible organic body (Henry, 1973, p. 606 ff.) He does not deny that we feel *in* our bodies; whereas sensation and perception are localizable in body parts, he denies that the foundation of the feeling aspect lies there too. The reason is that feeling of self or self-affectivity is not extended: "it results from the fact that the original revelation of feeling to itself constitutive of its affectivity consists in its very affectivity which, considered in itself and as such, is nothing extended" (Henry, 1973, p. 607, see also

p. 609). Although played out in (organic) space, feeling itself is not spatial; it is a dynamic, invisible phenomenon. Pain, for example, is never in the first place "there," in my organic body (although I can localize it in organic space because of the aspect of sensation/perception), but it sticks to my subjectivity as something I cannot escape (on pain see Henry, 1973, pp. 621–2).

Together, the four characteristics of subjectivity and Henry's consequential refusal to found affectivity on sensibility form an important challenge for recent approaches that situate the origin of subjectivity and awareness in interoception. In the second half of this chapter, we examine two recent prominent accounts in the light of the phenomenological interpretation of basic subjectivity and its characteristics.

16.3 Subjectivity: A modified neuroscience account

16.3.1 Neuroscientific accounts of awareness, consciousness, and the self

Seminal neuroscientific accounts formulated by Damasio (1999) and Craig (2002, 2003) situate the roots of awareness, consciousness, and the self in the topographic mapping of the inner dimension of the body. For example, Craig (2002) identifies the foundation of (self-) awareness in a homeostatic afferent pathway that conveys signals about the physiological status of all tissues of the body to the brain. This homeostatic afferent system constitutes a representation of the "material me," and includes not only the viscera, but also pain and temperature, mechanical stress, local metabolism, cell rupture, cutaneous parasite penetration, mast cell activation, and immune and hormonal activity (Craig, 2002, p. 657). In humans, these ascending pathways eventually lead to a re-representation in the anterior insular cortex (AIC). Both the re-representation in the AIC and intermediate representations topographically represent aspects of the "material me." For example, two rostrocaudally organized thalamic nuclei, representing all homeostatic afferent inflow project in a rostrocaudally topographic fashion to a field of the (dorsal) insular cortex (Craig, 2002, p. 659). According to Craig, evidence suggests that the final representation of the sentient self in the AIC consists of "one coherent somatotopic map" (Craig, 2009, p. 68). He considers the AIC, as the locus of a somatotopic-interoceptive map of the body, as the potential neural correlate of consciousness (Craig, 2009, p. 65), indicating, however, that the associations between body parts and emotions need further investigation (Craig, 2009, p. 68).

Craig's account has both strengths and weaknesses. First, he offers a plausible account of the bodily roots of the self, explaining how a self comes about, but leaping over the issue of sentience. How a *sentient* self is constructed remains unexplained in his model. That is problematic because it is not clear how sentience and consciousness differ in Craig's account. Second, Craig's focus seems rather on the coming about of the *self* of self-awareness, and on the idea that the basis of this self (the "material me") is to be found in the brain's topographic representations of the inner body. That is notable where he refers to the fact that some species are capable of self-recognition in the mirror. Whereas one can recognize oneself in a mirror, basic subjectivity is not "something" that is recognizable in a mirror image but rather underlies this capability. Craig, however, does not differentiate between self and subjectivity, and focuses, for example, on the demonstration that the AIC is engaged during self-recognition in the mirror test (Craig, 2009, p. 65). Third, whereas there is no objection to the idea that a "material me" is founded on topographic (and thus spatially extended) representations of the in-depth body, it is unclear whether these representations could constitute a basic subjective perspective, which resists spatialization and is the point from where all spatial extension is laid out. Fourth, the issue of self-awareness in the sense of self-affectivity remains untouched. Craig's approach of an embodied self is consistent with Henry's idea of sensibility, but not with the idea of affectivity. Although Craig's account refers to a "feeling of self," the self involved does not seem to address the basic form of subjective and non-relational self-awareness that underlies sensibility.

Interestingly, this basic form of subjectivity is approached by Damasio (in terms of consciousness). In his account, the deep roots of the self (the "proto-self") are also situated in brain representations of the homeostatic condition of the body. The "proto-self" is the non-conscious forerunner of consciously experienced levels of the self. It is "a coherent collection of neural patterns which constantly map, moment by moment, the state of the physical structure of the organism in its many dimensions" (Damasio, 1999, p. 154). Damasio's question is how this proto-self can become conscious (or, as we would say, (self-aware). Also, in his account as well as in others we need to assume a kind of inner sense based on the regulation and representation of the body's internal states. Consciousness is characterized here too as a kind of *feeling*. Although consciousness is not equated with the existence of a self, the problem is that here too, we cannot explain how a feeling arises (Damasio, 1999, p. 314). It turns out that what a feeling *is* cannot be solved in an account based on topographic, somatopic, or, in short, representational mapping of body dimensions. How we can get from a representational mapping of the inner body to a feeling remains mysterious.

To invoke a feeling or sentience actually repeats what needs to be explained: the coming about of subjectivity itself. Both Damasio and Craig face the fundamental problem that Henry clarified: in feeling or self-affectivity, there is no subject–object dichotomy. Recent neuroscience accounts have discovered exactly this: the topographic representation in the brain of inner body states installs a dichotomy between a representing pole (the brain) and a represented object (the inner body). Neuroscience accounts arrive at an impasse when they discover that feeling does not fit in this dichotomy, and that it is in feeling that subjectivity resides. What becomes manifest in these neuroscience accounts is that feeling is the phenomenon where subjectivity manifests itself (to itself), and that any objectification of subjectivity (such as happens in the topographic mapping of inner bodily processes) estranges subjectivity from itself and makes it evasive. An explanation in which the subject–object dichotomy is not installed may approach the non-relational nature of subjectivity.

The remainder of this chapter therefore explores whether a modified neuroscience model of subjectivity could preserve the role of interoception, but without the mediation of spatially extended, topographic representations of the inner body.

16.3.2 **Homeostasis and subjectivity**

Subjectivity as the basic trait that sets subjects apart from objects may be a phylogenetically primitive phenomenon arising quite early in animal life, since the physiological parameters of any animal organism have to be maintained within a narrow homeostatic range. This homeostatic dimension offers an organism criteria for assessing whatever is relevant for its own maintenance and survival. In other words, the homeostatic dimension establishes a perspective from which the environment is continually assessed. That requires a living system to be interoceptively informed about its internal milieu and how this deviates from the setpoints for maintenance and survival. Being a perspective is inseparable from the struggle between life and death, but does this imply subjectivity? Is each perspective established on an interoceptive-homeostatic basis a *sentient* perspective?

In these and similar discussions, sentience or feeling often slips in in an unnoticed manner. For example, discussing the coming about of a self, Christoff and colleagues (2011) refer to homeostatic regulation, in which self-specifying reafferent/efferent processes would be central. Homeostatic regulation would give rise to a distinction between I and not I on the very basic level of life preservation. Their central idea is that "afferent signals conveying information about the organism's internal state are continually coupled with corresponding efferent regulatory processes that keep afferent parameters within a tight domain of possible values" (Christoff et al., 2011, p. 106). These reafferent/efferent processes would not only specify a perspective but this perspective is also affective or based on feeling: "homeostatic regulation specifies a unique affective perspective based on the inner feeling of one's body" (Christoff et al., 2011, p. 107). This idea presents the problem nicely: homeostatic processes are deemed to specify a perspective proper to an organism. However, the reason why this perspective is subjective or sentient is much harder to capture. Would one say, for example, that the immune system specifies a *subjective* perspective? Certainly, it could be said to establish a perspective (and it also contributes to homeostasis), but the system is much less present in attempts to explain feeling or sentience. It seems, once more, that *feeling* is the bedrock of subjectivity, but it remains difficult to point out its exact relation with homeostatic-interoceptive processes. In Henry's terms, the current approaches to homeostatic-interoceptive processes rely on the idea of sensibility (see section 16.2.4). For homeostatic bodily life to be (self-)aware, self-affectivity needs to be present too. The central question therefore is how homeostatic bodily life and interoception can be intertwined with self-affectivity.

16.3.3 **Interoception, body representations in the brain, and feeling**

If interoception is indispensable for subjectivity, interoceptive processes should not only result into topographic representations of the in-depth body in the brain but they should also make up the basis of a true subject pole (cf. feeling or sentience). In other words, interoception should at least partly remain on the side of subjectivity itself and not wholly be turned into representations in the brain. As long as interoception is exclusively approached in terms of topographic representations of the in-depth body in the brain, we need the magical transition from the representation of body states to feelings. A solution may lie in a different processing of interoceptive material on its way from the in-depth body to subjectivity, avoiding an appeal to a miracle in the face of an infinite regress of non-conscious representations. We turn to Damasio's influential account to clarify this in more detail and to highlight the possibility of a modified approach to interoception and subjectivity.

Damasio uses the metaphor of the brain as a skilled cartographer, creating topographic maps of objects and actions, and also of the body, including the internal milieu and the viscera. The first whole-body maps would be situated in two upper-brainstem nuclei. Next to mapping the whole body, their activity also corresponds to so-called primordial *feelings*. These are elementary feelings of being alive (including feelings like pain and pleasure, comfort and discomfort), and they are closely connected to homeostatic processes. Those elementary feelings are based on the mapping of the internal milieu and viscera. However, Damasio (2010) is well aware that these felt aspects are not explicable on the basis of the mapping activity of the brain. The reason is that cartographic maps or representations inevitably take the body as an object of representation, blocking the way for the induction of subjectivity on the basis of interoception. Again, "object" or "objectification" does not mean that the body is represented as any inanimate object whatsoever. It means that aspects of bodily life become the content of an act of representation, and that in this relation between an act representing (brain activity) on the one hand and a content represented (bodily aspects) on the other hand, they hold the position not of the subject but of an object (given to a subject) (see also section 16.2.4).

In an attempt to solve this problem, Damasio (2010) considers primordial feelings as a *byproduct* of mapping activity of the brain, and accordingly, he switches from the metaphor of the cartographer to the terminology of "treating" of body signals. How "treating" differs from "mapping" remains unclear. Both the mapping and the "treating" happen at the level of the proto-self, the forerunner of the core self. According to Damasio, and importantly for what follows, the level of the proto-self already manifests a form of consciousness in numerous living species because of the qualitative, *felt* aspects that arise as byproducts of the mapping of the in-depth body. Damasio calls this primitive form of subjectivity present in the proto-self "sentience." Here again, we see the divide between sensibility (interoceptive mapping) and affectivity (feeling). Moreover, as in Henry's phenomenological approach, both are distinguishable but coupled.

Let us first focus on his proposal about the "treating" of body signals. In spite of the vague terminology, what happens in the treating of body signals is particularly interesting. Despite Damasio's initial and guiding metaphor of the brain as cartographer, the "treating" of body signals does not take the in-depth body as the *content* of representations in the brain. At this point, Damasio abandons his metaphor of the cartographer-brain. In more philosophical terms, the dichotomy of mapping/mapped, representing/represented, sensing/sensed, or subjectivity/object (body) is left behind. That is exactly what we were looking for (see section 16.3.1): the possibility of approaching the non-relational nature of subjectivity on the basis of an explanation in which the subject–object dichotomy is not installed. More concretely, we were looking for a model of subjectivity without the mediation of spatially extended, topographic representations of the inner body. The contours of such a modified model become visible where Damasio says that in the "treating" of body signals, the brain mapping of the in-depth body state on the one hand and the actual in-depth body state on the other hand are intimately associated such "that the signals conveyed would not be merely *about* the state of the flesh but literally extensions of the flesh" (Damasio, 2010, p. 294). Also, "the information from the body's interior is conveyed directly to the brain by numerous chemical molecules that course in the bloodstream and bathe parts of the brain that are devoid of blood-brain barrier" (Damasio, 2010, p. 297). The borders between brain mapping and actual bodily state, between mapping and what is being mapped, are blurred here. Body and body maps become virtually fused (Damasio, 2010, p. 121). It is from this unique, peculiar arrangement where there is no divide between subject and object that primordial feelings, or sentience, are said to arise. Remarkably, Damasio's way out of the difficulty to explain feelings closely corresponds to Henry's characterization of self-affectivity. Feelings seem to have a non-relational origin: what is mapped and what is mapping is no longer a matter of a relation between two poles.

16.3.4 Interoception, body representations in the brain, and the self

However, the story does not end here, because the notion of "self" enters the scene again. Sentience, on the level of the proto-self, is a sense of pure experience, which is on a next level—the level of the core self—claimed by an owner. This owner is the self, the protagonist in the play of consciousness. For Damasio, a sense of self is indispensable for consciousness; the self is the protagonist of experience, no matter how subtle this "self-sense" may be. Clearly, Damasio is not willing to consider the idea that subjectivity without a self is possible. However, on the level of Damasio's proto-self, there already is a sentient perspective from which an organism feels and acts. Somehow, his account fails to acknowledge the consequences of his newly introduced primordial level on which the boundaries between brain (mapping) and body (mapped) are blurred, for it is exactly here that there seems to be a level of basic subjectivity that does not include a self but "merely" instantiates a subjective perspective. This sentient subjective perspective is not based on a topographic representation of the in-depth body, but originates on a level where the dichotomy between subjectivity and object pole collapses, such that another mode of appearing—the mode proper to subjectivity—is possible. What happens on this level where sentience arises is remarkably similar to the self-manifestation of subjectivity in Henry: an immediate, non-objectifying, and passive occurrence. Similarly to the self-manifestation of subjectivity, the "treating" is non-relational (cf. the blurring of the boundaries between mapping and mapped) and is not *mediated* by an interoceptive sense that then transmits its signals to the brain. The receptors are parts of the brain itself. Consequently, it is also non-objectifying, because the body is not taken as an object of representation or mapping. Finally, it is a passive occurrence in the sense that this bond cannot be broken without resulting in the death of the organism.

In a more recent contribution, Damasio and Carvalho (2013) explicitly hold onto the idea that awareness is related to topographic maps of the body. "[I]n keeping with the notion that feelings are likely to arise from maps of body states, it is sensible to focus the search for neural substrates of feelings on the regions exhibiting *topographically* organized somatic maps" (Damasio and Carvalho, 2013, p. 145–6, emphasis added). If we keep in mind the basic characteristics of subjectivity, however, topographically organized maps of the body may exactly be where we should not look. On the contrary, those functions in the brain where body and brain are so intimately interwoven at the point of homeostasis and interoception that it is difficult to tell where the boundaries between mapping and mapped are, may be of particular interest for the coming about of subjectivity.

16.3.5 A non-topographic basis for subjectivity

The metaphor of the cartographer-brain thus neglects the fact that dozens of transmitters and hormones from the blood immediately activate neurons in the brain. They reach the brain not via nerves but via the blood. The bloodstream is a chemical mirror of the internal milieu in which all body cells bathe. Cardiovascular, pulmonary, respiratory, and gastrointestinal dimensions of the body are not exclusively topographically mapped in the brain via neural mechanisms. In-depth bodily dimensions should also be conceived in terms of non-neural and non-spatially laid out parameters, which are normatively organized around certain setpoints. After all, homeostasis is primarily about maintaining physical parameters of the internal milieu, including temperature, pH, and nutrient levels. Deviations from these setpoints can only happen within the small range of survival and integrity of the organism. Some chemoreceptors (including receptors that respond to osmotic changes) and some thermoreceptors also reside within the central nervous system (Cameron, 2002, p. 60) and do not lead to topographic mapping. Moreover, some nerve endings of interoceptors are often diffuse and do not differentiate one organ from another (Cameron, 2002, p. 60). A differentiation of organs is not always necessary in a non-topographic account. What is more important, is high fidelity for the measured physiological parameter—probably a dynamic one fluctuating with biological rhythms (e.g. circadian rhythms) (see Cameron, 2002, p. 75). In short, substances circulate through our bodies and the brain is sensitive to these substances and exerts homeostatic control through chemical and other interoceptors not only in the body but also in the brain itself. It might be this tight coupling between in-depth body and brain functioning in the maintenance of a set of physiological parameters within a narrow range of values that is at the heart of sentience. Therefore, it seems that an alternative for explaining basic subjectivity is situated where the dichotomy between subjectivity and the object (body) pole collapses, keeping in mind that interoception is not wholly reducible to cartographic mapping and neural transmission but should also be thought in terms of a set of non-topographically laid out physiological parameters that need to be kept within the small range of norms for integrity and survival of the organism.

16.4 Conclusion

This chapter offered a philosophical account of the most basic form of subjectivity and discussed four characteristics inherent to it: it is a sentient perspective, it does not necessarily imply the existence of a self, it resists spatial extension, and it is marked by self-affectivity. Whereas these four basic characteristics are conceptually distinguishable, a subjective perspective is only conceivable when we consider them as different facets of the same phenomenon. Together, they are necessary but perhaps not sufficient conditions for the more articulate form of subjectivity that is called "consciousness."

Philosophy, and phenomenology in particular, has a rich and complex tradition of considering the phenomenon of subjectivity. The drawback of that is that it requires time and effort from other disciplines to get acquainted with philosophical interpretations of subjectivity. In addition, phenomenology has always been wary of the familiar but tricky notion of representations in the mind or the brain. The metaphysics of representation most often implies a subject–object dichotomy, and stepping out of this dichotomy goes against common sense. Phenomenology has argued that such a dichotomy is especially hindering in discussions of awareness and subjectivity, and this chapter tried to show this for recent accounts of subjectivity in neuroscience. Equipped with the four basic characteristics of subjectivity from phenomenology, two related proposals about the interoceptive origin of awareness or sentience from the side of neuroscience have been discussed. Their heavy reliance on the notions of self and representation has been criticized, and their potential for developing an alternative has been highlighted. This chapter offered a first but limited idea of how the basic characteristics of subjectivity are in accordance with the non-topographic dimension of interoception. A further investigation of the normative, non-representational intertwining of body and brain and its consequences for the coming about of basic subjectivity might open up new avenues in this exciting domain of research into interoception.

References

Cameron, O. G. (2002). *Visceral Sensory Neuroscience—Interoception*. Oxford: Oxford University Press.

Christoff, K., Cosmelli, D., Legrand, D., and **Thompson, E.** (2011). Specifying the self for cognitive neuroscience. *Trends in Cognitive Sciences*, *15*(3), 104–12

Craig, A. D. (2002). How do you feel? Interoception: The sense of the physiological condition of the body. *Nature Reviews Neuroscience*, *3*(8), 655–66.

Craig, A. D. (2003). Interoception: The sense of the physiological condition of the body. *Current Opinion in Neurobiology*, *13*(4), 500–5.

Craig, A. D. (2009). How do you feel—now? The anterior insula and human awareness. *Nature Reviews Neuroscience*, *10*(1), 59–70.

Damasio, A. (1999). *The Feeling of What Happens: Body and Emotion in the Making of Consciousness*. New York, NY: Harcourt Brace.

Damasio, A. (2010). *Self Comes to Mind: Constructing the Conscious Brain*. New York, NY: Pantheon Books.

Damasio, A. and **Carvalho, G. B.** (2013). The nature of feelings: Evolutionary and neurological origins. *Nature Reviews Neuroscience*, *14*(2), 143–52.

De Preester, H. and **Knockaert, V.** (2005). *Body Image & Body Schema—Interdisciplinary Perspectives on the Body*. Amsterdam: John Benjamins Publishing Company.

De Preester, H. (2007). The deep bodily origins of the subjective perspective: Models and their problems. *Consciousness and Cognition*, *16*(3), 604–18.

Frank, M. (2007). Non-objectal subjectivity. *Journal of Consciousness Studies*, *14*(5–6), 152–73.

Frankfurt, H. (1988). *The Importance of What We Care About: Philosophical Essays*. Cambridge: Cambridge University Press.

Gallagher, S. (2000). Philosophical conceptions of the self: Implications for cognitive science. *Trends in Cognitive Sciences*, *4*(1), 14–20.

Gurwitsch, A. (1941). A non-egological conception of consciousness. *Philosophy and Phenomenological Research*, *1*(3), 325–38.

Henry, M. (1963). *L'essence de la manifestation*. Paris: PUF.

Henry, M. (1973). *The Essence of Manifestation* (trans. G. Etzkorn). The Hague: Martinus Nijhoff.

James, W. (1893). *The Principles of Psychology*. New York, NY: H. Holt and Company.

Husserl, E. (1966). *Zur Phänomenologie des inneren Zeitbewusstseins*. The Hague: Martinus Nijhoff.

Husserl, E. (1991). *On the Phenomenology of the Consciousness of Internal Time (1893–1917)*. Dordrecht: Kluwer Academic Publishers.

Kortooms, T. (2002). *Phenomenology of Time, Edmund Husserl's Analysis of Time Consciousness*. Dordrecht: Kluwer Academic Publishers.

Legrand, D. (2007). Pre-reflective self-as-subject from experiential and empirical perspectives. *Consciousness and Cognition*, *16*(3), 583–99.

Shoemaker, S. (1996). *The First-Person Perspective and Other Essays*. Cambridge: Cambridge University Press.

Strawson, G. (1999). The self and the SESMET. In: S. Gallagher and J. Shear (eds), *Models of the Self*. Thorverton: Imprint Academic, pp. 483–518.

Zahavi, D. (2005). *Subjectivity and Selfhood: Investigating the First-Person Perspective*. Cambridge, MA: The MIT Press.

Zahavi, D. (2007). Subjectivity and Immanence in Michel Henry. In: A. Grøn, I. Damgaard, and S. Overgaard (eds), *Subjectivity and Transcendence*. Tübingen: Mohr Siebeck, pp. 133–47.

Chapter 17

Inside insights: A phenomenology of interoception

Drew Leder

17.1 The phenomenological notion of the lived body

Phenomenology is a philosophical method, also employed within other disciplines, that begins by "suspending" conventional understandings of the world derived from science and metaphysical systems. This opens up the possibility of exploring without preconceptions (or at least with fewer preconceptions) the structure of human experience from which arises our sense of self, and of the "life-world" in which it is embedded (Moustakas, 1994).

In this regard, Husserl (1989), Merleau-Ponty (1962), Straus (1963, 1966), and many others have explored a conception of embodiment that differs from that conventionally presented within modern science. The "lived body," that is, the body as both experiencer and experienced, is not just an object in the world like any other. It is *that by which we have an experienced world* (life-world) to begin with. As I sit here in my chair, the scene I apprehend is organized around my corporeal position: my cup of tea to the left, my computer mouse to the right, ceiling above, and so on. Husserl calls the body a "null-point" (1989) like the zero point on a graph, around which is organized our up and down, front and back, above and below, left and right.

This is more than a world of oriented space and objects, however. These things take on specific meaning in relation to my bodily capabilities and desires. I made the cup of tea and placed it within my reach to provide a little pleasure and stimulation for my weary morning self. The computer mouse is on my right because I am right-handed, and it is shaped to my hand, as is my keyboard, so that I might write these words that we can then see with our eyes. Husserl and Merleau-Ponty speak of the lived body as involving the principle of the *I can* (Merleau-Ponty, 1962, p. 137), an interwoven system of capabilities. All that I can apprehend and can do, actually or potentially, arises out of the integrated modes of perception, desire, movement, language, sexual expression, social interaction, and so on, that my body makes possible.

This lived body does not float free like an immaterial soul. Rather, to perceive and act in the world it must be embedded within it, partaking of the same materiality that it apprehends. As such, the lived body is also an object body, with size, weight, and other such physical attributes. For example, I can stare at my image in a mirror, and see my half-lidded greenish eyes looking back at me, yet there remains an experiential gap, a non-coincidence, between my eyes lived out as a power-of-vision, orienting, and giving rise to the visible world around me, and the eyes I find in the mirror, one small element within that visual landscape. The lived body ever manifests this two-leaved structure, both subject and object, experiencer and experienced (Merleau-Ponty, 1962, 1968).

Such phenomenological explorations have tended to focus on our sensorimotor grasp of the world, paying some but relatively little attention to the field of interoception. Then too, as taken up in psychology and the neural sciences, the term "interoception" has been used in a variety of ways, leading to crucial ambiguities. Sherrington (1906) introduced the notion of "interoceptors" to refer specifically to receptors on, and perceptions of, the *visceral* region (as opposed to proprioception and exteroception). Over time, though, the term has also been given an expanded meaning and used to refer to *all* perceptions of our own body, including those with a musculoskeletal or skin origin (Ceunen, 2016). Different usages can be justified in relation to the physiology of the body; for example, distinctions between smooth and striated muscle, types of receptors, and the afferent and efferent pathways that innervate different organs (Ceunen, 2016).

However, proceeding phenomenologically we find that the lived body operates as an integrated whole, often undermining any clear and fast distinction between the fields of visceral interoception, proprioception, body-surface sensation, even exteroception. For example, when feeling low in blood sugar there is a bit of ache in my stomach, a generalized feeling of trembling weakness, a craving for food, a fuzziness to my thinking such that the words on my computer screen no longer make sense, a tendency toward irritability, and so on (I'll return to this example in section 17.4). Sharp distinctions between what would count as visceral or non-visceral, even between the interoceptive and exteroceptive realms, blur. We should not allow categories derived from the dissection of corpses, and the accumulation of laboratory data, however scientifically useful, to obscure the unities of the lived body in action. Still, the threads that woven together form the tapestry of experience can, to a degree, be pulled apart and separately examined—as long as we don't lose sight of their interweavings.

It would be impossible in a short chapter like this to examine all the variegated forms that interoception, broadly defined as perception of one's own body, can take. That said, I will often place a special focus on *visceral* interoception, and for four reasons. This accords with Sherrington's original coining of the term; this allows us to explore a region of experience that has been relatively neglected by phenomenology with its historical focus on the outer-directed senses; the visceral dimension will prove to have important medical relevances; and finally, examining the most "internal" realm of experience will allow us to challenge the very distinction between inner and outer: even visceral sensations will prove to be intertwined with the life-world in multiple ways. At times my focus will be on sensation arising from visceral organs, such as those in the thorax and abdomen. More broadly, however, I am exploring functional systems with a prominent visceral dimension, such as digestion, respiration, and circulation, which yet surface in various ways both experientially and anatomically.

17.2 The personal, pre-personal, and impersonal

Initially, one attribute that distinguishes "interoceptive" from "exteroceptive" experience is that the former is private and personal. To a degree, one might say the same of outer-directed experience. If I gaze at a tree across an open plaza I have my own perception of it that no-one else exactly shares. I see it from a certain angle at a certain moment, and it may summon up meanings, emotions, associations, particular to me—yet the tree does remain publicly available. Others view it, and we can compare, and for the most part agree upon, many of our perceptions: for example that it is a green, roughly 20-foot tall, maple tree. The interoceptive world is not shared in the same way. You cannot experience the queasiness I feel in my stomach. Only I directly apprehend it. What Scarry writes about pain, noting an epistemic divergence, could be generalized to the interoceptive field:

> Pain enters into our midst as at once something that cannot be denied and something that cannot be confirmed (thus it comes to be cited in philosophic discourse as an example of conviction, or alternatively as an example of skepticism). To have pain is to have *certainty*; to hear about pain is to have *doubt*. (Scarry, 1985, p. 13)

That interoception constitutes a private, personal field of experience has a number of ramifications. Research has shown that there is a good deal of variability in the levels of sensitivity and vigilance individuals have relative to their inner body (Herbert and Pollatos, 2012). We cannot assume that the same processes will elicit similar inner experiences for different individuals, or even for the same individual at different times. In a medical context, this contributes to the difficulty of deducing the nature and severity of disease simply from a patient's report of interoceptive symptoms.

Moreover, the personal nature of interoception can make it hard for a patient even to communicate these experiences. When seeing a clinician I might point toward the relevant bodily region, and describe interior sensations—"there's a kind of dull aching I feel around here, now and then, and sometimes a sharp pain"—but this all verges on the incommunicable (Scarry, 1985, p. 162). The other cannot directly share the object of reference as they could if I were pointing toward that maple tree we both see. He or she must "take my word for it," but the words I have at my disposal are disappointingly crude. "Aching," "sharp," "bloated," "crampy": such language seems to lack precision. Contrast this, for example, with the ability of a paint store to present hundreds of slightly different color shades, each with its own designator, such as "teal," "turquoise," "aqua," "jade," "sage," "edgewater," "valley mist," and so on. This kind of subtlety of discrimination and verbal labelling is possible because these colors manifest in a shared world. We can see and name them together. By comparison, our speech about the interoceptive field, private to each person, remains relatively impoverished. (In section 17.3 I will discuss how this is also an offshoot of the vague and generalized nature of much interoceptive experience, especially that drawn from visceral regions.)

While *personal* to each individual, interoception also gives us glimpses of a *pre-personal* level of embodiment. Organismic functions of circulation, respiration, digestion, production of blood cells, filtering of toxins, and so on, largely proceed without the need, and often the possibility, of conscious perception and control (Leder, 1990, pp. 36–68; Ricoeur, 1966). Our life arose from a pre-personal process of embryological organ growth, and each night we lapse back into a blind reliance upon these organs to sustain us even when we fall into a deep sleep.

Interoception, particularly of visceral regions (organs of the thorax/abdomen) or functions (circulation, digestion, respiration) provides hints and reminders of the pre-personal dimension that subtends our existence. I might, for example, experience a fullness or burning that indicates it is time to find a bathroom, and quick. This may not have been part of my "personal" agenda—perhaps I am in the middle of an engrossing movie—but embodied messages can override personal wishes. The pre-personal organism demands my attention.

This way of speaking can sound dualistic. Paradoxically, interoceptive experience can both subvert and reinforce a sense of self-body dualism (Leder, 2016a). On the one hand, the embodied self radically *coincides* with itself through interoceptive experience in a way it doesn't through exteroception. Vis-à-vis exteroception, as mentioned earlier, the round, small eyes I see looking back at me in the mirror don't experientially coincide with my eyes-as-lived, the power of sight that organizes the visible world. Similarly, Merleau-Ponty discusses how, when touching one hand with another, we still experience each hand as *either* the one doing the touching *or* the fleshy object being touched; right and left hands can switch off roles, but there is always a non-coincidence, a gap, between the part of the body used as perceiver and the part perceived (1962, p. 92; 1968, 147–8). *This is not so in the same way for the interoceptive field.* When I have a cramp in my midsection I feel it from within. There may be no clear divergence of perceiving and perceived body, but simply the sensation of cramping. While there are modes of meditation that welcome and focus on such "non-dual" experiences (Loy, 1988), these can also take on a threatening quality. Inner pain and discomfort can feel trapping, overwhelming, inescapable. It is hard to establish distance from that which seizes you from within.

While exhibiting our inescapable embodiment, paradoxically visceral interoception can also provoke a sense of *self–body dualism*. In the West we tend to identify our core self as somewhere up in our head, where our brain and certain exteroceptive senses reside. From this vantage point what unfolds in the stomach can seem distant, something non-I. Moreover, we are receiving messages from a pre-personal, organismic level. The bodily *I can* Merleau-Ponty refers to is here replaced by a kind of *it can* (e.g. my stomach can digest food), or in some cases, an *it cannot*—(this food won't go down right; I am about to throw up).

The conscious self can thus feel separate from what it apprehends, neither fully understanding nor in control of visceral signals and functions. The pre-personal world is then revealed as having an estranging *impersonal* character. The Latin word, *impersonalis*, is derived from the roots *in*, meaning "not" and *personalis* (personal, relating to an individual). Visceral sensations can seem radically non-personal, almost anti-personal, foreign to our individual agenda. This is true not only in deeply disruptive cases, like that of a kidney stone or congestive heart failure, but even with something as innocuous as the gurglings of a hungry stomach. (I hope these are not audible to my co-workers because they are embarrassing, they undercut my self-presentation.)

Philosophical dualisms, such as Descartes' famous mind/body split, may have their origins, or at least part of their appeal, in such experiences of divergence between the intellectual, volitional self and our necessary, but often burdensome, viscerality. As I explore elsewhere (Leder, 1990, pp. 126–48), the Western philosophical tradition often valorizes faculties such as reason and will associated with an immaterial, immortal soul. In contrast, the body can surface to awareness at times it presents an impediment, as the source of lethargy, distraction, lust, and illusion, and that part of us that must necessarily die.

This dualist split is not present within all cultures. Nor must the volitional and pre-personal levels of the embodied self necessarily clash or coexist uneasily. Physiologically, they are in a communicative relationship which can certainly take positive form. For example, the meditator practicing abdominal breathing and progressive muscle relaxation can increase oxygenation, slow the heart, lower blood pressure, improve digestion, and provoke other salutary effects mediated through the parasympathetic nervous system. One can not only send messages to, but be receptive to signals from, the inner body. To head for bed when fatigued; lay off a food that always causes stomach upset; notice the signs of a building anxiety, and take remedial measures; all these are ways of positively attending to and learning from interoceptive cues—about which I will say more in section 17.5.

17.3 The inaccessible, indistinct, and intermittent

I will now turn more explicitly to what is distinctive about visceral interoception, as opposed to surface sensations and exteroceptive experience. Of course, it is impossible in a short chapter to do full justice to the range of visceral experience: how different, for example, is the feeling of being overfull from a big meal; the light-headedness induced by inadequate oxygenation; the sharp pain of an appendicitis; and so on. I will note a few general features, however, that are often characteristic and distinctive concerning visceral experience.

First, there are regions of *inaccessibility*, a kind of organismic null-point at the heart of our biological life. This is not exactly the same null-point mentioned in section 17.1: there I discussed how the eyes do not themselves appear within the visual field they create but form an absent center. This sensorimotor surface-body effaces itself in the act of projecting toward an experienced world. I gaze upon the computer screen; my hand reaches for the teacup. Yet my eyes, my hands, are not what I focus *on*, but what I focus *from* as I interact with the world around me (Polanyi, 1969). As I will discuss in section 17.5, this can sometimes be true of our visceral states as well, but our visceral body is often less projective than it is "recessive" (Leder, 1990, pp. 36–68). Hidden in the depths of pre-personal anonymity, certain organs, tissues, and functions, may disappear almost entirely from conscious perception. Important regions of the visceral body, such as the alveoli of the lung or the parenchyma of the liver, are virtually insensate and unavailable to direct experience.

This constitutes a different kind of experiential "null-point" within one's own body; parts are so pre-personal as to be inaccessible.

In some ways, this recessive absence is salutary. It frees us up to focus on our conscious projects as vital processes are silently managed by our body. In other ways, such interoceptive gaps can prove problematic. For example, certain cancers are more deadly because they progress asymptomatically. By the time a patient experiences problems, the growth of a large mass, and metastases to distant regions, may already have occurred.

While the inner body is not entirely inaccessible, what interoceptive awareness we have, when compared to exteroception, is often marked by a variety of forms of *indistinctness*. We scan the outer world with our classical five senses, each with modes of acuity which synesthetically supplement one another (Merleau-Ponty, 1962; Jonas, 1966; Straus, 1963). Through vision we survey a world of objects seamlessly arrayed in depth. We can gaze at galaxies billions of light years away or hone in on the minute patterns and colors of a single flower. Hearing alerts us in all directions to passing events; I hear the whispering of leaves in the wind behind me, or distinguish the subtle complexities of spoken language. With touch I experience with precision the proximate; our fingertips can distinguish stimuli to the accuracy of a millimeter. By contrast, the inner body yields a far more indistinct landscape. Physiologically, our bodily interior is replete with a host of specialized sensors that minutely monitor the slightest variations of the inner milieu. However, on the subjective level we remain largely unaware of most of these measurements and adjustments.

What surfaces to consciousness can also be indistinct in the sense of spatial ambiguity. Having a "stomach-ache" we may point toward our midsection but this hardly coincides with the outlines of a particular organ. Neither does the "ache" have anything like the qualitative precision that exteroceptive senses, used singly and in combination, yield (Leder, 1990, pp. 39–42). Moreover, due to the complexity of our organs' spatial and physiological relationships, and neural distortions like referred pain, we may not even be sure if what we experience reliably correlates with the "what" and "where" of organic processes. In clinical situations the patient and doctor alike are involved in a hermeneutic process, trying to decode and supplement through laboratory tests and diagnostic imaging, indistinct interoceptive messages (Svenaeus, 2001; Gogel & Terry, 1987; Leder, 2016, pp. 87–105).

Then too, interoceptive experience often exhibits what Ricoeur calls the "strange mixture of the local and the non-local" (1966, p. 412) that attends vital functions. A chest pain may be "right here" in a certain sense but also be experienced as reverberating throughout the discomforted body, and even, as I will discuss in section 17.5, distorting the outer world. Proust, that consummate literary phenomenologist, poses an interesting question in *The Guermantes Way*: "Is there not such a thing as diffused bodily pain, radiating out into parts outside the affected area, but leaving them and disappearing completely the moment the practitioner lays his finger on the precise spot from which it springs?" (2002, p. 114). The interoceptive field may combine specific pains, tickles, and spasms with diffused, even confusing, regional effects.

This sensory field is often not only spatially and qualitatively indistinct in the ways mentioned, but temporally *intermittent*. By way of contrast, the world of vision exhibits a sense of constancy and completion. As long as our eyes are open and our vision intact the world fills in around us, continuous in time. Within that world we can see our external body, also always there, yet interoception yields a more intermittent register, surfacing to and disappearing from awareness at different times. For example, though I take more than 20,000 breaths a day I do not consciously attend to the vast majority, nor to my shifting oxygen/carbon dioxide balance. This can be altered to a degree by deliberate attention—with discipline and practice, the *vipassana* (insight) meditator learns to focus on the breath and other subtle bodily sensations for hours, but for most of us, most of the time, visceral interoception remains intermittent, often reaching awareness mostly at times of demand. "I'm really hungry," or "need to find a bathroom," or "am having an allergy attack," or "may be getting my period."

Interoceptive cues thus do at times grab hold of the conscious mind. Taking an evolutionary viewpoint, it seems logical that this would be particularly the case when conscious awareness and volition are needed to aid in the preservation of bodily homeostasis. By way of contrast, although we may occasionally notice sensations of unusual health and vigor—"I feel really energetic today"—often states of health manifest in a lack of interoceptive focus. We are freed up by our well-functioning body to focus outward on life-world activities (Leder & Jacobson, 2014).

Interoception is "intermittent" also vis-à-vis the life-course insofar as it is more or less prominent at different developmental stages: for example, puberty, pregnancy, old age. To take the latter example, the system failures associated with old age and dying can provoke strong, often unpleasant, inner experiences. Hence the "organ recitals" of certain older individuals who share tales of their latest visceral pains and procedures, and attend minutely to the particulars of digestion and bowel movements—yet this enhanced inner awareness is not only a negative thing. In later life one may (out of maturity or necessity) become more cognizant of the wisdom of the inner body which guides one toward healthier patterns of eating, rest, activity, and substance use. The young can blithely ignore or override such messages. This is harder to do as the years go by and we pay heavier prices for inattention.

17.4 **The exterior interior: Interpretive, emotive, purposive, projective**

My treatment heretofore is somewhat provisional and oversimplified. I have portrayed visceral interoception as involving the "inaccessible, indistinct, and intermittent." It has been taken up as a sensory field, and a rather deficient one at that.

While useful to a degree, this analysis needs to be expanded to address the complexity of the relationship between sensations and cognitive interpretations, emotive responses, action-oriented purposes, that is, all the ways in which visceral processes arise from and return to the life-world. I will treat these as aspects of the "exterior interior" which together challenge the very notion of a pure "interoceptive" field.

One popular mode of research on interoception explores the degree to which individuals apprehend their own heartbeat and/or can be trained to do so (Herbert & Pollatos, 2012, p. 693). While interesting results ensue, this is an example of a case of visceral interoception treated qua sensation, largely isolatable from the rest of the sensory field, and more importantly, from the interpretive and practical contexts of everyday life. This does allow for protocols that can be standardized and yield measurable results. However, the interoceptive field-as-lived is more than just an amalgam of individual sensations.

Let us consider instead a life-world context in which heartbeat sensitivity might naturally rise. A woman has a light breakfast with coffee and goes to the gym for an early morning swim. By the end she notices that her heart is racing. What is going on? Perhaps it was too much coffee—if so, better cut back on the caffeine buzz. Or she might interpret this as the sign of a good aerobic workout—you're supposed to get your heart rate up. Perhaps she is worried—is this pounding in her chest a sign of how out of shape she is? She might even fear that this is truly a cause for alarm—could this be an arrhythmia, or even the start of a heart attack?

In all cases she is not simply experiencing a pure sensation but a sensation-as-interpreted and thereby resonant with a certain quality and meaning. The elevated heart rate, when taken as signifying a healthy aerobic workout, feels very different from that associated with danger, even if the interoceptive stimulus is the same. In the latter case, the heart pounds with an ominous, distressing quality like a stranger knocking on the door in the middle of the night. This is *heartbeat-as-threat*, each pulsation feeling like a potential assault.

A number of points might here be made. First, and most obviously, interoceptive experience is never "pure sensation" but always shaped by interpretation. In this it is not different from exteroception; as Heidegger (1962) and Gadamer (1984) suggest, *all experience* is necessarily "hermeneutical," that is, interpretive (Palmer, 1969). The swimmer's various interpretations of her heartbeat are not purely personal but draw upon Western understandings of anatomy and physiology. She may have seen pictures of the heart, studied it in classes, and understands that life depends on its mechanical pump function. Cultural training feeds into our interoceptive experience. (Phenomenology itself has moved in this existential, hermeneutical direction, realizing that cultural presumptions can never be fully suspended, but we can do our best to be aware of and examine them.)

This is part of what I have in mind when referring to the "exterior interior." Our body is turned inside out, so to speak. Interoception is shaped by information we receive from outside sources. Moreover, in the West, the body (even the bodily interior) is largely thematized *qua* externalized object, that thing which can be opened on the pathologist's table, or imaged through magnetic resonance imagery (MRI) (Foucault, 1973, pp. 124–72; Leder, 1990, pp. 146–8.) Hence the swimmer does not simply feel a series of sensory impressions; rather, she feels *her heart*, that quasi-external object residing within her chest.

Sensations not only provoke such interpretations, but interpretations can provoke sensation. A vivid example is provided by Groopman, himself an oncologist who, in being treated for a hand problem, received a bone scan which seemed to show metastatic rib cancer. "I generally think of myself as reasonably well put together psychologically, but within moments my chest began to ache. When I touched my ribs, they hurt" (2007, pp. 265–66). Even when further tests showed he was cancer-free, the pain continued for several hours afterwards. Fortunately, he recovered from this distressing experience which mimicked the disease he feared. Certain individuals, often labeled hypochondriacs, suffer from an over-vigilant and catastrophizing turn of mind which can make the interoceptive field nightmarish in a continuing way.

For sensation is not only *interpretive* but also *emotive*. For the swimmer, we have seen that her pounding heart may be suffused with an aura of elation, worry, or terror. At times, this emotional tone is even the predominant quality and significance of inner-body experience. For example, we speak of having a "heavy heart," "heartache," or even a "broken heart." These expressions relate to real sensations in the chest area that can accompany grief. The heart is often experienced/understood as the emotional center of love; we say "you're in my heart," or send a heart-shaped Valentine's Day card. The heart is also viewed as a place of intuitive knowledge, as in "I know in my heart." Others might refer to having a "gut feeling," or a "gut-wrenching" experience. Where cognitive/emotional responses are felt can differ among individuals and cultures. For example, the Chinese refer to *xin*, the "heart-mind," and to the lower *dantian*, below the navel, as crucial energy centers. Hindus describe a series of *chakras* (energy wheels) running up and down the spine, mediating, for example, sexual urges or interpersonal love.

These examples also suggest that interoceptive experience is not only *interpretive* and *emotive* but also *purposive* (Herbert & Pollatos, 2012), that is, generative of urges and actions. Depending on her processing of the heartbeat, the swimmer may feel the need to catch her breath, moderate her caffeine intake, swim a few more laps to get in better shape, or immediately exit the pool and phone her doctor. She may later talk with friends, conduct Internet searches, and in other ways arrive at a rational plan, but the sense of a pre-reflective *call to action*, a push or pull in certain directions, is felt right within interoceptive experience itself. Fatigue beckons us to sit down. Heartburn calls out for a glass of milk. Here, too, we see the principle of the "*exterior interior*" at play, for the inner body is both affected by, and motivates actions in, the external world.

Taken collectively, this suggests the *projective* nature of interoception. This word is derived from the Latin *jacere*, "to throw," and *pro*, "forth." Interoception is not simply internal sensation but also "throws us forth" into the life-world and its projects. Earlier, in section 17.3 I contrasted the recessive features of visceral experience with the richness of exteroception, yet we should be careful not to overemphasize such splits. The lived body is not simply a collection of discrete regions and organs but operates in an unified fashion vis-à-vis the life-world. Interoceptive experience is shaped by that world, and helps determine how we perceive and respond to our surroundings.

Let me return to another example mentioned in section 17.1, that of a mild hypoglycemic state (to which I am prone). Working too long on this chapter I begin to feel fatigued. My head swims; the words I am writing no longer come easily. I begin to feel a bit distracted and irritable. I have some stomach queasiness from the tea I've been drinking. Am I hungry? Not sure. What time is it? Past noon. Though confused, tired, and a bit depressed, I don't want to knock off before finishing a section—but I'm having trouble even parsing the words on the computer screen. Time to take a break; better have some lunch.

In this example, I note certain interoceptive cues (queasy stomach, fatigue, irritability, depression), yet these are blended with alterations in my life-world. To use Heidegger's term, the world is always experienced through a certain *mood* (1962, pp. 172–9)—in this instance, irritation and confusion. We encounter the world filtered not only through our external senses but through our inner-body states as well. In many cases one comes to know one's internal states only indirectly through noting changes in how the world around oneself appears. As Sartre writes, "'coenesthesia' rarely appears without being surpassed toward the world by a transcendent project" (1966, p. 436). For example, the fact that the words on the computer screen no longer make sense clarifies to me that I am growing hypoglycemic. Again, this is a manifestation of how the internal body *pro-jects*, is thrown forth into the surrounding world.

This involves a temporal, not merely a spatial self-transcendence, casting us into past and future. When regarded as a collection of isolable sensations interoception seems to manifest as pure presence. I feel a tickle *now*. A pain *now*. Everything is simply *now*. In the life-world, however, interoceptive experience has a thick temporality—my hypoglycemic state gradually developed, imperceptibly unfolding until it pushed through into self-awareness. Moreover it refers to the past—when did I last eat?—and the future—what should I have for lunch? If my issues were more serious than transitory low blood sugar, the horizon of futurity might take on even greater meaning. For example, the return of pain for someone with a chronic condition can raise the specter of continued disability, deterioration, even death. Again, these resonances are not simply subsequent to the sensation but felt within it, adding ominous weight to what otherwise might be a minor tug.

A projective temporality manifests even on the pre-personal interoceptive level, composed of habits and anticipations. For example, prone to acid reflux, I have noticed that simply *thinking* of drinking a glass of orange juice will provoke acid release and a burning sensation in my throat. On a visceral level, my body has been shaped by past experiences, anticipates the citric bolus it is about to receive, and responds accordingly. The visceral body has its own sensorimotor *pro-jects*, cast forth across space and time.

17.5 The inferior interior: Overlooking, overriding, and gaining insight

The previous analyses have hovered ambiguously between the universal and the culturally/historically specific. Some features, such as the inaccessiblity to consciousness of certain bodily regions due to the limited nature of their sensory innervation, would presumably apply to humans in general. Other aspects of the interoceptive landscape—for example, our degree of awareness, the places in the body we most sense, and the interpretive models we use—not only differ among individuals but also among different cultures and historical periods. This is a job for medical anthropologists, cultural historians, and others, to investigate. I have focused on contemporary Western experience, yet it is valuable to reflect on how this itself was historically shaped, and therefore what may be peculiar to it, and even problematic.

Beginning in the seventeenth century a new conception of the material world, and the human body, was proposed and gained a certain ascendency. This has been referred to as "the death of nature"(Merchant, 1980)—that is, nature, and most particularly the human body, comes to be understood according to the analogy of a lifeless *machine.* For Descartes, the mind or soul (*res cogitans*) is the repository of conscious thought, including perceptual experience, imagination, rationality, memory, and the like. The body (*res extensa*), like the rest of the natural world, simply operates as a machine, according to material properties and forces (Burtt, 1952; Descartes, 1911). For example, the heart eventually comes to be understood as a mechanical pump, using muscular force triggered by electrical impulses. This soul/body dualism also gave rise to a monistic variant, popular in contemporary science, in which the mind or soul disappears entirely, or is considered simply as an epiphenomenon of mechanistic processes. *L'Homme Machine* (*Man-the-Machine*) by La Mettrie, eighteenth century French physician and philosopher, is one famous example of this position (1996). Foucault comments,

> The great book of Man-the-Machine was written simultaneously in two registers: the anatomico-metaphysical register, of which Descartes wrote the first pages and which the physicians and philosophers continued, and the technico-political register, which was constituted by a whole set of regulations and by empirical and calculated methods relating to the army, the school and the hospital, for controlling or correcting the operations of the body. (1979, p. 136)

Once the body is reconceived as a machine, its placement and action can be minutely controlled, made to serve the end of military, educational, medical, or industrial institutions.

To an extent we still live in such an era, and this shapes our interoceptive experience in crucial ways. First, it fosters a tendency to *overlook* the inner-body's sensory field. Insofar as we inhabit something like a body-machine, we need not attend to its messages. Again, wisdom and experience are the possession of the mind, while the body is a mechanism devoid of higher consciousness. Thus we are acculturated to overlook interoceptive experience; that is, look elsewhere, look above, in our hierarchy of value, to messages from the external world or from our own intellect.

For the interoceptive field comes to be regarded as what I will term the *inferior interior.* Descartes and other philosophers valorized the rational powers of the mind. Theologians looked to the soul that human beings uniquely possess, with its capacity to worship the Divine, read Scripture, exercise moral judgment. Here, then, is the *superior interior*, that belonging to "mind," or "soul." This is where rational reflection takes place, meditative prayer, and the deliberative processes now necessary to function well in our complex, bureaucratized, and technologized world. In school, we are trained to think much, and think better. All the input we receive from the external world—a ceaseless flow of language, data, images, needing absorption and processing––leads us back into that thinking mind, rehearsing its sub-vocalized language, memories, and symbolic representations.

By contrast with this *superior interior*, that of the "mind," messages arising from our bodily interior take on secondary status. Schools do not teach us, for the most part, to pay attention to our interoceptive sensations. They are not publicly available, nor do they contribute to the required studies and activity patterns. Employers are not interested in hearing about our aches and twinges. They wish us to be present for and focused on outward tasks.

Without coaching and validation, it is difficult to pick up on and understand interoceptive messages. They are non-verbal, private, and, as we have seen, often subtle, intermittent, ambiguous. It is not necessarily that we lack knowledge per se about our inner physiology—for example, we may have learned a lot about diet, digestion, and gut bacteria from classes and Internet searches. At the same time, however, we may lack the practices and training that help us notice and utilize signals from within.

In addition to overlooking inner-body messages, we often energetically *override* them. Foucault, in the quote earlier mentioned in this section, writes of the "technico-political register" according to which man-the-machine is disciplined. School attendance is mandatory, as are the rooms you occupy at which times, the chairs you should sit in, and how to face and address your teachers. Prisons engage in their own modes of intensive surveillance and bodily restriction. So too, workplaces filled with time clocks to be punched, phone conversations to be recorded, work spaces to be divided, and productivity to be measured. The body, as Foucault writes, is micromanaged, rendered docile in the face of power, even while its utility is maximized (1979, pp. 135–69).

Discipline, according to Foucault, is most effective when it is internalized such that the individual manages one's own body in accordance with the larger systems in which one is embedded. Again, this leads many of us not only to *overlook* but actively *override* interoceptive messages. True, we may have thoughts like "I'm tired of sitting in this office chair—I need to go for a run," or "My stomach is cramping, I don't want to go to work," or "I have a headache; this project is stressing me out," but such interoceptive messages threaten one's conformity to a role and thus are overridden in the name of being a good worker, parent, or volunteer. Even our consumerist modes of entertainment—also mandatory for the capitalist engine to hum at full throttle—involve overriding internal messages. We drink too much, exhaust ourselves in travel to distant destinations where we seek relaxation, get too little sleep and are too sedentary as we interface with our electronic screens, even over-exercise, trying to "get back in shape." (This of course refers to the shape of our *outer* body, whose appearance is viewed as of paramount importance, especially for women in our sexist culture.) All the while we "lose touch" with the inner body, and whatever wisdom could be derived from its messages.

Hence the import of gaining, or recovering, what I will call *inside insight.* There are interoceptive cues that suggest what will support or deplete our energy and spirit, what assists or impairs digestion, the effects of different types of breathing, with their potential to increase or relieve stress, and on and on. In clinical research, a pattern of "body awareness" and "somatic awareness" has sometimes been associated with anxiety, bodily hypervigilance, and catastrophizing, of a sort that can intensify pain and distress, but there are *positive* modes of body awareness that should be distinguished from those that are dysfunctional (Mehling et al., 2012). If we develop in-sight—learn to look within—— the inner-body offers up a wealth of information and requests valuable for our health and welfare. Yes, this body itself has insights, often "knowing" more than our preoccupied, driven mind. As Nietzsche writes, "There is more reason in your body than in your best wisdom" (1954, pp. 146-147).

But to do us any good we have to recover the capacity to attend to these bodily messages, even if intermittent and indistinct. There are many cultures and traditions more focused on this than ours, and their methods have now become available in the West. To name but a few, there is Buddhist *vipassana* meditation which teaches careful, sustained attention to the breath and other bodily sensations; this has given rise to mindfulness protocols now popular in integrative medicine (Kabat-Zinn, 2013). There are Chinese medical practices such as acupuncture, and meditative/martial art/exercise/dance forms like *qigong* and *taiji* (Jahnke, 2002) that work with the bodily *qi* (vital energy). Hinduism has given rise to *hatha yoga* poses, and *pranayama*—breath-control techniques (Rosen, 2002)—to render the body strong and flexible, tone inner organs, and move *prana* (vital energy) through the different *chakras* (energy centers).

Admittedly, such systems may map the inner body in ways that differ from Western anatomy and physiology. Some may or may not be shown to have direct medical benefit; studies are beginning to explore the mechanisms and clinical efficacy of "alternative" treatments such as acupuncture and yogic practices. It is unclear whether "*qi*" or the "*chakras*" will ever register as anatomico/physiological realities in the Western sense. But they do speak to the phenomenological experience of the inner body as interpreted by different cultures, and for those interested, increasingly within our own. This is accompanied by a proliferation of Western holistic body-centered therapies such as Alexander Technique, Feldenkreis, Healing Touch, massage therapy, and reflexology. Again, regardless of their medical efficacy, such treatment systems are indications of a growing desire to get back "in touch" with the body rather than ignoring and overriding its messages (Mehling et al., 2011).

Whether through these systems, or in ways more personal and informal, gaining *inside insight* might do a good deal to assist the health of both individuals and society. It was actually health concerns that motivated Descartes to develop his mechanical view of the body:

> They caused me to see that it is possible to attain knowledge which is very useful in life . . . principally because it brings about the preservation of health, which is without doubt the chief blessing and the foundation of all other blessings in this life . . . we could be free of an infinitude of maladies both of body and mind, and even also possibly of the infirmities of age, if we had sufficient knowledge of their causes, and of all the remedies with which nature has provided us. (1911, pp. 119–20)

While it is true that Cartesian-style medicine, with its diagnostic technologies, chemical pills, and surgical repairs or transplants, has offered great relief of suffering and helped prolong the human lifespan, this model also has its shadow side. In addition to contributing to a depersonalized style of medicine, the Cartesian notion of the body-machine, and the repairs thereto, can distract focus from the development of an inner-body awareness that could prevent certain disease processes for which medicine offers end-stage treatment (Leder, 2016b, 56–83). There is a temptation, when downing another cheeseburger and fries, to believe that one can always take a cholesterol-lowering statin, or have a cardiac procedure to open up or replace clogged arteries. This is symptomatic of an exaggerated cultural fantasy of a fix-all medicine. Greater awareness and valuing of inner-body signals (I feel sickish when I eat that burger and fries) might forestall the need for some of those pills and procedures.

To pay greater attention to interoceptive messages—what kind of foods sit well, how much sleep and movement we need, what subtle symptoms of imbalance are manifesting that might lead to chronic problems if left unattended—constitutes an ever-available resource in preventive medicine. Such inside insights are free; they demand no costly insurance premiums and co-pays. These might forestall expensive and burdensome doctor visits, invasive laboratory studies, prescription drugs laden with side effects, emergency organ repairs and transplants. Even those already struggling with chronic diseases or age-related debilities may find ways to monitor and moderate these, improving quality of life and reducing medical services. Those who are healthy may remain so longer, and improve the texture of day-to-day life; such are potential benefits of inside insights.

Some of what I assert here is common sense, some more speculative or challengeable. The debate concerning the relative benefits of preventive science and curative healthcare is complex and contentious and ultimately beyond the scope of this chapter. For certain diseases, a personal preventive approach is crucial but may be less effective with ones where a genetic trigger predominates, or an environmental factor the individual is powerless to alter. Ideally, we can incorporate the best of what Western medicine has to offer, distributed through a rational, affordable healthcare system. Twenty-first century medicine surely offers miracles of healing. (I myself have benefitted dramatically from two surgeries, including an innovative process involving a cadaver nerve-sheath transplant.) We need also address the environmental and social causes of many disease such as obesity, diabetes, asthma, lead-poisoning, certain cancers, etc. But we should not overlook the medical and personal import of our inside insights. Our inner body can sometimes be a stranger, or a threat—but we may also discover it to be a close friend and wise counselor.

References

Burtt, E. A. (1952). *The Metaphysical Foundations of Modern Science*. Atlantic Highlands, NJ: Humanities Press.

Ceunen, E., Vlaeyen, J. W. S., and **Van Diest, I.** (2016). On the origin of interoception. *Frontiers in Psychology*, *7*, 743.

de La Mettrie, J. O. (1996). *Machine Man and Other Writings*. Cambridge: Cambridge University Press.

Descartes, R. (1911). *The Philosophical Works of Descartes*, Vol. 1 (E. Haldane and G. R. T. Ross, eds). Cambridge: Cambridge University Press.

Foucault, M. (1973). *The Birth of the Clinic*. New York, NY: Vintage Books.

Foucault, M. (1979). *Discipline and Punish: The Birth of the Prison*. New York, NY: Vintage Books.

Gadamer, H.-G. (1984). *Truth and Method*. New York, NY: Crossroad.

Gogel, E. and **Terry, J.** (1987). Medicine as interpretation: The uses of literary metaphors and methods. *Journal of Medicine and Philosophy*, *12*, 205–17.

Groopman, J. (2007). *How Doctors Think*. New York, NY: Houghton Mifflin.

Heidegger, M. (1962). *Being and Time*. New York, NY: Harper & Row.

Herbert, B. M. and **Pollatos, O.** (2012). The body in the mind: On the relationship between interoception and embodiment. *Topics in Cognitive Science*, *4*, 692–704.

Husserl, E. (1989). *Ideas Pertaining to a Pure Phenomenology and to a Phenomenological Philosophy. Second book: Studies in the Phenomenology of Constitution*. Dordrecht: Kluwer Academic Publishers.

Jahnke, R. (2002). *The Healing Promise of Qi: Creating Extraordinary Wellness through Qigong and Tai Chi*. New York, NY: McGraw-Hill.

Jonas, H. (1966). *The Phenomenon of Life: Toward a Philosophical Biology*. Chicago, IL: University of Chicago Press.

Kabat-Zinn, J. (2013). *Full Catastrophe Living: Using the Wisdom of your Body and Mind to Face Stress, Pain, and Illness*. New York, NY: Bantam.

Leder, D. (1990). *The Absent Body*. Chicago, IL: University of Chicago Press.

Leder, D. and **Jacobson, K.** (2014). Health and disease: The experience of health and illness. In: B. Jennings (ed.), *Bioethics*, Vol. **3**, 4th edn. Farmington Hills, MI: Macmillan Reference, pp. 1434–43.

Leder, D. (2016a). *The Distressed Body: Rethinking Illness, Imprisonment, and Healing*. Chicago, IL: University of Chicago Press.

Leder, D. (2016b). The experiential paradoxes of pain. *Journal of Medicine and Philosophy*, *41*(5), 444–60.

Loy, D. (1988). *Nonduality: A Study in Comparative Philosophy*. Atlantic Highlands, NJ: Humanities Press.

Mehling, W. E., **Wrubel, J.**, **Daubenmier, J. J.**, **Price, C. J.**, **Kerr, C. E.**, **Silow, T.**, et al. (2011). Body awareness: A phenomenological inquiry into the common ground of mind-body therapies. *Philosophy, Ethics, and Humanities in Medicine*, *6*, 6

Mehling, W. E., **Price, C.**, **Daubenmier, J. J.**, **Acree, M.**, **Bartmess, E.**, and **Stewart, A.** (2012). The multidimensional assessment of interoceptive awareness (MAIA). *PLoS One*, *7*(11), e48230.

Merchant, C. (1980). *The Death of Nature*. San Francisco, CA: Harper and Row.

Merleau-Ponty, M. (1962). *Phenomenology of Perception*. London: Routledge and Kegan Paul.

Merleau-Ponty, M. (1968). *The Visible and the Invisible*. Evanston, IL: Northwestern University Press.

Moustakas, C. (1994). *Phenomenological Research Methods*. Thousand Oaks, CA: Sage Publications.

Nietzsche, F. (1954). Thus Spoke Zarathustra. In: W. Kaufman (ed.), *The Portable Nietzsche*. New York: Viking Press, pp. 112–442.

Palmer, R. (1969). *Hermeneutics: Interpretation theory in Schleiermacher, Dilthey, Heidegger, and Gadamer*. Evanston, IL: Northwestern University Press.

Polanyi, M. (1969). *Knowing and Being*. Chicago, IL: University of Chicago Press.

Proust, M. (2002). *Guermantes Way*. New York, NY: Penguin.

Ricoeur, P. (1966). *Freedom and Nature: The Voluntary and the Involuntary*. Evanston, IL: Northwestern University Press.

Rosen, R. (2002). *The Yoga of Breath: A Step-by-Step Guide to Pranayama*. Boston, MA: Shambhala Press.

Sartre, J.-P. (1966). *Being and Nothingness*. New York, NY: Pocket Books.

Scarry, E. (1985). *The Body in Pain: The Making and Unmaking of the World.* New York, NY: Oxford University Press.

Sherrington, C. S. (1906). *The Integrative Action of the Nervous System.* New Haven, CT: Yale University Press.

Straus, E. (1963). *The Primary World of Senses: A Vindication of Sensory Experience.* (trans. J. Needleman) New York, NY: The Free Press of Glencoe.

Straus, E. (1966). *Phenomenological Psychology.* New York, NY: Basic Books.

Svenaeus, F. (2001). *The Hermeneutics of Medicine and the Phenomenology of Health: Steps Towards a Philosophy of Medical Practice,* 2nd edn. Dordrecht: Kluwer Academic Publishers.

Author Index

Subject Index

Notes
vs. indicates a comparison
Tables and figures are indicated by an italic *t* or *f* following the page number.